Modern Approaches to
Endometriosis

Modern Approaches to Endometriosis

Edited by

Eric J. Thomas, MD

Professor, Department of Human Reproduction and Obstetrics,
University of Southampton, Southampton, UK

and

John A. Rock, MD

Professor, Department of Obstetrics and Gynecology,
Johns Hopkins University Hospital, Baltimore,
Maryland, USA

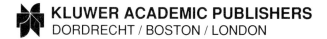

KLUWER ACADEMIC PUBLISHERS
DORDRECHT / BOSTON / LONDON

Distributors

for the United States and Canada: Kluwer Academic Publishers, PO Box 358, Accord Station, Hingham, MA 02018-0358, USA
for all other countries: Kluwer Academic Publishers Group, Distribution Centre, PO Box 322, 3300 AH Dordrecht, The Netherlands

British Library Cataloguing in Publication Data

Modern approaches to endometriosis.
   1. Women. Endometriosis
   I. Thomas, Eric J. II. Rock, John A.
   618.14

   ISBN 0-7923-8901-8

Library of Congress Cataloguing in Publication Data

Modern approaches to endometriosis/edited by Eric J. Thomas and John A. Rock.
      p.   cm.
   Includes bibliographical references and index.
   ISBN 0-7923-8901-8 (case)
   1. Endometriosis. I. Thomas. Eric J. II. Rock, John A.
   RG483.E53M63 1991   90-22965
   618.1—dc20   CIP

Published in the United Kingdom by Kluwer Academic Publishers, PO Box 55, Lancaster, UK.

Kluwer Academic Publishers BV incorporates the publishing programmes of D. Reidel, Martinus Nijhoff, Dr W. Junk and MTP Press.

Printed in Great Britain by Butler and Tanner Ltd., Frome and London.

Contents

v

List of contributors

R. L. Barbieri
Department of Obstetrics and
    Gynecology
Health Sciences Center
SUNY at Stony Brook
Stony Brook
New York 11794-8091
USA

A. Bergqvist
Department of Obstetrics and
    Gynecology
University of Lund
Malmö General Hospital
S-214 01 Malmo
Sweden

D. Braun
Departments of Internal Medicine and
    Immunology/Microbiology
Rush Medical College
1725 W. Harrison
Chicago, IL 60614
USA

I. A. Brosens
Division of Obstetrics and Gynaecology
Faculty of Medicine
Catholic University of Leuven
B-3000 Leuven
Belgium

W. P. Dmowski
Department of Obstetrics and
    Gynecology
Rush Medical College and Institute for the
    Study and Treatment of Endometriosis
Chicago, IL 60614
USA

H. Gebel
Departments of Immunology/Microbiology
    and General Surgery
Rush Medical College
1725 W. Harrison
Chicago, IL 60614
USA

T. R. Groff
2455 N.E. Loop 410, Suite 242
San Antonio, TX 78217
USA

A. F. Haney
Duke University Medical Center
PO Box 2971
Durham, NC 27710
USA

A. F. Henderson
King's College Hospital
Denmark Hill
London
UK

B. S. Hurst
Department of Obstetrics and
    Gynecology
Division of Reproductive Endocrinology
The Johns Hopkins Hospital
Baltimore, MD 21205
USA

S. M. Markham
Division of Reproductive Endocrinology
Department of Obstetrics and
    Gynecology
Georgetown University School of
    Medicine
3800 Reservoir Road NW
Washington DC 20007
USA

L. Mettler
University Frauenklinik u.
Michaelsis 316
Hebammenlehranstalt
2300 Kiel
Federal Republic of Germany

J. A. Rock
Department of Obstetrics and
   Gynecology
Division of Reproductive Endocrinology
The Johns Hopkins Hospital
Baltimore, MD 21205
USA

R. W. Shaw
Academic Department of Obstetrics and
   Gynaecology
Royal Free Hospital School of Medicine
Pond Street
London NW3 2QG
UK

S. K. Smith
Department of Obstetrics and
   Gynaecology
University of Cambridge
Rosie Maternity Hospital
Cambridge CB2 2SW
UK

J. W. W. Studd
Consultant Gynaecologist
120 Harley Street
London W1N 1AG
UK

C. J. G. Sutton
Consultant Gynaecologist
Department of Obstetrics and
   Gynaecology
Royal Surrey County Hospital
Guildford, Surrey
UK

E. J. Thomas
Department of Human Reproduction and
   Obstetrics
Princess Anne Hospital
Coxford Road
Southampton
SO9 4HA
UK

J. M. Wheeler
Department of Obstetrics and
   Gynecology
Baylor College of Medicine
6550 Fannin, #801
Houston, Texas
USA

Preface

Endometriosis provides a unique clinical and scientific challenge. It is being diagnosed with increasing frequency and yet we are unsure of the significance of this in many patients. Its appearance varies from a tiny focus of disease to a potently destructive phenomenon. We are still unsure of the relative value of medical or surgical treatment. The pathogenesis and control of the cellular function of the disease provide many scientific problems. The presence of a comparative normal epithelium, namely endometrium, provides a unique research opportunity. It is probable that only through basic science research will we be able to solve the clinical dilemmas that endometriosis presents.

We felt that it was important to create a book that explored the important scientific and clinical problems. We therefore invited acknowledged experts from both Europe and the United States of America to review their fields. The purpose of these reviews is not only to provide a resource for clinicians and scientists but also to stimulate thought and new ideas for research and treatment. To fulfil that aim we have asked that the authors be more speculative than normal for a volume such as this. We thank them for responding to their task so well and hope that you will feel as stimulated by their efforts as we have been.

Eric Thomas   **John Rock**

Section A
Scientific Aspects of Endometriosis

1
The pathogenesis and aetiology of endometriosis

A. F. Haney

INTRODUCTION

Despite being one of the most frequently encountered gynaecological diseases requiring surgery and medical treatment, the pathophysiology of endometriosis remains controversial. Since the turn of the century, there has been substantial interest in this fascinating disease, but relatively little objective scientific data are available concerning its cause, natural history and, particularly, its relationship to infertility. It has been estimated that approximately 10–15% of all premenopausal women have endometriosis, albeit not all the women are symptomatic[1]. As a consequence, this represents a major clinical problem and consumes a significant proportion of the health care expenditures for gynaecological care. Until a better understanding of the pathophysiology of this disease is reached, effective therapy and, hopefully, prevention will elude us. This article attempts to review the relevant literature regarding the pathophysiology of endometriosis in an effort to identify those areas that may prove profitable for future research endeavors.

INCIDENCE

In order to obtain the true incidence of endometriosis in a population of unselected premenopausal asymptomatic women, the most sensitive diagnostic test, i.e. laparoscopy, would need to be performed prospectively. Obviously, such a trial is unethical and will never be completed. An alternative, although less accurate, approach is to estimate the incidence of this disease in women presenting with one of several symptoms justifying laparoscopy, i.e. pelvic pain, dysmenorrhoea and infertility. There are basically three types of studies in this category. The first is that group of trials using women undergoing gynaecological procedures in general and identifying the subset that have endometriosis. Approximately 10–15% of women undergoing diagnostic laparoscopy for some symptom have this diagnosis confirmed. The second group of studies involves women undergoing laparoscopies for tubal ligation. These are obviously fertile women and thus have some selection bias. The incidence of the disease has been estimated to be 2–5% in this population[2]. The last group of studies involves women undergoing laparoscopies for infertility. They carry the highest probability of having endometriosis, varying from 30% to 40%[2–4]. These wide ranges probably reflect the heterogeneous population studied with inherent selection bias, including presenting symptomatology, educational level, socioeconomic status, cultural attitudes towards medical care, contraceptive use and delayed childbearing. Despite these considerations, it seems reasonable to estimate a gross clinical incidence of endometriosis in an unselected population of premenopausal women of approximately 2–5%.

EPIDEMIOLOGY OF ENDOMETRIOSIS

In an attempt to understand the nature of this disease, the first logical step is to identify the population at risk for having endometriosis, as that should provide insights into the pathophysiology of the process. To some extent, the questions asked by the epidemiologist will reflect the current understanding of the disease. As a result, the historical development of our understanding of endometriosis contains the biases of the investigators at the time of the studies.

An example of this bias involves the originally identified racial preponderance of the disease in white women. The initial studies demonstrated that only rarely was the disease identified in black women, and consequently it was thought that endometriosis had a racial predilection[5,6]. Initially, the potential confounding variables such as the availability of health care, access to contraception, cultural patterns of childbearing, and the attitudes toward menses were not considered[7–9]. It is now known that these factors significantly influence the likelihood of developing this disease. Once these variables were controlled for, the difference in the frequency between caucasian and black patients disappeared[10–12]. The only documented racial predilection of endometriosis, given comparable cultural and socioeconomic status, is that of the Japanese. Japanese women have twice the incidence of the disease of caucasian women[9].

Another example involves the ascertainment bias of selection by presenting symptoms. If one simply selects those women with infertility[3,4], finding endometriosis is far more likely than in those women with more non-specific gynaecological signs or symptoms such as the presence of an adnexal mass, dyspareunia, dysmenorrhoea, dysfunctional uterine bleeding and pelvic pain[13–29]. Infertile women, by definition, have not fulfilled their childbearing desires and, as a consequence, typically have a lower number of children, are older when first seen, and have a higher probability of delayed childbearing either voluntarily or otherwise.

Because of the above considerations, it is unclear how seriously to consider the earlier epidemiological studies in the understanding of this disease. If one simply accepted an incidence of endometriosis in a fertile population at 2–5% and made an assumption that endometriosis was associated with delayed childbearing secondary to infertility by other aetiology, the incidence in an infertile population of 25–50% would neither be surprising nor necessarily be a reason to consider it aetiological in their infertility. The strongest data to suggest that endometriosis is associated with a lower probability of conception come from couples who are infertile because of azoospermia undergoing therapeutic donor insemination. When these women were evaluated prior to insemination and found to have endometriosis, their subsequent cycle fecundity with donor insemination was found to be substantially lower than in the women without endometriosis[30]. This constitutes the strongest data to date suggesting that some aspect of the pathophysiology of endometriosis is at least contributory, if not causal, in the patient's infertility.

PATHOGENESIS

Pathologists as well as gynaecologists have been interested in the phenomenon of ectopically implanted endometrium since its description in the mid-1800s. Several theories of pathogenesis were put forth prior to the era of objective scientific inquiry. Unfortunately, several of these theories have continued to enjoy popularity with clinicians despite the absence of scientific data. These misconceptions as to the nature of this disease have had a major effect on the therapeutic recommendations up to the present time. The unfortunate consequence has been the perpetuation of non-efficacious 'therapy' that compounds the problem by discouraging couples from participating in randomized clinical trials with appropriate untreated control arms. Until it is appreciated what constitutes efficacious treatment, appropriately controlled clinical trials that are at variance with the current unsubstantiated dogma will continue to be difficult to perform.

Before considering the various proposed mechanisms of development of endometriosis, it is appropriate to establish some criteria to evaluate these theories. First, there must be a uniformly accepted definition of the disease. The gold standard for diagnosis is having histologically documented endometrial glands and stroma outside the uterus, with evidence of menstrual cyclicity with haemosiderin-laden macrophages. This is an empirical definition arrived at by consensus in the early part of this century when only a minimal amount was known about the reproductive cycle in women and this description was used to ensure uniform reporting. Identification of glands and/or stroma as endometrial in origin, on the basis of morphology, is certainly tenuous. This is particularly true without specific biochemical markers of endometrium and in the presence of an inflammatory reaction that may substantially modify the histological appearance. With the emphasis today on endoscopy, the diagnosis of endometriosis is based almost exclusively on the visual appearance of the peritoneal implants. In the future, a more exacting definition may be forthcoming, with antibodies directed against unique endometrial antigens being used to document unequivocally the tissue of origin.

The finding of endometrial glands and stroma deep within the myometrium, i.e. adenomyosis, constitutes a disease with entirely different epidemiology and clinical profile. This disease cannot be considered 'endometriosis' despite the old nomenclature of 'endometriosis interna', referring to adenomyosis, and 'endometriosis externa', referring to what we now consider endometriosis.

Second, the disease must be able to be re-created using an experimental design equivalent to an inoculum of endometrium. Obviously, some modification to adapt to the theories of autologous transplantation, congenital cell rests and coelomic metaplasia must be made. Lastly, the experimentally created disease must be equivalent in virtually all respects to the spontaneously developing entity both morphologically and functionally. While these criteria may seem overly stringent, they seem appropriate given the wide variance of the proposed pathophysiological mechanisms.

COELOMIC METAPLASIA

The first widely considered theory of histogenesis was that of coelomic metaplasia, and it was initially advocated by Dr Robert Meyer, the Dean of Gynaecologic Pathology, at the turn of the century. According to this proposal, under certain unspecified stimuli, cells might undergo a metaplastic process that changes their character and physiological function from that of peritoneal mesothelium to endometrium[31]. This concept underwent some expansion, with other investigators suggesting inductive influences on the coelomic membrane, and menstrual detritus and hormones have been most prominently mentioned. In the 1920s other theories of pathogenesis were proposed and a bitter debate raged. The disciples seemed to carry the intensity of the debate beyond that of the original proposer. There is clear evidence that Dr Meyer did not intend the coelomic metaplasia theory to exclude consideration of other ideas[31].

Experimental data supporting the coelomic metaplasia theory are meagre at best. The most prominently mentioned study is that of Merrill who noted 'endometrium-like' cells adjacent to Millipore filter chambers containing endometrium implanted in the peritoneum of rabbits[32,33]. These experiments were designed to investigate the inductive influence of menstrual detritus on the peritoneal mesothelium. Despite some morphological similarity to endometrial glands, no evidence of endometrial stroma or functional characteristics of endometrium could be appreciated. Other inductive influences have been postulated, such as gonadal steroids and follicular fluid contents, all without experimental evidence.

A firm scientific basis for the concept of coelomic metaplasia has yet to be established. There are several questions that need to be addressed if this pathophysiological mechanism is to be seriously entertained. The first would be that endometriosis could develop in the absence of endometrium, i.e. in women with congenital absence of the uterus. Although there are case reports purporting to demonstrate endometriosis in these women[34], the situation is

6

confusing. There are invariably fallopian tube remnants present and occasionally small blind uterine horns that may be the source of endometrium. Second,
if peritoneal epithelium has the potential to undergo metaplasia, this
phenomenon would be expected to occur in men as well as women. While
there are case reports of endometriosis in men, each involves the treatment
of metastatic prostate cancer with high-dose oestrogens[35–38]. This probably
represents hyperplasia of the endometrial cell rests in the prostatic utricle, the
remnant of the Mullerian ducts in men. Third, coelomic metaplasia should
occur in those sites where the coelomic membranes are present. While there
is embryological evidence that the coelomic membrane covers both the
abdominal and thoracic cavities[39,40], endometriosis is rare outside the pelvis
or its contiguous structures. Lastly, if coelomic metaplasia is similar to
metaplasia elsewhere, it should occur with increasing frequency with advancing
age. The clinical pattern of endometriosis is distinctly different, with an abrupt
halt in the disease with cessation of menstruation. While endometriosis has
been observed in postmenopausal women[41,42], it is probably associated with
oestrogen replacement therapy or an endogenous oestrogen source.

Until the above-noted concerns are addressed, there is little justification
for considering coelomic metaplasia as a serious candidate as the aetiology
of endometriosis.

EMBRYONIC CELL RESTS

It has been speculated that embryonic cell rests could explain the presence
of ectopic endometrium. This is based on the assumption that in areas adjacent
to the Mullerian ducts, rudimentary duplications of the Mullerian system
might be present, allowing cells of Mullerian origin to develop into functioning
endometrium, particularly in peritoneal pockets or defects at the base of the
broad ligaments[43].

There are disconcerting questions regarding this concept. First, the
embryonic distribution of the urogenital ridges is from the pelvis into the
thoracic activity. The distribution of ectopic endometrium would be expected
to correspond to the distribution of these putative precursors[39,40]. Such
incidental cell rests have not been identified in the pelvis or thoracic cavity.
Furthermore, the rare endometriosis found in the thoracic cavity is in the
distribution of the vasculature, consistent with blood-borne transplanted
endometrial cells[31]. Second, if the embryonic cell rest hypothesis is to
be seriously entertained, one would anticipate finding the endometriosis
immediately after menarche, when hormonal stimulation is initiated. By
contrast, endometriosis has its greatest incidence in the fourth decade of
life[3,44]. On the basis of these considerations the likelihood that endometriosis
has its origin in remnants of embryonic structures is highly improbable.

TRANSPLANTATION OF EXFOLIATED ENDOMETRIUM

A scientific approach to understanding the aetiology of endometriosis began
with the pioneering efforts of a private practitioner from Albany, New York,

Dr J. A. Sampson. Based on his clinical experience, he proposed that the menstrual effluent contained viable endometrial cells that could be transplanted to ectopic sites[45-48]. He reasoned that since the oviducts communicate freely between the peritoneal and uterine cavities, regurgitation of menstrual debris through the oviducts was the likely source of these cells in the vast majority of patients. A substantial clinical data base exists to support this hypothesis. Several other routes of dissemination have been observed, including lymphatic and vascular channels and by iatrogenic deposition. Transtubal dissemination appears to be the most common route of dissemination, by far, with the preponderance of endometriosis being found on the peritoneal surfaces of the pelvis and on the pelvic viscera.

Specific scientific evidence that supports the ability of endometrial cells to be transplanted, regardless of route, includes:

1. Viable endometrial cells have been demonstrated in the menstrual effluent[49,50].

2. Endometrium can be implanted experimentally and grow within the peritoneal cavity[51].

3. Endometrial cells obtained from the menstrual effluent are transplantable to the abdominal wall fascia[31,52].

4. Neither oestrogen nor progesterone is required for implantation and early growth of endometrial cells, although there does appear to be some long-term necessity for these gonadal hormones to maintain the viability of endometrial implants[53].

Retrograde menstruation

Dr Sampson concluded that from his clinical experience it was most likely that endometrial cells were regurgitated through the fallopian tubes at the time of menses. In order to understand this situation, one must consider the physiology of menstruation. Following ovulation, unique histological and functional changes occur in the endometrium in preparation for implantation. In a non-conceptive menstrual cycle, luteolysis is marked by declining oestrogen and progesterone levels, resulting in a breakdown of the surface layer of the endometrium. The menstrual effluent is thus composed of extracellular fluid, blood, and clusters of shed endometrial cells[54,55]. This decline in gonadal steroids triggers the release of uterine prostaglandins[56], which appear to be involved in arterial spasm in the superficial layers of the endometrium as well as in stimulating rhythmic uterine contractions, elevating the pressure within the uterus and aiding in the expulsion of menses[56].

There are three possible routes of egress for the menstrual effluent from the uterine cavity — the cervix and both fallopian tubes. As the cervical canal generally has the largest calibre and the lowest resistance, the majority of flow is in that direction. There is a paucity of information on the physiology on the uterotubal junction in humans with respect to directional flow of the menstrual debris. The rarity of spontaneous endometriosis in monkeys may be related to the small calibre of the uterotubal junction[57,58] and the difficulty in demonstrating reflux of dye through the uterotubal junctions with hysterosalpingography[51]. Unfortunately, little is known of the physiology of the uterotubal junction in humans. Uterotubal junction 'spasm' is thought to occur in response to irritating solutions, stress, smoking and even general anaesthesia. Paradoxically, the general anaesthetic halothane, as well as glucagon (known to relax smooth muscles), is used in an attempt to overcome uterotubal junction 'spasm'[59–61]. Evidence to support an 'incompetent' uterotubal junction allowing increased menstrual regurgitation in women with endometriosis comes from Ayers and Friedenstab, who observed relative hypotonia of the uterotubal junction in women with endometriosis[62]. Similarly, cervical stenosis has been suggested to increase the probability of endometriosis by creating relative uterine outflow obstruction, allowing the normal uterine pressure to overcome the uterotubal junction during menses, although there are no data aside from those for women with congenital anomalies[14,63,64].

Some degree of regurgitation of menses via the oviducts appears to be a universal event in women in virtually every menstrual cycle. This is supported by evidence of bloody peritoneal dialysates at the time of menses in women undergoing peritoneal dialysis[65] and bloody peritoneal fluid observed at laparoscopy during menses[66,67]. Even on non-menstrual days, the aspiration of peritoneal fluid reveals a greater probability of having endometrial tissue in women with endometriosis than in control women[68]. While a slower clearance of 'normally' regurgitated menses cannot be excluded, these data do support the concept of increased retrograde menstruation in women with endometriosis.

In order to consider retrograde menstruation the prime mechanism for development of the bulk of endometriosis, several observations must be present. First and foremost, viable endometrial cells must be present in the fallopian tubes. Second, viable endometrial cells must be present in the menstrual debris and have the ability to be transplanted. Third, the anatomic distribution of the disease should be compatible with the tenets of transplantation biology and be more common at the site of entry into the pelvis, i.e. the fimbrial ostia. The following evidence exists to support these points:

1. Viable endometrial cells have been demonstrated in the fallopian tube by perfusing excised segments of the human oviducts[69] as well as in histological segments of the fallopian tubes during menses[70].

2. Endometrial cells have been noted by cytology of the peritoneal fluid with the peritoneal fluid being collected either by culdocentesis[71] or laparoscopy[68].

3. The natural position of the fallopian tube ostia is near the insertion of the uterosacral ligament into the uterus at the base of the broad ligament. This is an extremely common site of endometriosis[72].

4. Gravity should affect free-floating endometrial cells in the peritoneal cavity. When either supine or upright, the pelvic cavity is the most dependent portion of the abdominal cavity and represents, by far, the most common site of endometriosis. In addition, when the pelvic cavity is bisected by an anteflexed uterus, endometriosis is commonly found in

both the anterior and posterior dependent compartments, i.e. the uterovesicle fold in the cul de sac. When the uterus is retroflexed and does not bisect the pelvic cavity and no dependent anterior compartment exists, implants on the uterovesicle fold are extremely uncommon[72].

5. Attachment of free-floating endometrial cells is influenced by the mobility of the pelvic structures. Those that are fixed in the pelvis have a much higher rate of transplantation than mobile structures. The actively peristalsing small bowel and mobile fallopian tube are rarely involved, in contrast to the non-mobile structures such as the ovary, pelvic peritoneum and fixed portion of the sigmoid colon[72].

6. Transplantation is predictable on the basis of the suitability of the surface epithelium, vascularity, and the local hormone environment. The pelvic peritoneum would seem ideal, being thin, well vascularized and bathed in high levels of gonadal steroids after ovulation. This is in distinct contrast to the remainder of the epithelium in the genital tract, with ciliated fallopian tube epithelium, mucus secreting endocervical epithelium, and squamous epithelium of the exocervix, vagina and vulva. As the endometrium is dependent upon ovarian hormones and the ovary is adjacent to the fallopian tube ostia, it is no surprise that the most common site of endometriosis is the ovary[6,72].

It is obvious from the above that a substantial amount of hard evidence supports the pathophysiological process of retrograde menstruation and transplantation of endometrial cells on the peritoneum of the pelvis. No comparable data base exists for any other proposed mechanism of development.

Lymphatic and haematogenous dissemination

Dissemination of endometrial cells through lymphatic or vascular channels has long been considered. This would account for the rare finding of endometrial tissue at sites distant from the pelvis. Endometrial tissue in lymphatic spaces was first noted by Halban in 1925 when he reported five cases with lymphatic spread[73]. Endometrial tissue has been noted microscopically in lymphatic channels[74] and lymph nodes[73,74] as well as the umbilicus[75], known to be rich in the lymphatics of pelvic origin.

Dissemination through the vascular system was initially suggested by Sampson[47] and subsequently confirmed by Javert[74]. There have been many reports since, demonstrating endometriosis in well-vascularized organs such as the lungs, skin and muscles[31]. The circumstances leading to the shedding of endometrial cells in the venous system are unknown. This must be an extremely unusual event or, alternatively, the viability of cells within the vascular system is extremely low.

Iatrogenic dissemination

It has long been appreciated that gynaecological surgical procedures, particularly when the endometrial cavity is entered, have been associated with iatrogenic transplantation of endometrial cells. Typically, these are caesarean sections, myomectomies, and hysterotomies for non-obstetric indications[76,77]. As the development of endometriosis involves the transplantation of autologous cells, the exfoliated cells would be expected to have a relatively high transplantation rate. This is supported by the experiments transplanting human endometrial tissue to the upper vagina[72] and anterior abdominal wall[52].

The squamous epithelium of the lower genital tract (exocervix, vagina and vulva) probably protects these areas from implantation of endometrial cells. Whether the likelihood of transplantation varies with the time of the cycle in which the surgery is performed remains unclear. It has been suggested that the probability of attachment is highest in the interval phase of the menstrual cycle, diminishing in the secretory luteal and premenstrual phase, and being least likely during pregnancy[78]. In the monkey, the survival of endometrial grafts derived from the basalis region is much higher than that of the functionalis region (80% vs 20%)[54,79]. This may explain the relatively low iatrogenic dissemination rate, as infrequently will the full thickness of the endometrium be surgically dislodged.

Summary of the transplantation hypothesis

From the above information, it is apparent that the aetiology of endometriosis involves transplantation of exfoliated endometrial cells. There is a substantial data base to support this with the vast majority of disease being accounted for by retrograde menstruation and intraperitoneal implantation. While lymphatic and haematogenous or iatrogenic routes have been demonstrated, the clinical pattern strongly supports the retrograde menstrual process in the vast majority of patients.

OTHER FACTORS

While virtually all cycling women menstruate retrogradely to some degree, not all develop endometriosis. The prevalence of the disease in the general female population of reproductive age is difficult to establish. Only women with clinical problems or desirous of voluntary sterilization have their pelvis visualized. Even with this selection bias, it becomes apparent there are some factors that influence any individual's probability of developing the disease.

Genetics

A familial probability of developing endometriosis has long been suspected on the basis of case reports[80] and retrospective reviews[81]. More formal genetic studies have demonstrated endometriosis in approximately 7% of first-degree female relatives of affected individuals[82,83] with a 2% risk for second-degree female relatives[82]. This appears to be through a maternal inheritance pattern[82], and those women with a first-degree relative with endometriosis are more likely to have severe disease[84]. The pattern appears to be one of polygenetic or multifactorial inheritance, and no relationship to HLA cell surface antigens has been noted[85,86].

Race

As noted earlier, endometriosis was originally believed to have a strong racial preponderance. However, once the confounding variables, such as availability of health care, access to contraception, cultural differences regarding childbearing patterns, and attitudes toward dysmenorrhoea and menses were considered, these differences disappear. Only in Japanese women does an increase in the incidence of endometriosis persist when corrected for confounding variables[9].

Menstrual factors

While no cases of endometriosis have been reported prior to the onset of puberty, the disease has certainly been noted in the teenage years[87]. There is a disproportionally large number of cases of endometriosis in this early interval attributable to Mullerian anomalies with absolute or relative uterine outflow obstruction. As our diagnostic tools have improved (e.g. laparoscopy), increasing numbers of young women have been detected with endometriosis, urging further efforts in preventing and controlling the disease in an attempt to minimize the effect on future fertility.

As retrograde menstruation is the predominant mechanism of development of endometriosis, women with menstrual patterns offering a greater opportunity for contamination of the peritoneal cavity by menstrual debris are likely to be at greater risk for development of the disease. This concept is supported by a controlled study of women with endometriosis-associated infertility, in which women with short menstrual lengths (less than 27 days) and longer menstrual flow (more than 7 days) had twice the risk of developing endometriosis compared with women with longer cycle lengths and shorter durations of flow[88]. Essentially, the more days of menstrual bleeding per year, the greater the probability of developing the disease. A greater incidence of menorrhagia and earlier average age of menarche have also been associated with endometriosis[89], but this has also been disputed[67], so no clear consensus is apparent.

The symptom of dysmenorrhoea has long been associated with endometriosis and has been proposed to be a consequence of the disease. Alternatively, prostaglandin-induced elevations in uterine pressure are thought to cause dysmenorrhoea[90] and may increase uterine pressure sufficiently to alter the volume of retrograde menstruation. This is particularly true if relative uterine outflow obstruction is present, and nulliparous women may be considered to have some degree of outflow obstruction in the absence of a vaginal delivery. According to this concept, dysmenorrhoea may be a clinical characteristic associated with higher pressures and increased tubal regurgitation rather than a consequence of the disease. While dysmenorrhoea has been reported to increase the risk of endometriosis, fertile women undergoing tubal sterilization have paradoxically been found to have no significant differences in the occurrence of dysmenorrhoea whether or not they had endometriosis[67]. Until further information is available about the pressure relationships between the uterotubal junction and cervix, this will remain a clouded area.

Delayed childbearing

Childbearing has long been recommended as a protective measure against the development of endometriosis[5]. Delayed childbearing, either by choice or as the result of infertility, has been implicated as a risk factor for the development of the disease. The finding to support this concept is that the risk of developing the disease correlates with a cumulative menstrual exposure (menstrual frequency and volume over time)[88,91]. Whether the protective hormones produced during pregnancy or an irreversibly enlarged cervix after a vaginal delivery alters the ultimate likelihood of retrograde menstruation remains to be clarified.

Uterine outflow obstruction

Development of endometriosis in the first few years after menarche has been associated with a high rate of obstructing genital tract anomalies including non-communicating rudimentary uterine horns, cervical stenosis, cervical atresia, vaginal agenesis, or an imperforate hymen[87]. As a general rule, those lesions at the level of the cervix have a higher incidence of the endometriosis than those lower in the genital tract (imperforate hymen). This explains the observation that in women with Mullerian anomalies, those with outflow obstruction were more likely to have endometriosis than those without outflow obstruction (77% vs 37%)[92,93].

Modest degrees of relative uterine outflow obstruction may play a role in development of endometriosis, but empiric cervical dilatation has never been shown to be preventative or therapeutic. Until better diagnostic methods are available to determine the direction of menstrual flow, this will remain a controversial issue. It has been suggested that contraceptive methods such as diaphragms or the use of tampons may obstruct outflow of the genital tract[13]. No convincing demonstration of an increased risk of endometriosis with the use of tampons, douching, cervical caps, or coitus during menses has been forthcoming.

Dependence on reproductive hormones

While endometriosis is found virtually exclusively in menstruating women, a clear picture of the hormonal dependence of these implants is still not available. While menopausal women may develop the disease[41,42], it is probably related to activation of pre-existing disease by oestrogen replacement therapy or increased endogenous hormone production because of obesity. The vast majority of women after menopause will have atrophic implants, consistent with the loss of gonadal hormone support. The specific hormonal conditions required for maintenance of endometrial implants has yet to be clearly defined.

It has been proposed that the cyclic use of monophasic oral contraceptive tablets may prevent or assist in management of endometriosis[94]. This is based on the lighter menstrual flow associated with these formulations and decreased dysmenorrhoea, presumably leading to decreased retrograde menstruation. The use of oral contraceptives is supported by the finding that only 13% of women with histologically proven endometriosis had taken oral contraceptives in the 2 years prior to diagnosis, substantially fewer than in the control group[89]. Caution should be exercised, as these data are potentially biased by the use of laparoscopy for detecting endometriosis in women with infertility. The length of oral contraceptive use tends to be inversely related to the severity of the disease as well[95]. Controversy continues, however, as women who are infertile may have less oral contraceptive use than expected[96]. Furthermore, the risk of developing endometriosis may be greater with the use of the older contraceptive tablets containing more than 50 μg of oestrogen. No increased risk has been observed with currently available lower-dose pills, but this requires a substantially greater data base to provide secure observation.

The use of pseudo-pregnancy (continuous high-dose oral contraceptives) has long been advocated because of the beneficial effects of pregnancy on existing endometriosis[97,98]. The behaviour of endometriosis during pregnancy is extremely variable and endometriosis clearly cannot be considered to be 'cured' by pregnancy[99].

Prenatal exposure to diethystilboestrol (DES) has been noted to cause a variety of anomalies of the genital tract and has been suggested to be associated with infertility[100–103]. No association between endometriosis and prenatal DES exposure has been established. The cause of infertility in this population is not clear, but, as increasingly subtle degrees of endometriosis are being identified, the possibility of an association still remains.

Immunological phenomena

As endometriosis represents an autologous tissue graft, the possibility of an aberrant immunological response has fascinated many investigators. Cell-mediated immunity, as measured by lymphocyte cytotoxicity *in vitro*, has been demonstrated in women[104] and in a rhesus monkey model of endometriosis[105]. Despite this interest, no clinically significant immune system abnormalities have been observed in women with endometriosis, and there are no differences in individual subsets of circulating lymphocyte populations[106].

It has been apparent recently that there is a localized intraperitoneal inflammatory reaction associated with endometriosis[107–110]. The likely stimulus responsible for eliciting this response is retrograde menstruation rather than endometrial implants. Women who have ovulation suppressed, or do not have patent fallopian tubes, have much lower intraperitoneal leukocyte counts[111]. A variety of secretory products of these inflammatory cells (i.e. proteolytic enzymes and cytokines), are also present and may have adverse influences on sperm or embryos. It has further been suggested that growth factors in the peritoneal fluid of women with endometriosis may enhance the likelihood of transplantation. How significant this inflammatory response is in the development of endometriosis is unclear. It is more likely a response to the regurgitated menstrual debris rather than the stimulus for developing endometriosis.

SUMMARY

The probability that an individual woman will develop endometriosis can be viewed in quantitative terms. Familial factors, delaying childbearing and increasing the cumulative menstrual exposure appear to enhance the development of the disease. The nearly universal phenomenon of retrograde menstruation and the inherent ability of pelvic tissues to support endometrial transplantation allow virtually any woman the opportunity to develop the disease. Factors that determine the degree of retrograde menstruation remain to be elucidated, and immunological factors may affect a woman's susceptibility to the implantation of exfoliated endometrial cells.

REFERENCES

1. Hassan, H.M. (1976). Incidence of endometriosis in diagnostic laparoscopy. *J. Reprod. Med.*, **16**, 135
2. Strathy, J.H., Molgaard, C.A. and Coulman, C.B. (1982). Endometriosis and infertility: a laparoscopic study of endometriosis among fertile and infertile women. *Fertil. Steril.*, **38**, 667
3. Norwood, G.E. (1960). Sterility and fertility in women with pelvic endometriosis. *Clin. Obstet. Gynecol.*, **3**, 456
4. Dmowski, W.P. (1981). Current concepts in the management of endometriosis. *Obstet. Gynecol. Annu.*, **10**, 279
5. Meigs, J.V. (1953). Endometriosis. Etiologic role of marriage, age and parity: Conservative treatment. *Obstet. Gynecol.*, **2**, 46
6. Scott, R.B. and Telinde, R.W. (1950). External endometriosis: Scourge of the private patient. *Ann. Surg.*, **131**, 697
7. Chatman, D.L. (1976). Endometriosis and the black woman. *J. Reprod. Med.*, **16**, 303
8. Meigs, J.V. (1949). The medical treatment of endometriosis. *Surg. Gynecol. Obstet.*, **106**, 516
9. Miyazawa, K. (1976). Incidence of endometriosis among Japanese women. *Obstet. Gynecol.*, **48**, 407
10. Lloyd, F.P. (1964). Endometriosis in the Negro woman. *Am. J. Obstet. Gynecol.*, **89**, 468
11. Cavanagh, W.V. (1951). Fertility in the etiology of endometriosis. *Am. J. Obstet. Gynecol.*, **61**, 539
12. Weed, J.C. (1955). Endometriosis in the Negro. *Ann. Surg.*, **141**, 615
13. Sensky, T.E. and Liu, D.T.Y. (1980). Endometriosis: associations with menorrhagia, infertility and oral contraceptives. *Int. J. Gynecol. Obstet.*, **17**, 573
14. Hanton, E.M., Malkasian, G.D. Jr and Dockerty, M.B. (1967). Endometriosis in young women. *Am. J. Obstet. Gynecol.*, **98**, 116
15. Fallus, R. and Rosenblum, G. (1940). Endometriosis: a study of 260 private hospital cases. *Am. J. Obstet. Gynecol.*, **39**, 964
16. Buttram, V.C. Jr (1979). Conservative surgery for endometriosis in the infertile female: a study of 206 patients with implications for both medical and surgical therapy. *Fertil. Steril.*, **31**, 117
17. Haydon, G.B. (1942). A study of 569 cases of endometriosis. *Am. J. Obstet. Gynecol.*, **43**, 704

18. Ranney, B. (1971). Endometriosis. III. Complete operations: reasons, sequelae, treatment. *Am. J. Obstet. Gynecol.*, **109**, 1137
19. Holmes, W.R. (1942). Endometriosis. *Am. J. Obstet. Gynecol.*, **43**, 255
20. Smith, G.V.S. (1929). Endometrioma. *Am. J. Obstet. Gynecol.*, **17**, 806
21. Sturgis, S.H. and Call, B.J. (1954). Endometriosis peritonei — relationship of pain to functional activity. *Am. J. Obstet. Gynecol.*, **68**, 1421
22. Noble, A.D. and Letchworth, A.T. (1979). Medical treatment of endometriosis: a comparative trial. *Postgrad. Med. J.*, **5**(suppl.), 55
23. Novak, E.R. (1960). Pathology of endometriosis. *Clin. Obstet. Gynecol.*, **3**, 413
24. Radwanska, E., Rana, N. and Dmowski, W.P. (1984). Management of infertility in women with endometriosis and ovulatory dysfunction. *Fertil. Steril.*, **41**, 77S
25. Soules, M.R., Malinak, L.R., Bury, R. *et al.* (1976). Endometriosis and anovulation: a coexisting problem in the infertile female. *Am. J. Obstet. Gynecol.*, **125**, 412
26. Abeshouse, B.S. and Abeshouse, G. (1960). Endometriosis of the urinary tract: a review of the literature. *J. Int. Coll. Surg.*, **34**, 43
27. Bates, J.S. and Beecham, C.T. (1969). Retroperitoneal endometriosis with ureteral obstruction. *Obstet. Gynecol.*, **34**, 242
28. Davis, C., Jr. and Trueheart, R. (1964). Surgical management of endometrioma of the colon. *Am. J. Obstet. Gynecol.*, **89**, 453
29. Sen, S.K., Treherne, C.A. and Perry, F.A. (1967). Endometriosis of the ureter in a post-hysterectomy patient. *J. Natl. Med. Assoc.*, **59**, 327
30. Jansen, R.P.S. (1986). Minimal endometriosis and reduced fecundability: Prospective evidence from an artificial insemination by donor program. *Fertil. Steril.*, **46**, 141
31. Ridley, J.H. (1968). A review of facts and fancies. *Obstet. Gynecol. Surv.*, **23**, 1
32. Merrill, J.A. (1963). Experimental induction of endometriosis across millipore filters. *Surg. Forum*, **14**, 397
33. Merrill, J.A. (1966). Experimental induction of endometriosis across millipore filters. *Am. J. Obstet. Gynecol.*, **94**, 780
34. Acien, P. (1986). Endometriosis and genital anomalies: Some histogenetic aspects of external endometriosis. *Gynecol. Obstet. Invest.*, **22**, 102
35. Melicow, M.M. and Pachter, M.R. (1967). Endometrial carcinoma of the prostate utricle (uterus masculinus). *Cancer*, **20**, 1715
36. Olikar, A.F. and Harns, A.E. (1971). Endometriosis in the bladder in a male patient. *J. Urol.*, **106**, 858
37. Pinkert, T.C., Catlow, C.E. and Strauss, R. (1979). Endometriosis of the urinary bladder in a man with prostatic carcinoma. *Cancer*, **43**, 1562
38. Schrodt, G.R., Alcorn, M.D. and Ibanez, J. (1980). Endometriosis of the male urinary system: A case report. *J. Urol.*, **124**, 722
39. Filatow, D. (1933). Uber die Bildung des Anfangstadium bie der Extremitatenentwhchlung. *Roux Arch. Entwicklungsmechnd. Organ.*, **127**, 776
40. Maximow, A. (1927). Uber der Mesothel (Deckzellen der serosen Exudate: Untersuchungen an entzundetem Gewebe und and Gerwebskulturen. *Arch. Exp. Zellforsch.*, **4**, 1
41. Kempers, R.D., Dockerty, M.B. and Hunt, A.B. (1960). Significant postmenopausal endometriosis. *Surg. Gynecol. Obstet.*, **111**, 348
42. Punnonen, R., Klemi, P. and Nikkanen, R. (1980). Postmenopausal endometriosis. *Eur. J. Obstet. Gynecol. Reprod. Biol.*, **11**, 195
43. Batt, R.E., Smith, R.A., Buck, G.M., Maples, J.D. and Severino, M.F. (1989). A case series — Peritoneal pockets and endometriosis: Rudimentary duplications of the Mullerian system. *Adolesc. Pediatr. Gynecol.*, **2**, 47
44. Olive, D.L., Franklin, R.R. and Gratkins, L.V. (1982). Association between endometriosis and spontaneous abortions: a retrospective clinical study. *J. Reprod. Med.*, **27**, 333
45. Sampson, J.A. (1922). Ovarian hematomas of endometrial type (performing hemorrhagic cysts of the ovary) and implantation adenomas of endometrial type. *Boston Med. Surg. J.*, **186**, 445
46. Sampson, J.A. (1925). Heterotopic of misplaced endometrial tissue. *Am. J. Obstet. Gynecol.*, **10**, 649
47. Sampson, J.A. (1927). Metatasis of embolic endometriosis due to menstrual dissemination of endometrial tissue into the venous circulation. *Am. J. Pathol.*, **3**, 93

48. Sampson, J.A. (1927). Peritoneal endometriosis due to the menstrual dissemination of endometrial tissue to the peritoneal cavity. *Am. J. Obstet. Gynecol.*, **14**, 422
49. Cron, R.S. and Gey, G. (1927). The viability of cast-off menstrual endometrium. *Am. J. Obstet. Gynecol.*, **13**, 645
50. Keetel, W.C. and Stein, R.J. (1951). The viability of the cast-off menstrual endometrium. *Am. J. Obstet. Gynecol.*, **61**, 440
51. Allan, E., Peterson, L.F. and Campbell, Z.B. (1954). Clinical and experimental endometriosis. *Am. J. Obstet. Gynecol.*, **68**, 356
52. Ridley, J.H. and Edwards, K.I. (1958). Experimental endometriosis in the human. *Am. J. Obstet. Gynecol.*, **76**, 783
53. Dizerega, G.S., Barber, D.L. and Hodgen, C.D. (1980). Endometriosis: Role of ovarian steroids in initiation, maintenance and suppression. *Fertil. Steril.*, **33**, 649
54. Markee, J.E. (1948). Morphological basis for menstrual bleeding. *Bull. N.Y. Acad. Med.*, **18**, 159
55. Flowers, D.E. Jr. and Wilborn, W.H. (1978). New observations on the physiology of menstruation. *Obstet. Gynecol.*, **51**, 16
56. Vijayakumar, R. and Walters, W.W.W. (1977). Myometrial prostaglandins during the human menstrual cycle. *Am. J. Obstet. Gynecol.*, **141**, 313
57. Scott, R.B., Telinde, R.W. and Wharton, L.R. (1953). Further studies on experimental endometriosis. *Am. J. Obstet. Gynecol.*, **66**, 1101
58. Scott, R.B. and Wharton, L.R. (1957). The effects of estrone and progesterone on the growth of experimental endometriosis in Rhesus monkeys. *Am. J. Obstet. Gynecol.*, **74**, 852
59. Gerloch, A.H. and Hooser, C.W. (1976). Oviduct response to glucagon during hysterosalpingography. *Radiology*, **119**, 727
60. Beller, R.M. and Hochner-Celnikier, D. (1982). The effect on uterine cornual spasm during general anesthesia. *Int. J. Fertil.*, **27**, 187
61. Winfield, A.C., Pittaway, D. and Maxson, W. (1982). Apparent cornual occlusion in hysterosalpingography. Reversal by glucagon. *Am. J. Radiol.*, **13**, 525
62. Ayers, J.W.T. and Friedenstab, A.P. (1985). Uterotubal hypotonia associated with pelvic endometriosis [abstract 519] presented at the *41st Annual Meeting of the American Fertility Society*, Chicago, September 28–October 2
63. Baker, E.R., Horger, E.O. and Williamson, H.O. (1982). Congenital atresia of the uterine cervix: two cases. *J. Reprod. Med.*, **27**, 156
64. Schifrin, B.S., Erez, S. and Moore, J.G. (1973). Teenage endometriosis. *Am. J. Obstet. Gynecol.*, **116**, 973
65. Blumenkrantz, M.J., Gallagher, N. and Bashore, R.A. (1981). Retrograde menstruation in women undergoing chronic peritoneal dialysis. *Obstet. Gynecol.*, **57**, 667
66. Halme, J., Hammond, M.G. and Hulka, J.F. (1984). Retrograde menstruation in healthy women and in patients with endometriosis. *Obstet. Gynecol.*, **64**, 141
67. Liu, D.T.Y. and Hitchcock, A. (1968). Endometriosis; Its association with retrograde menstruation, dysmenorrhea and tubal pathology. *Br. J. Obstet. Gynaecol.*, **93**, 859
68. Bartosik, D., Jacobs, S.L. and Kelly, L.J. (1986). Endometrial tissue in peritoneal fluid. *Fertil. Steril.*, **46**, 796
69. Geist, S.F. (1979). The viability of fragments of menstrual endometrium. *Am. J. Obstet. Gynecol.*, **125**, 751
70. Novak, E. (1926). The significance of uterine mucosa in the fallopian tube with a discussion of the origin of aberrant endometrium. *Am. J. Obstet. Gynecol.*, **12**, 484
71. Manning, J.O. and Shaver, E.R. Jr. (1937). The demonstration of endometrial cells by Papanicolaou and supravital techniques obtained by culdocentesis. *Bull. Tulane Univ. Med. Fac.*, **18**, 159
72. Jenkins, S., Olive, D.L. and Haney, A.F. (1986). Endometriosis: Pathogenic implications of the anatomic distribution. *Obstet. Gynecol.*, **67**, 335
73. Halban, J. (1925). Metastatic hysteradenosis: lymphatic organ of so-called heterotopic adenofibromatosis. *Arch. Gynak.*, **124**, 475
74. Javert, C.T. (1949). Pathogenesis of endometriosis based on endometrial homeoplasia, direct extension, exfoliation and implantation, lymphomatic and hematogenous metastasis. *Cancer*, **2**, 399

75. Scott, R.B., Nowak, R.M. and Tindale, R.M. (1958). Umbilical endometriosis and Cullen's sign: Study of lymphatic transport from pelvis to umbilicus in monkeys. *Obstet. Gynecol.*, **11**, 556

76. Chatterjee, S.K. (1980). Scar endometriosis: A clinicopathologic study of 17 cases. *Obstet. Gynecol.*, **56**, 81

77. Lewin, E. (1954). Artificial endometriosis of vagina. *Geburtshilfe Frauenheilkd.*, **14**, 550

78. Scott, R.B. and Telinde, R.W. (1954). Clinical external endometriosis. *Obstet. Gynecol.*, **4**, 502

79. Brenner, R.M., Sternfeld, M.D. and West, N.B. (1987). Subcutaneous endometrial grafts in rhesus monkeys as a model of endometriosis [abstract 16]. Presented at the *43rd Annual Meeting of the American Fertility Society*, Reno, Nevada, September 28–30

80. Frey, C.H. (1957). The familial occurrence of endometriosis. *Am. J. Obstet. Gynecol.*, **73**, 418

81. Ranney, B. (1971). Endometriosis. IV. Hereditary tendencies. *Obstet. Gynecol.*, **37**, 374

82. Lamb, K., Hoffman, R.G. and Nichols, T.R. (1986). Family traits analysis: A case-control study of 43 women with endometriosis and their best friends. *Am. J. Obstet. Gynecol.*, **154**, 596

83. Simpson, J.L., Elias, S. and Malianak, L.R. (1984). Heritable aspects of endometriosis. I. Genetic studies. *Am. J. Obstet. Gynecol.*, **137**, 327

84. Malinak, L.R., Buttram, V.C. Jr. and Elias, S. (1980). Heritable aspects of endometriosis. II. Clinical characteristics of familial endometriosis. *Am. J. Obstet. Gynecol.*, **137**, 332

85. Moen, M., Bratile, A. and Moen, T. (1984). Distribution of HLA-antigens among patients with endometriosis. *Acta Obstet. Gynecol. Scand.*, **123** (suppl.), 25

86. Simpson, J.L., Malinak, L.R. and Elias, S. (1984). HLA associations in endometriosis. *Am. J. Obstet. Gynecol.*, **148**, 395

87. Huffman, W. (1981). Endometriosis in young teenage girls. *Pediatr. Annu.*, **10**, 44

88. Cramer, D.W., Wilson, E. and Stillman, R.J. (1986). The relation of endometriosis characteristics, smoking and exercise. *J. Am. Med. Assoc.*, **255**, 1904

89. Sensky, T.E. and Liu, D.T.Y. (1980). Endometriosis: Association with menorrhagia, infertility and oral contraceptives. *Int. J. Gynecol. Obstet.*, **17**, 573

90. Schulman, H., Duvivier, R. and Blattner, M.S. (1983). The uterine contractility index: A research and diagnostic tool in dysmenorhea. *Am. J. Obstet. Gynecol.*, **145**, 1049

91. Olive, D.O. and Hammond, C.B. (1986). Endometriosis and mechanisms of infertility. *Postgrad. Obstet. Gynecol.*, **5**, 1

92. Olive, D.L. and Henderson, D.Y. (1987). Endometriosis and mullerian anomalies. *Obstet. Gynecol.*, **69**, 412

93. Ranney, B. (1980). Etiology, prevention and inhibition of endometriosis. *Clin. Obstet. Gynecol.*, **23**, 875

94. Novak, E.R. and Woodruff, J.D. (1979). *Novak's Gynecologic and Obstetric Pathology*, 8th edn. p. 561. Philadelphia: W.B. Saunders

95. Buttram, V.C. (1979). Cyclic use of combination oral contraceptions and the severity of endometriosis. *Fertil. Steril.*, **31**, 347

96. Cramer, D.W., Wilson, E. and Stillman, R. (1986). The association of endometriosis with oral contraceptive use [abstract 328]. Presented at the *42nd Meeting of the American Fertility Society*, Toronto, Ontario, Canada, September 27–October 2

97. Andrews, M.C., Andrews, W.C. and Strauss, P. (1959). Effects of progestin-induced pseudopregnancy on endometriosis: Clinical and microscopic studies. *Am. J. Obstet. Gynecol.*, **78**, 776

98. Kistner, R.W. (1958). The use of newer progestins in the treatment of endometriosis. *Am. J. Obstet. Gynecol.*, **75**, 264

99. McArthur, J.W. and Ulfelder, H. (1965). The effects of pregnancy upon endometriosis. *Obstet. Gynecol. Surv.*, **20**, 709

100. Berger, M.J. and Goldstein, D.P. (1980). Impaired reproductive performance in DES exposed women. *Obstet. Gynecol.*, **55**, 25

101. Kaufman, R.H., Adam, F. and Binder, G.L. (1980). Upper genital tract changes and pregnancy outcome in offspring exposed to diethylstilbestrol. *Am. J. Obstet. Gynecol.*, **137**, 299

102. Stillman, R.J. and Miller, L.C. (1984). Diethylstilbestrol exposure in utero and endometriosis

in infertile females. *Fertil. Steril.*, **41**, 369
103. Senekjian, E.K., Pokul, R.K., Frey, K. and Herbst, A.L. (1988). Infertility among daughters either exposed or not to diethylstilbestrol. *Am. J. Obstet. Gynecol.*, **158**, 493
104. Steele, R.W., Dmowski, W.P. and Marmer, D.J. (1984). Immunologic aspects of human endometriosis. *Am. J. Reprod. Immunol.*, **6**, 33
105. Dmowski, W.P., Steele, R.W. and Baker, G.F. (1981). Deficient cellular immunity in endometriosis. *Am. J. Obstet. Gynecol.*, **141**, 377
106. Gleicher, N., Dmowski, W.P. and Siegel, I. (1984). Lymphocyte subsets in endometriosis. *Obstet. Gynecol.*, **63**, 463
107. Drake, T., O'Brien, W. and Grunert, G. (1980). Peritoneal fluid volume in endometriosis. *Fertil Steril.*, **34**, 280
108. Haney, A.F., Muscato, J.J. and Weinberg, J.B. (1981). Peritoneal fluid cell populations in infertility patients. *Fertil. Steril.*, **35**, 696
109. Halme, J., Becker, S. and Hammond, M.G. (1983). Increased activation of pelvic macrophages in infertile women with mild endometriosis. *Am. J. Obstet. Gynecol.*, **145**, 333
110. Badawy, S.Z.A., Cuenca, V. and Marshall, L. (1984). Cellular components of peritoneal fluid in infertile patients with and without endometriosis. *Fertil. Steril.*, **41**, 20S
111. Haney, A.F. and Weinberg, J.B. (1988). Reduction of the intraperitoneal inflammation associated with endometriosis by treatment with medroxyprogesterone acetate. *Am. J. Obstet. Gynecol.*, **159**, 450

2
The endometriotic implant

I. A. Brosens

Endometriosis is classically defined by the presence of endometrial glands and stroma in regions remote from the uterine cavity. Evidence is increasing that different types of implants may represent different stages in the evolution of the disease and be associated with a different pathophysiology. The question has also been posed whether these types have different laparoscopic appearances. This chapter discusses the concept of endometriosis as a progressive disease, but self-limiting and therefore producing multiple appearances. A classification system for the morphological and laparoscopic appearances is attempted.

MICROANATOMICAL STRUCTURE

Using a combination of scanning electron microscopy (SEM) and histology, Vasquez *et al.*[1] described three microanatomical types of peritoneal endometriosis (Table 2.1). The first type is characterized by multiple or single endometriotic polyps measuring 200–700 µm in largest diameter, although one polyp of 1800 µm was observed. The polyps are sited under a mesothelial vesicle, which usually ruptures when the biopsy is taken. The surface of the polyp is covered by rounded to cuboidal non-ciliated cells bearing microvilli

Table 2.1 Histological characteristics of three micro-anatomical types of endometriotic implants

Relation to peritoneum	Endometrial components		
	Surface epithelium	*Glands*	*Stroma*
Submesothelial	+	−	+
Intraperitoneal	+	+/−	+/−
Subperitoneal	−	+	+/−

and a few isolated ciliated cells. Glandular openings are not seen. Histological sections of the polyps revealed the presence of a highly vascularized stroma beneath the surface epithelium. The stroma occasionally extends further in the neighbouring subperitoneal tissue so that the endometriotic implant is larger than the polyp seen by scanning electron microscopy. Additional serial sections revealed that these polyps were in continuity with glands at the base of the polyp (Figure 2.1). The surface epithelium of the polyp is, as in eutopic endometrium, an extension of the glandular epithelium.

The second type presents endometrial surface epithelium replacing the mesothelium. Ciliated cells can be identified by SEM (Figure 2.2). At the transition with the surrounding mesothelium the epithelial cells tend to become flattened. In contrast with the first type, this type is a true intraperitoneal implant. Glandular structures can be present or absent. Murphy et al.[2] have shown that this type of implant can be found by SEM in areas where no lesions are seen at laparoscopy.

A third type of implant cannot be detected by SEM as it is enclosed in the subperitoneal tissue. The endometriotic elements include glands and stroma but no surface epithelium (Figure 2.3). This endometrial lesion represents the classical definition of endometriosis.

These three microanatomical types of endometriotic implants are distinguished on the basis of their relationship with the peritoneum and their endometrial components (Table 2.1). In a series of 30 biopsies, Vasquez[1] found 16 (53%) implants with a surface epithelium (Type I or II).

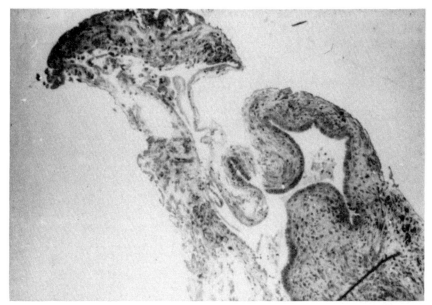

Figure 2.1 Polyp type of peritoneal endometriotic implant. The polyp arises from a glandular structure and was covered by mesothelium. The biopsy was taken from a haemorrhagic vesicle

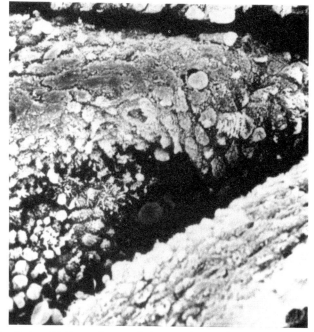

Figure 2.2 Endometriotic surface epithelium replacing the mesothelium. The area is identifiable by the presence of ciliated cells in scanning electron microscopy.

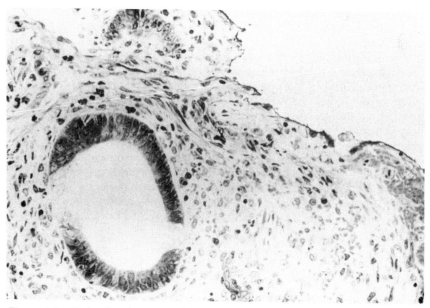

Figure 2.3 Enclosed endometriotic lesions with glandular and stromal elements but no surface epithelium. The area is covered by normal peritoneum

COMPARISON WITH ENDOMETRIUM

Cyclic histological changes in ectopic implants have been reported by Roddick et al.[3]. Enzyme histochemical studies also supported the concept that endometriotic foci undergo cyclic changes similar but not identical to those of the uterine glands. Schweppe et al.[4] have shown by histological and electron-microscopic studies that functional changes in endometriotic glands do not proceed as clearly and uniformly as in the uterine mucosa. The selection of implants for biopsy may have influenced their result, and as their material included glands only it is very likely that their study was largely based on the classical type of lesion.

In 1962 Nieminen[5] examined the vascular changes in large pathological specimens of pelvic endometriosis in correlation with endometrial changes and distinguished three histological types of implants: the free, enclosed, and healed implants.

The free-growing implants have a polyp or cauliflower structure, and are growing along the surface or covering a cystic structure. They are characterized by the presence of a surface epithelium supported by endometrial stroma. Endometrial glands can be present or absent. Cyclical changes corresponding with superficial endometrium changes, including advanced secretory changes and menstrual bleeding, are noted in free-growing implants.

The enclosed implants have no surface epithelium and are located within tissue or are part of a free-growing lesion. They may also present as wedge-like extensions of stroma, often deep in local tissue connecting lesions with each other. Cyclical changes during the menstrual cycle occur only in the minority of the cases and late secretory changes or menstrual bleeding are not seen in these implants. Capillary and venous dilatation are seen during the luteal phase but no arterial necrosis or bleeding occurs at the time of menstruation.

The healed lesion is characterized by cystically enlarged glands with a thin glandular epithelium supported by small, fusiform stromal cells and surrounded by connective tissue.

The endometriotic implant reacts differently during the menstrual cycle according to the presence or absence of surface epithelium. In the presence of surface epithelium, the implant compares with the superficial endometrium, where at the end of the cycle the secretory changes are associated with arteriolar changes leading to necrosis and bleeding at the time of menstruation. In the absence of surface epithelium, the implant compares rather with basal endometrium, where proliferation, some secretory changes and vasodilatation occur but no necrosis of the arterioles at the time of menstruation. In the absence of stroma, the atrophic cystic gland is enclosed in connective tissue, resulting in scar formation.

LAPAROSCOPIC APPEARANCES

During recent years the different laparoscopic appearances of peritoneal endometriosis have been studied and correlated with their morphological characteristics[1,2,6,7]. More than 15 laparoscopic appearances have been described. On the basis of the appearance and cellular activity, the following correlation between laparoscopic appearance and the morphological structure can be proposed.

The classical implant is a *nodular lesion* characterized by a variable degree of fibrosis and pigmentation (Figure 2.4). The colour can vary from white to blue, brown or black. On histological examination the biopsies of such lesions show glandular tissue in approximately 50% of the biopsies. The endometrial tissue is represented by glandular epithelium surrounded by stroma. The glandular epithelium shows a variable degree of activity but is frequently inactive or even involutionary during the menstrual cycle.

The *vesicular implant* is a small lesion with a diameter of less than 5 mm and occurs singly or in clusters. The implant is characterized by a prominent vascularization and is frequently red in appearance because of haemorrhagic admixture (Figure 2.5). The surrounding peritoneum also shows an increased vascularization. In the absence of bleeding, the vesicle contains a straw-yellow fluid. On biopsy, endometrial tissue is found in 95% of the biopsies. The endometrial tissue frequently shows the presence of surface epithelium covering a highly vascularized stroma. Fluid is accumulated between the surface of the implant and the overlying peritoneum, resulting in a blister or vesicle formation.

The *papular implant* is also a small lesion with a diameter of less than 5 mm and occurs singly or in clusters. The colour is whitish or yellow. On histology, the implant represents a cystic glandular structure with stroma and is enclosed

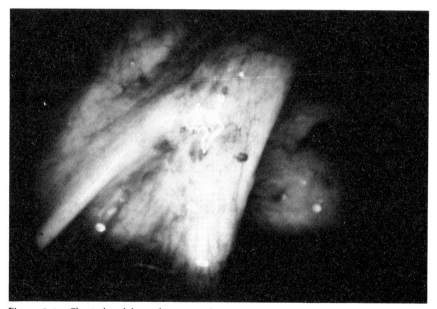

Figure 2.4 Classical nodular endometriotic lesion with pigmentation, fibrosis and retraction. Histologically this lesion is characterized by the presence of a variable degree of glandular and stromal components and a variable degree of cellular activity (proliferation)

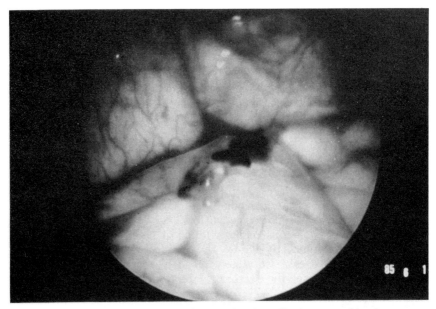

Figure 2.5 Haemorrhagic vesicle. The lesion is histologically characterized by the presence of surface epithelium and stroma. The fresh bleeding is accumulated in a vesicle covered by mesothelium

in the subperitoneal tissue. The vascularization of the peritoneum can be seen overlying the implant (Figure 2.6). Accumulation of secretory products results in a cystic structure of the implant with a whitish or yellow opaque colour protruding on the surface of the peritoneum.

Table 2.2 summarizes the proposed correlation between the morphological type of implant and the laparoscopic appearance. Haemorrhagic lesions are found when the implants have a surface epithelium studded by stroma and its vascular supply. These lesions are flourishing and show proliferation, secretion, vesicle formation and haemorrhage at the time of menstruation. They can be identified at laparoscopy by their fresh haemorrhagic appearance. Papular and nodular lesions have no surface epithelium and their components show proliferation and vasodilatation only during the menstrual cycle. Full secretory changes and menstrual bleeding are not seen in these implants. Healed implants with cystic glands and scanty or no stroma but surrounded by connnective tissue present as nodular or fibrotic scar tissue. Laparoscopic criteria for distinguishing between the active and the inactive or healed nodular implant have not been established.

EVOLUTION OF PERITONEAL ENDOMETRIOSIS

Endometriotic implants have been shown to respond in a variable degree to the hormones of the ovarian cycle and to have steroid receptors, but to a lesser degree than eutopic endometrium. This variation may depend largely

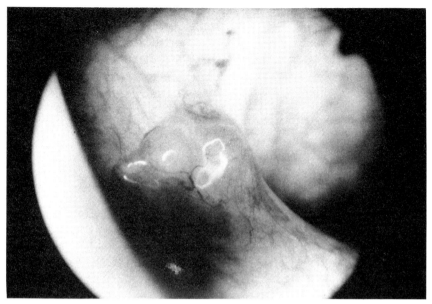

Figure 2.6 Subperitoneal papular lesion. The lesion is produced by a cystic glandular structure and is surrounded by peritoneum with its vascular network. No surface epithelium is present. Proliferative changes but no haemorrhage are found in this lesion

Table 2.2 Histological characteristics of endometriotic implants and their laparoscopic appearance

Histological type	Components			Hormonal response			Laparoscopic appearance
	Surface epithelium	Glands	Stroma	Proliferation	Secretion	Menstruation	
Free	+	+/−	+	+	+	+	Haemorrhagic vesicle or spot
Enclosed	−	+	+	+	+/−	−	papule (early lesion) nodule (late lesion)
Healed	−	+	−	−	−	−	Nodule, scar

on the type and evolution of the implant.

The peritoneal implants are likely to represent different stages of the disease and further studies are needed to clarify the evolution of these implants. What was an active enclosed lesion may become a healed, inactive lesion depending on the regression of the stromal component and the increase in connective tissue and fibrosis. Flattening and involutionary changes in the glandular epithelium are characteristics of a healed lesion. It is therefore no surprise that frequently glandular tissue is not found in white, fibrotic, healed lesions.

Redwine[8] has shown the colour of the implant evolving from clear to red to black with the increasing mean age of the patients. The haemorrhagic vesicle is indeed likely to be derived from the whitish or opaque papular implant. Epithelial tuffs of the active gland can form polypoidal structures emerging on the surface of the implant and producing the haemorrhagic vesicle. The highly vascularized polyp responds like superficial endometrium to the ovarian hormones leading to vascular necrosis and bleeding at the time of menstruation. Inflammatory changes and fibroreactive tissue can modify the free haemorrhagic implant into an active enclosed implant that may either continue to grow as a deep implant or lead to spontaneous healing (Table 2.3).

OVARIAN ENDOMETRIOSIS

In the ovary, endometriosis presents usually either in the form of a superficial haemorrhagic lesion or in the more severe form as a haemorrhagic cyst.

The *superficial lesions* can occur on all sides of the ovary. There is a strong tendency for adhesion formation, sometimes covering most of the ovary. These adhesions can be missed at laparoscopy when they are avascular and transparent.

The term 'chocolate cyst' has been applied to describe the endometrial cyst of the ovary. The term is descriptive but can be misleading if one notices only the chocolate-coloured content of the cyst. Haemorrhagic cysts of functional origin are a frequent finding in the presence of pelvic endometriosis and the diagnosis of ovarian endometriosis by the chocolate content of the cyst can be misleading. Other features such as the site of the cyst on the lateral surface of the ovary, the haemorrhagic adhesions and the puckering scar formation are indicative of an endometriotic cyst. However, not infrequently and particularly following ovarian surgery, these characteristics can be lacking, making the exact diagnosis of the endometrial origin impossible.

The histopathology of ovarian endometriosis is characterized by a wide variation in the amount of endometrial tissue. The endometrial cyst can be lined by free endometrial tissue that histologically and functionally cannot be distinguished from eutopic endometrium. On the other hand, all traces of endometrial tissue can be lost and the wall of the cyst covered by fibrotic

Table 2.3 Proposed evolution of the endometrial peritoneal implant

Laparoscopic appearance	Morphological process
Subperitoneal papule (whitish, opaque) ↓	Active, dilated gland covered by peritoneum. Epithelial tuffs leading to polyp formation with surface epithelium
Haemorrhagic vesicle (red) ↓	Subperitoneal polyp with haemorrhage
Classical endometriotic nodule (black, brown, blue, white)	Inflammatory reaction and fibrosis leading to enclosed lesion. Continuing growth of glands and stroma or scarification

and reactive tissue. No specific pathology can be found in up to one-third of clinically typical endometriosis cases, and these cysts are classified as haemorrhagic cysts (compatible with endometriosis). The haemorrhagic content of these cysts is likely to originate from chronic bleeding of small areas of free endometriosis, and occasionally from bleeding of an haemorrhagic corpus luteum within the endometrial cyst. Hughesdon[9] has pointed out that in most endometrial cysts the inside of the chocolate cyst is the outside of the ovary. The inverted ovarian cortex is frequently adherent to the parametrium or fossa ovarica. It is a well-known clinical observation that frequently such a chocolate cyst cannot be mobilized from its fixed position in the ovarian fossa or on the back of the broad ligament without rupturing its content.

THE EVALUATION OF MEDICAL THERAPY

Clinical studies of medical therapy of endometriosis are faced with major difficulties in evaluating the effect of treatment. Laparoscopy has been used to evaluate the effect of medical treatment and a variable degree of resolution has been described after long-term therapy. However, the observations made at the time of the second-look laparoscopy at the end of a medical treatment can be subject to erroneous interpretations. In such circumstances the foci of endometriosis are compared under two different hormonal conditions, i.e. under conditions of normal versus suppressed ovarian activity. Suppression of the ovarian activity by medical treatment may allow resorption of the serous or haemorrhagic vesicles. Therefore, a so-called 'clean' pelvis at the end of therapy is no proof of disappearance of the implant in terms of endometrial tissue. Second-look laparoscopy at 2 months after therapy has not shown a significant difference in the size and number of implants with preoperative laparoscopy[10].

Histological and ultrastructural studies have shown that medical therapy with danazol, gestrinone or GnRH agonists has a marked involutionary effect on many endometriotic glandular epithelial cells[11]. Lysosomal degradation, especially within the apical cytoplasm, is a striking morphological event. Lysosomes are numerous and usually they are of large size. Most of them are of the telelysosome type and contain amorphous cell debris, while a few others include a lipidic moiety and thus resemble lipofuscin vacuoles. Simultaneously, the cell nucleus may be heavily indented, its chromatin being clumped. Loss of apical microvilli and extrusion of cytoplasmic lysosomes resulting in a concentration of damaged mitochondria within the thin supranuclear area are observed. In the endometrium, an activation of the lysosomal system is usually observed towards the end of the cycle when autophagic vacuoles are numerous and some of them are of a large size (giant lysosomes). Apoptic bodies are also described. This endometrial intracellular lysosomal involution seems to be a physiological hormonal withdrawal effect. It seems reasonable to suggest that lysosomal involution of endometriotic cells may be enhanced due to competitive binding of danazol or gestrinone to cellular progesterone receptors or steroid deprivation by GnRH agonists.

The low number, or even the absence, of progesterone receptors in some foci may thus explain why not all lesions respond to this activation of the lysosomal system. Furthermore, since in most implants growth and differentiation of endometriotic cells are usually less pronounced than in the endometrium, the subsequent endometriotic involution is less dramatic and less organized. Therefore, apoptosis is rather uncommon while the number of intra-epithelial phagocytes is not substantially increased. It may thus be concluded that epithelial cellular involution mainly proceeds by autophagy.

This cellular involution can be achieved by a short-term medical therapy. There is no evidence that a long-term therapy will significantly enhance the regressive changes. On the contrary, a 2-month therapy with a daily dose of 1.25 mg gestrinone was shown to have a stronger effect than a 4-month therapy of 2.5 mg gestrinone twice or thrice weekly or danazol (600 mg daily)[12].

THE AFS CLASSIFICATION SYSTEM

The extent of endometriosis is usually staged by the American Fertility Society Classification System. It evaluates the sequelae of endometriosis in terms of fibrosis, adhesions or cyst formation but not the implants in terms of cells or evolution[13]. This system was devised to evaluate the results of surgical treatment. What is called a stage I or minimal endometriosis may represent a pelvis full of active, atypical endometriosis as well as a single inactive healed implant. Adhesions and scar formation can represent progression of the disease as well as a healing process. The size of an endometrioma has never been correlated with the amount of endometrial tissue. The chocolate content can result from menstrual shedding of free endometrial implants as well as from bleeding of congested vessels or from a haemorrhagic corpus luteum in the endometrial cyst.

The pathophysiology of endometriosis may change during its evolution and this explains the changing clinical faces of this disease. Haemorrhagic implants have been shown to modify the prostaglandin content of peritoneal fluid[14]. Free endometrial implants may be more related to infertility, and active enclosed implants to pelvic pain. Therefore, a more functional classification system of endometriosis is urgently needed for the benefit of basic and clinical research in this enigmatic disease.

REFERENCES

1. Vasquez, G., Cornillie, F. and Brosens, I.A. (1984). Peritoneal endometriosis: scanning electron microscopy and histology of minimal pelvic endometriotic lesions. *Fertil. Steril.,* **42**, 696–703
2. Murphy, A.A., Green, W.R., Bobbie, D., de la Cruz, Z.C. and Rock, J. (1986). Unsuspected endometriosis documented by scanning electron microscopy in visually normal peritoneum. *Fertil. Steril.,* **46**, 522–524
3. Roddick, J.W., Conkey, G. and Jacobs, E.J. (1960). The hormonal response of endometrium in endometriotic implants and its relationship to symptomatology. *Am. J. Obstet. Gynecol.,* **79**, 1173–117

4. Schweppe, K.W., Wynn, R.M. and Beller, F.K. (1984). Ultrastructural comparison of endometriotic implants and eutopic endometrium. *Am. J. Obstet. Gynecol.*, **148**, 1024–1039

5. Nieminen, U. (1962). Studies on the vascular pattern of ectopic endometrium with special reference to cyclic changes. *Acta Obstet. Gynecol. Scand.*, **41** (suppl. 3), 1–81

6. Jansen, R.P. and Russel, P. (1986). Nonpigmented endometriosis: clinical, laparoscopic, and pathologic definition. *Am. J. Obstet. Gynecol.*, **155**, 1154–1159

7. Stripling, M.C., Martin, D.C., Chatman, D.L., Vander Zwaag, R. and Poston W.M. (1988). Subtle appearance of pelvic endometriosis. *Fertil. Steril.*, **49**, 427–431

8. Redwine, D.B. (1987). The distribution of endometriosis in the pelvis by age groups and fertility. *Fertil. Steril.*, **47**, 173–175

9. Hughesdon, P.E. (1957). The structure of the endometrial cyst of the ovary. *J. Obstet. Gynaecol. Br. Empire*, **64**, 481–487

10. Evers, J.L.H. (1987). The second-look laparoscopy for evaluation of the result of medical treatment of endometriosis should not be performed during ovarian suppression. *Fertil. Steril.*, **47**, 502–504

11. Cornillie, F.J., Vasquez, G. and Brosens, I. (1985). The response of human endometriotic implants to the anti-progesterone steroid R2323: a histologic and ultrastructural study. *Pathol. Res. Pract.*, **180**, 647–655

12. Brosens, I.A., Verleyen, A. and Cornillie, F. (1987). The morphologic effect of short-term medical therapy of endometriosis. *Am. J. Obstet. Gynecol.*, **157**, 1215–1221

13. Brosens, I.A., Cornillie, F., Koninckx, P. and Vasquez, G. (1985). Evolution of the Revised American Fertility Society Classification of Endometriosis (letter). *Fertil. Steril.*, **44**, 714–716

14. Vernon, M.W., Beard, J.S., Graves, K. and Wilson, E.A. (1986). Classification of endometriotic implants by morphologic appearance and capacity of synthesize prostaglandin F. *Fertil. Steril.*, **46**, 801–806

3
Steroid receptors in endometriosis

A. Bergqvist

THE STEROID RECEPTOR CONCEPT

Target organs bind and retain steroids against a high concentration gradient. The presence of an intracellular steroid receptor is considered as a prerequisite for hormonal response. The existence of specific oestrogen-binding proteins in oestrogen target tissues was first described by Jensen and Jacobsen[1], and a quantitative assay of oestrogen receptors (ER) was first performed by Toft and Gorski[2]. Since then, steroid receptors have been extensively studied (for review and references see Edwards *et al.*[3]). The traditional steroid receptors are acid proteins, which are characterized by high steroid-specificity of the binding, high binding affinity to the ligand and limited binding capacity at near physiological concentrations of the ligand. They are found only in tissues sensitive to steroid hormones. For several years the steroid receptors were regarded as localized mainly to the cytoplasm, where they were thought to bind to the hormone. The steroid–receptor complex was then transported to the nucleus, where it bound the chromatin chain. Thus, initially most studies on steroid receptors were performed in cytosol.

In recent years, our knowledge in steroid receptors has changed and today we know that steroid receptors, both in the presence and in the absence of steroids, reside mainly in the nuclear compartment of target cells[4–6]. The receptors assayed in the cytosol derive partly from the nuclear compartment and have come into the cytosol after mechanical destruction during preparation. The nuclear receptor appears in two forms, one more loosely bound to the chromatin chain than the other, and it is this receptor form that comes into the cytosol during preparation. The findings of nuclear steroid receptors indicate a functioning receptor mechanism. Steroid receptors transmit the hormonal message to the chromatin chain, and extensive studies, mainly on breast cancer, have shown a strong correlation between ER level, hormone sensitivity of the tumour and disease-free survival (DFS) after hormonal treatment. Breast tumours positive for both ER and progesterone receptors (PR) appear more likely to be hormone sensitive than those that are positive for only ER[7]. Both ER and PR synthesis are stimulated by oestrogen and inhibited by progesterone. The finding of PR thus indicates the presence of biologically active ER.

STEROID RECEPTOR ASSAY TECHNIQUES

Several assays for quantitation of steroid receptors have been developed through the years (Figure 3.1). The most widely used methods have been biochemical binding techniques using different types of ligands, usually radioactively labelled synthetic steroids. Most common is the dextran-coated charcoal (DCC) method, originally described by Korenman in 1968[8], but modified several times since then for various hormone receptor determinations[9]. Data are usually plotted according to Scatchard[10], to obtain the quantitative and kinetic characteristics of the binding. Isoelectric focusing in polyacrylamide gel (IFPAG), combined with limited proteolysis, described by Gustafsson and collaborators[11], is an extensive refinement of the DCC-method, and is used for quantitative assay of oestrogen cytosolic receptors (ERc). Other binding techniques have also been used such as the sucrose gradient method and the hydroxyapatite method. Binding techniques only assay receptors unoccupied by endogenous hormones, and, after an exchange procedure, some previously occupied receptors.

Biochemical receptor assays in general are time-consuming and include several steps where mechanical, temperature and time factors as well as the levels of endogenous hormones, proteins, DNA, salt, charcoal and pH may affect the results[12-16]. Moreover, the synthetic hormones used as ligands may to some degree bind to more than one type of steroid receptor. For example, R1881 that is used for androgen receptor (AR) assay binds to some degree to PR, and R5020 and ORG2058, that are used for PR assay, also bind to AR and to the glucocorticoid (CR) receptor[7,17]. Whereas interassay variations within the same laboratory are usually within an acceptable range, variations from one laboratory to another tend to be greater[18-20].

In 1977 Greene and co-workers[21] reported the isolation of specific anti-oestrophilin (ER) antibodies, and specific monoclonal antibodies to ER of

I.	Biochemical ligand binding techniques
	A. Dextran-coated charcoal (DCC) method
	B. Isoelectric focusing in polyacrylamide gel (IFPAG)
	C. Sucrose gradient centrifugation
	D. Hydroxylapatite method
II.	Immunochemical techniques
	A. Enzyme-linked immunochemical assay (EIA)
	B. Immunoradiometric assay (IRMA)
III.	Immunohistochemical techniques
	A. Immunocytochemical assays (ICA)

Figure 3.1 Different techniques used for steroid receptor assays

MCF-7 breast cancer cells have lately been isolated, representing unique epitopes on the receptor molecule[22]. These antibodies have been used in an enzyme-linked immunochemical assay (EIA) for direct antigenic recognition of the steroid receptor[22]. Thirteen different specific monoclonal antibodies to human oestrophilin have been prepared, each one recognizing a different antigenic determinant on the receptor molecule. A combination of two such antibodies can be used in a sandwich technique. One antibody (D547Spy) serves to immobilize the receptor on a supporting surface, such as a polystyrene bead; a second antibody (D75P3y), labelled with horseradish peroxidase, is used to measure the amount of receptor bound to the first antibody. The second antibody may also be labelled with ^{125}I for an immunoradiometric assay (IRMA) determination. Recently, monoclonal antibodies to PR have been developed as well. The monoclonal antibodies are capable of recognizing receptors of which the steroid-binding sites are either occupied or unoccupied by steroid hormones, but give no information on whether the receptors assayed are biologically active or not. The method may be used for quantitative assays in both the cytosol and the nuclear fraction. It has shown a good correlation to the ligand-binding techniques[23]. These specific monoclonal antibodies make it possible to perform steroid receptor assays in very small tissue samples. This means that isolated endometriotic tissue with high purity can be studied.

Recently, techniques have been developed for histochemical steroid receptor localization using monoclonal antibodies[24] in a sandwich technique (Figure 3.2). The monoclonal rat antibodies H226Spy and H222Spy cross-react with ER derived from human uterus. The binding sites are localized by PAP (peroxidase antiperoxidase) technique. This immunohistochemical technique has shown a good correlation to binding assays[5,7,25].

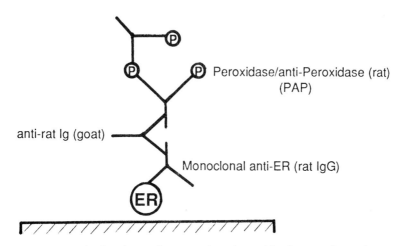

Figure 3.2   A sandwich technique for immunohistochemical localization of steroid receptors (Abbott Laboratories, Diagnostic Division)

ER AND PR IN UTERINE ENDOMETRIUM

The interpretation of ER and PR in uterine endometrium has been extensive[26–31]. The ERc level increases during the proliferative phase, reaching a maximum at late follicular phase, after which it steadily falls throughout the luteal phase. The PRc level reaches a maximum at midcycle and decreases in midsecretory phase. The receptor level in the nuclear compartment has its maximum somewhat later than in the cytosol fraction. The amount of steroid receptors varies in different parts of the endometrium, being highest in the functional layer in the fundal region and declining towards the cervix region[31,32] and also declining in the basal layer.

STEROID SENSITIVITY OF ENDOMETRIOTIC TISSUE

Endometriosis is almost exclusively found in women in the reproductive ages, indicating an oestrogen dependence of the tissue. Animal experiments[33,34] have shown that endometriotic tissue in most cases is dependent on oestrogen for proliferation and for long-time survivial. After a few weeks, endometrial and endometriotic grafts in untreated nude mice became atrophic, but in oestrogen-treated animals the tissue was highly proliferative[34]. This oestrogen dependence of endometriotic tissue is the basis for hormonal treatment that leads to ovarian inactivation and oestrogen deprivation of the endometriotic tissue. However, about 20% of endometriotic patients are clinically non-responders to hormonal treatment, which means that the endometriotic tissue in these cases is not dependent on the endogenous hormones and not influenced by exogenous hormones.

The histological resemblance between endometriotic tissue and uterine endometrium is well known, but there are also histological differences between the two tissue types that indicate a deficient response to progestogen influence on endometriotic tissue. Extensive light- and electron-microscopic studies have revealed that endometriotic tissue reacts in a different manner from endometrium to the endocrine milieu[35–37]. Functional changes in endometriotic tissue do not always proceed as clearly and uniformly cyclicly as in endometrium. A poor differentiation is found in 20–25% of endometriotic samples. These findings suggest an incomplete response of endometriotic tissue to the prevalent hormonal milieu and indicate that the endometriotic tissue is more or less autonomous, not governed by the normal control mechanisms regulating the uterine endometrial glands and stroma.

OESTROGEN AND PROGESTERONE BINDING IN ENDOMETRIOTIC TISSUE

ER and PR levels assayed biochemically have been studied by four different groups (Table 3.1). The first report on steroid receptors in endometriotic tissue was published by Tamaya and collaborators in 1979[38]. They compared ER and PR in ovarian endometriotic tissue and uterine endometrium from 7 women of whom one was on hormonal contraception. They found that in 5 cases, where tissue samples were obtained from both localizations, the ER

Table 3.1 The number of endometriotic and endometrial samples containing ER and PR in the five studies published where ligand techniques have been used

Author	Number of samples	Endometriotic tissue (n)		Endometrium (n)	
		ERc + [a]	PRc + [a]	ERc +	PRc +
Tamaya et al.[38]	7[b]	6/7	6/7	6/6	5/6
Bergqvist et al.[40]	20	8/20	2/9	10/12	8/8
Jähnne et al.[42]	47	ca. 40%	ca. 80%	9/9	9/9
Vierikko et al.[43]	52	38/52	49/52	—	—
Lyndrup et al.[44]	14	9/14	12/12	12/14	13/14

[a]ER = oestrogen receptor; PR = progesterone receptor; c = in cytosol
[b]One woman on contraceptive pills

and PR levels were lower in endometriotic tissue than in endometrium. In particular, the PR levels were lower in endometriotic lesions, although measurable in 6 out of 7 samples.

In 1980 we presented data on ERc and PRc in endometriotic tissue from 14 patients compared to uterine endometrium obtained simultaneously from the same patient[39]. The complete study on 20 women, using biochemical ligand techniques (IFPAG for ER and DCC for PR), was published in 1981[40]. The concentrations of both ERc and PRc were markedly lower in endometriotic tissue than in uterine endometrium obtained simultaneously from 12 of the women. In some endometriotic samples the receptors were even not detectable (Figures 3.3 and 3.4). Fourteen of the 20 endometriotic samples consisted of pure endometriotic tissue scraped from the inside of ovarian endometriomas.

In 1980 Jänne and collaborators[41] published a study on ER and PR in malignant and benign ovarian tumours and tumour-like lesions including 13 samples of ovarian endometriosis. They found low or absent ER but a high PR level in endometriotic tissue. In 1981[42] they published the results of receptor assays of endometriotic tissue from 41 patients. The material included 9 cases from whom they had obtained uterine endometrium for comparison. In this study, ER in endometriotic tissue was often not measurable, and when measurable, the levels were lowest between cycle days 10 and 22. The PR level in endometriotic tissue was in this study much lower than in uterine endometrium, and in 20% of the samples the PR was even not detectable. Vierikko and co-workers[43] studied ER and PR in 52 untreated endometriotic samples and found ERc in 73% and PRc in 94% of the samples. The receptor levels are not given. Lyndrup and collaborators[44] published in 1987 a comparative study on 14 women in which they had found ERc in 9 out of 14 and PRC in 12 out of 12 endometriotic samples. Oestrogen receptors in the nuclear fraction (ERn) were detected in all of 4 endometriotic samples. Significantly lower values of both ERc and PRc were found in endometriotic tissue than in endometrium, but the PRc/ERc ratio was significantly higher in endometriotic tissue.

Thus the results from all study groups have consistently shown that the level of ERc was markedly lower in endometriotic tissue than in endometrium. Also the PRc assays showed lower levels in endometriotic tissue, but the results in one of the groups have been contradictory[41,42]. The low detection rate with these techniques and the contradictory results concerning PR levels

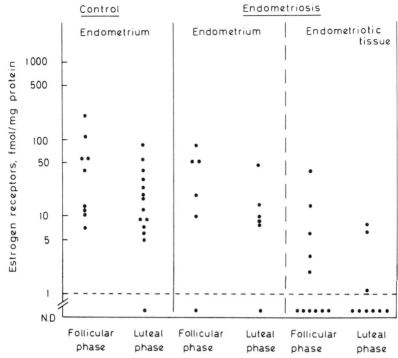

Figure 3.3 Cytosol oestrogen receptor levels in endometriotic tissue and uterine endometrium from 20 patients with endometriosis and endometrium from 30 control patients in the different cycle phases. Dashed horizontal line indicates the detection limit of the receptor assay

might depend on a detection limit differing at the different laboratories, methodological discrepancies and different tissue sampling techniques. However, the conclusion is that, when biochemical techniques are used, ER and PR levels in endometriotic tissue are lower than in the corresponding uterine endometrium and in some cases PRc are even not detectable. These findings indicate defects in the prerequisites for hormonal regulation in endometriotic tissue and a reduced cellular responsiveness to steroid hormones compared to uterine endometrium. However, the high frequency of negative samples was confusing as there are so many indications for a steroid sensitivity of the tissue.

The problems in detecting ER and PR in endometriotic samples with ligand binding techniques might be due to some disadvantage connected with these methods. In all these early studies the DCC method was used for PR assays and in five of them for ER assays[38,41-44]. However, different ligands were used. For the analyses rather big tissue samples are needed, which might be a problem when endometriotic samples are to be studied, often constituting only tiny volumes of endometriotic tissue with surrounding fibrotic tissue growing into it. As fibrotic tissue is receptor-poor, a dilution of the receptor concentrations in the endometriotic tissue might often be obtained, leading to falsely low receptor levels assayed. Sufficient volumes of pure endometriotic

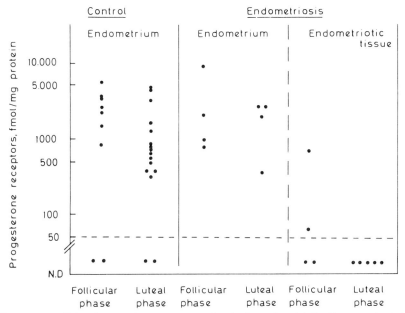

Figure 3.4 Cytosol progesterone receptor levels in endometriotic tissue and uterine endometrium from 9 patients with endometriosis and endometrium from 30 control patients in the different cycle phases. Dashed horizontal line indicates the detection limit of the receptor assay

tissue can only be obtained by scraping the inside of endometriotic cysts. However, as 70% of our endometriotic samples were pure endometriotic tissue, the low receptor concentrations found cannot be explained solely as caused by a dilution of endometriotic tissue by non-receptor containing tissue. Without microscopic visualization of the tissue, uncertainty exists as to whether one is actually measuring the steroid receptors within endometriotic tissue, and distinction between different cell types is impossible. The blood content in the tissue sample might interfere with the receptor levels found, as it usually is referred to the level of deoxyribonucleic acid (DNA) or protein. The levels of other steroid-binding proteins in the different tissue types might also interefere with the results. Moreover, as mentioned previously, the ligand techniques assay only receptors unoccupied by endogenous hormones and they might be inactivated if handled inappropriately, for example by being kept at too high a temperature.

Other methods have been used to study oestrogen binding in endometriotic tissue. Using *in vitro* steroid-autoradiography, Gould and collaborators[45] found that, unlike uterine endometrium, which displays cyclic changes in the oestrogen binding, the endometriotic foci showed no such changes in tissue samples from two women. However, when Eisenfeld and collaborators[46] in an experimental study administered [3H]oestradiol intravenously to rhesus monkeys, they found that the radioactivity in the endometriotic tissue was of the same level as in the endometrium.

In 1983 we used fluorochrome-labelled oestradiol and progesterone for localizing specific oestrogen and progesterone binding sites histochemically, again comparing endometriotic tissue and uterine endometrium obtained simultaneously from the same patient[47]. The steroid specificity of the binding had been shown to be acceptable[48]. Specific fluorescence was demonstrated in the cytoplasm only. We found that the sites of the specific fluorescence often varied in endometrium, being either mostly basal or apical in the cells while in endometriotic epithelial cells the whole cytoplasm was usually more uniformly fluorescent. The fluorochrome-labelled steroids were bound to the epithelial structures in most endometriotic samples. The different localization of the specific binding found with this method compared to that found with autoradiography and immunohistochemical methods (see next section) indicates that this method localizes another specific binding protein in the cytoplasm.

Gould and co-workers[45] postulated that in endometriotic tissue there is a change in the PR, making the amount, activation or function of the receptor abnormal. This would in turn allow for a failure of downregulation in the nuclear and/or cytoplasmic oestrogen receptor concentrations in the luteal phase. In conclusion, there are several indications that endometriotic tissue differs from that of endometrium in ERc and PRc content, in PRc/ERc ratio, and in capacity for secretory changes.

ER AND PR LEVELS IN ENDOMETRIOTIC TISSUE ASSAYED WITH IMMUNOLOGICAL TECHNIQUES

Because of the confusing results of the binding assays, we turned to the enzyme immuno technique, EIA (Abbott Laboratories, Diagnostic Division, North Chicago, Ill., USA) for studies on ER and PR in cytosol (ERc, PRc) and in the nuclear fraction (ERn, PRn) in endometriotic tissue. We have consequently made most quantitative receptor studies with monoclonal antibodies on ovarian endometriosis in order to obtain as pure endometriotic tissue as possible. Endometriotic samples were obtained from 31 women at laparotomy and uterine endometrium was simultaneously obtained by curettage from 24

Table 3.2 ER, PR and AR levels (mean and standard deviation) in cytosol and nuclear fraction in endometriotic tissue and endometrium assayed with biochemical and immunochemical assays[a]

	Endometriotic tissue		Endometrium	
	n	Mean ± SD	n	Mean ± SD
ERc IF	25	199 ± 216	20	942 ± 894
ERc EIA	31	879 ± 1033	24	2464 ± 1774
ERn EIA	24	179 ± 334	20	555 ± 545
PRc DCC	21	2355 ± 3011	20	4521 ± 4891
PRc EIA	15	4116 ± 5515	13	4943 ± 3780
PRn EIA	13	413 ± 472	13	827 ± 1115
ARc DCC	4	943 ± 969	5	1136 ± 861

[a]ER = oestrogen receptor; PR = progesterone receptor; AR = androgen receptor; c = cytosol; n = nuclear fraction; IF = isoelectric focusing in polyacrylamide gel; EIA = enzyme immunoassay; DCC = dextran-coated charcoal method.

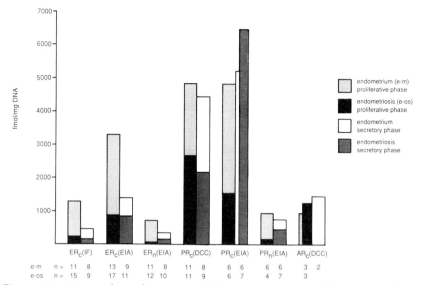

Figure 3.5 Mean values of oestrogen (ER) and progesterone (PR) receptors during proliferative and secretory phases assayed with ligand techniques and enzyme immunoassays. IF = isoelectric focusing in polyacrylamide gel; EIA = enzyme immunoassay; DCC = dextran-coated charcoal method; c = receptors in cytosol; n = receptors in nuclear fraction

of the women[49]. Table 3.2 and Figure 3.5 show the receptor levels. With this method, ER and PR were measurable in all endometriotic samples but the receptor levels were lower than in uterine endometrium. The PRc level is numerically higher than the ERc level, and this difference is more pronounced in endometriotic tissue than in uterine endometrium. The level of ERc did not change during the menstrual cycle in endometriotic tissue as pronouncedly as in endometrium and the highest level of ER and PR during the menstrual cycle appeared in endometriotic tissue later than in endometrium (Figure 3.6). It was also possible to study the receptor levels in primary and recurrent disease (Figure 3.7). We did not find any obvious difference in the receptor levels in these two groups, but the number of samples was very uneven.

As ER function is regarded as a prerequisite for the synthesis of PR, the PR level indicates biologically active ER in endometriotic tissue. The pronounced discrepancy between the low PRc levels found with ligand techniques and the PRc levels found with monoclonal antibodies, detecting a similar level in endometriotic tissue as in endometrium, might indicate that the PR assayed immunologically are not always biologically active. The PRn level found immunologically is significantly lower in endometriotic tissue than in endometrium. These data support the theory of a different steroid receptor regulation in endometriotic tissue from that in endometrium and might explain the sparsity of secretory changes seen histologically in endometriotic tissue.

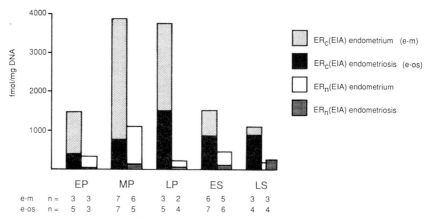

Figure 3.6 Mean values of ERc and ERn in endometrium and endometriotic tissue during the different menstrual phases. ERc = oestrogen receptors in cytosol; ERn = oestrogen receptors in nuclear fraction; EIA = enzyme immunoassay; EP = early proliferative; MP = mid-proliferative; LP = late proliferative; ES = early secretory; LS = late secretory

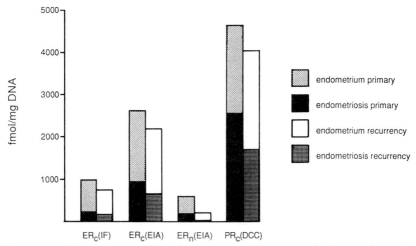

Figure 3.7 Mean oestrogen (ER) and progesterone (PR) receptor levels in endometriotic tissue and uterine endometrium from women with primary ($n = 26$) and recurrent ($n = 5$) endometriosis. IF = isoelectric focusing in polyacrylamide gel; EIA = enzyme immunoassay; DCC = dextran-coated charcoal method; c = receptors in cytosol; n = receptors in nuclear fraction

IMMUNOHISTOCHEMICAL LOCALIZATION OF ER AND PR IN ENDOMETRIOTIC TISSUE

Bur and co-workers[50] studied ER in trypsin-pretreated, formalin-fixed, paraffin-embedded endometrium and endometriotic tissue from 20 women. The monoclonal D75, the only one that yields consistent and strong staining for ER in tissue samples treated in this way, was used. It was possible to date histologically the endometriotic tissue in 10 cases (9 proliferative and 1 secretory). Five of the remaining samples were classified as inactive and 5 contained epithelium without glandular formation and could thus not be dated. In the 9 cases showing proliferation, with endometriotic tissue in phase with the endometrium, the ER staining was similar in the two tissue types. There was a marked heterogeneity in the binding pattern in both tissue types. In general, proliferative endometriotic tissue was associated with diffuse medium-to-strong nuclear staining of both glandular and stromal cells. Secretory type endometriosis showed much less staining that was mainly confined to the basalis-like portion of the glands. Staining of 'inactive' endometriotic samples was variable. Routine paraffin-embedded sections are not the ideal specimen for immunohistochemical localization of ER, since receptor protein appears to be very sensitive to the effects of prolonged fixation and tissue processing. This may explain the variation in staining intensity observed. The intensity of staining was more uniform in frozen sections in the same study. Nevertheless, the pattern of immunostaining observed in paraffin-embedded endometrium was strikingly similar to that observed previously in frozen sections of endometrium throughout the menstrual cycle.

Lessey and collaborators[51] studied frozen sections from 16 women of whom 4 were on hormonal therapy. Uterine endometrium was obtained simultaneously from 9 of the remaining 12 women. The specific monoclonal antibodies H222 developed against MCF-7 cell ER and JZB-39 developed against human PR, both of rat origin, were used. The ER and PR levels were assessed according to an HSCORE, which is related to the percentage of stained cells and the staining intensity. In all cases both ER and PR were localized within the nucleus in both endometriotic tissue and uterine endometrium. Also in this study there was a marked heterogeneity in the ER and PR binding pattern in endometriotic tissue. The mean HSCOREs in endometriotic tissue were not significantly lower than in the corresponding endometrium. However, in some samples no binding was obtained in glands or stroma. Two of the endometrial samples showed no ER binding in the glands and three no ER binding in the stroma, while the ER level was comparable in only 6 samples — 3 in proliferative phase and 3 in secretory phase. PR could be compared in the two tissue types in 8 cases — 5 in proliferative and 3 in secretory phase. These small numbers of samples do not allow statistical calculations. Moreover, the heterogeneous cellular pattern in endometriotic samples and the subjective appreciation of the staining intensity do not allow an exact quantitation of the steroid receptor content according to the HSCORE used in the study. Hitherto the histochemical methods could not be used for quantitative assays, only for qualitative and semiquantitative assays.

A multiparametric computerized system specifically developed for the analysis of coloured immunostained surfaces in tissue sections, referred to as SAMBA, has been developed[25]. This system seems to have a high reliability and reproducibility. When the SAMBA analyses of PR-ICA were compared to the immunocytochemical (ER-ICA) semiquantitative assay, a significant difference was found, but when the SAMBA analysis of PR-ICA was compared to the DCC assays, a high correlation was found.

In an immunocytochemical study using ER-ICA and PR-ICA (Abbott Laboratories) on 21 endometriotic samples, we found that the anti-ER and the anti-PR bound as distinctly in endometriotic tissue as in uterine endometrium, both in epithelial cells and in stroma cells, almost exclusively in the nuclei[52]. There was a heterogeneous binding pattern in endometriotic epithelial tissue, but this was also pronounced in the uterine endometrium where positive and negative glands were found side by side (Figures 3.8, 3.9 and 3.10). Also, the stroma cells showed a heterogeneous pattern concerning receptor positivity. In most women from whom endometrium was obtained, the positivity for ER and/or PR was higher in endometrium than in endometriotic tissue, both in epithelial cell nuclei and in stromal cell nuclei. The contrary case was less common. Thus in all three studies the binding of the specific antibodies was found to be almost exclusively to the nuclei both in the glandular epithelium and in the stroma in the two tissue types. The binding in endometriotic tissue was less pronounced than in endometrium.

In a well-performed study on nine rhesus monkeys a combination of two specific monoclonal rat antibodies (H222 and D75) against ER were used[53]. In this study, 300–400 cells per tissue compartment per tissue sample were counted, permitting a fairly good quantitative calculation. The study showed that the receptor levels in endometriotic lesions were lower than in endometrium in the proliferative phase and that there were no significant differences between the different cycle phases in the mean percentage of ER-positive epithelial or stromal cells. Furthermore, there was a great individual

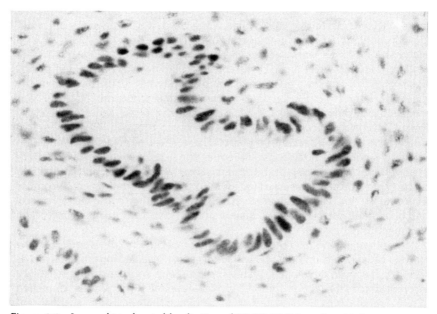

Figure 3.8   Immunohistochemical localization of ER (ER-ICA) in endometriotic tissue

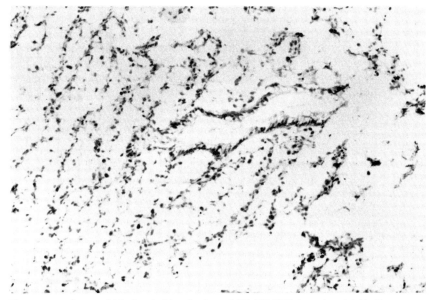

Figure 3.9 Immunohistochemical localization of PR (PR-ICA) in endometriotic tissue

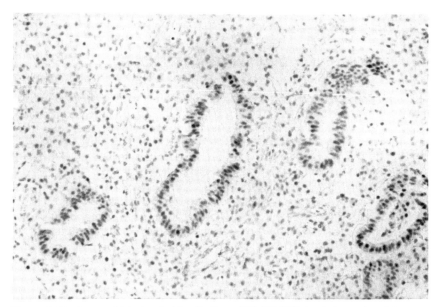

Figure 3.10 Immunohistochemical localization of ER (ER-ICA) in uterine endometrium

variability in the number of ER-positive epithelial cells and less variability in the number of ER-positive stromal cells throughout the cycle. However, there were significantly fewer positive stromal cells in the lesion than in the endometrium during the follicular phase. During the luteal phase, the mean percentage of ER-positive epithelial cells in many lesions was high despite high serum progesterone level. Neither biochemical receptor assay on the endometriotic samples showed any significant changes during the menstrual cycle.

The lack of change in the mean percentage of ER-positive stromal cells in the lesions during the cycle and their lower number during the follicular phase indicates consistent differences in ER regulation between the stromal cells of lesions and of endometrium. These data also suggest that the epithelial cells in many lesions have an insensitivity to the well-documented suppressive effect of progesterone on the levels of ER.

AR IN ENDOMETRIOTIC TISSUE

Testosterone and derivatives of the hormone have clinically shown a therapeutic effect on endometriosis. However, AR have been studied in only a few cases until now[38,49,54]. In all three studies, binding techniques have been used. Data from a total of 12 patients have been published (Table 3.3). No obvious differences in AR levels in endometriotic tissue compared to those in endometrium have been found, the receptor levels being low in both types of tissue.

OTHER DIFFERENCES IN STEROIDAL EFFECTS IN ENDOMETRIOTIC TISSUE AND UTERINE ENDOMETRIUM

The low levels of ER and PR in endometriotic tissue may indicate not only faulty regulation of steroid hormone receptors but also incomplete expression of other differentiated cellular processes. In a comparative study on total hydrolysis of oestrone sulphate as well as specific formation of oestradiol (E_2), we found a lower activity of both oestrogen sulphatase and 17β-hydroxysteroid oxidoreductase (17β-OHSD) in endometriotic tissue than in uterine endometrium (Figures 3.11 and 3.12)[55]. These results concerning E_2 formation in endometriotic tissue are in accordance with those reported by Vierikko and co-workers[43] who found that there was no significant increase in the activity of 17β-OHSD in endometriotic tissue under the influence of endogenous progesterone such as was seen in endometrium. Thus, if the oestrogen metabolic pattern in endometriotic tissue does respond to hormonal

Table 3.3 Studies on androgen receptors (AR) in endometriotic tissue and uterine endometrium

Author	Endometriosis	Endometrium
Tamaya et al.[38]	$n = 5$	$n = 4$
Punnonen et al.[54]	$n = 3$	$n = 0$
Bergqvist et al.[49]	$n = 4$	$n = 5$

46

Total hydrolysis of [³H] estrone sulfate,
fmol × min⁻¹ × mg protein ⁻¹

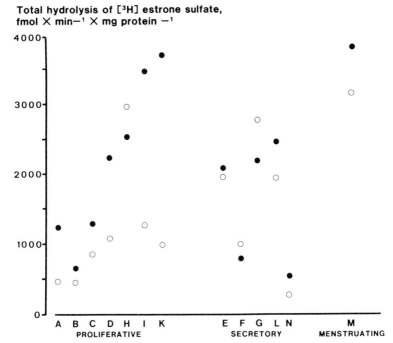

Figure 3.11   Total hydrolysis of [³H]oestrone sulphate to oestrone and oestradiol *in vitro* by homogenates of uterine endometrium (filled circles) and by endometriotic tissue (open circles)

stimuli, such a response is far less pronounced than in uterine endometrium.

Glycogen as well as acid and neutral mucopolysaccharides are synthesized in endometriotic tissue as in endometrium[56]. However, compared with uterine endometrium, where glycogen and mucopolysaccharides are more prominent in the secretory compared with the proliferative phase, there was no obvious difference in the amount of these substances in endometriotic tissue during the different menstrual cycle phases (Figures 3.13 and 3.14). Some endometriotic samples with an inactive phase pattern contained mucopolysaccharides, indicating that these endometriotic cells had been active previously. Even when the epithelial cells in the endometriotic samples were atypical or when fibrous tissue had replaced the specific stroma beneath the epithelium, positive granules could be seen. These studies indicate that at least part of the PR found in endometriotic tissue must be biologically active to express the hormonal message. However, the studies indicate a disturbance in the cyclic expression of progesterone activity in endometriotic tissue.

Prakash *et al.*[57] found that although there was no significant difference in activity of alkaline or acid phosphatase or oxidative enzymes in endometriotic tissue compared with uterine endometrium, the enzyme activity did not always change cyclically in endometriotic lesions as it did in endometrium. Another expression of hormonal effects in the uterine endometrium is the secretion of prostaglandins[58]. The production and content of prostaglandins

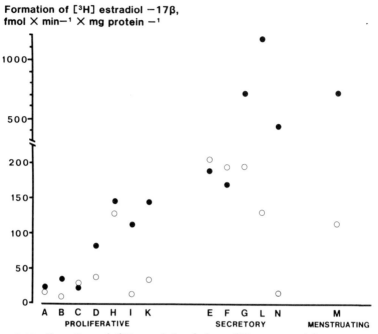

Figure 3.12 Formation of [³H]oestradiol-17β from [³H]oestrone sulphate *in vitro* by homogenates of uterine endometrium (filled circles) and of endometriotic tissue (open circles)

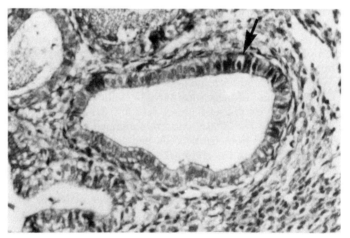

Figure 3.13 Periodic acid–Schiff-positive granules (arrows) in epithelial cells of endometriotic glands indicating the localization of mucopolysaccharrides

is lower in endometriotic tissue than in endometrium and the content is similar for all stages of endometriosis.

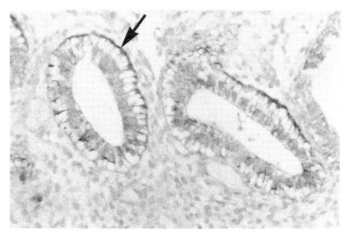

Figure 3.14 Best's carmine-positive granules (arrows) in epithelial cells of endometriotic glands indicating the localization of glycogen

THE IMPORTANCE OF THE STROMA IN ENDOMETRIOTIC TISSUE

The importance of the stroma in endometriotic tissue has been discussed. The stroma seems to be of vital importance for the survival of the endometriotic glands. When fibrotic tissue grows into endometriotic lesions in the healing process, it will eradicate the stroma but will never grow into the epithelial structures. However, when the stroma has disappeared, the epithelial structures will atrophy and may even change to atypical cellular patterns.

The significance of the higher PRc/ERc ratio found in endometriotic tissue than in endometrium is unclear, as are also the differences in ER and PR level changes in endometriotic glands and stroma during the menstrual cycle that are sometimes found[51]. In three implants from the secretory phase reported by Lessey, the characteristic low epithelial/stroma PR ratio also seen in normal secretory endometrium was observed. It might be due to differences in the stroma content in the two tissue types. Endometrial stroma contain equal concentrations of ERc but lower concentrations of PRc compared to glandular epithelium[59]. As the stromal component in endometriotic tissue is usually smaller than in uterine endometrium, this might indicate that the PRc level in the stroma is higher in endometriotic tissue than in endometrium. A cycle-dependent reversal in PR content between glandular epithelium and stromal cells in uterine endometrium has been shown. A selective elevation of PR content in stroma suggests an increased functional importance of this tissue during the secretory phase[51]. These findings might indicate that some of the therapeutic activity of gestagens on endometriotic tissue may be derived from their effects on the stromal nutrition via steroid receptors. Gould and

49

co-workers[45] found a marked degree of oestrogen binding in endometriotic stromal cells throughout the cycle, while in the endometrium stromal binding sites were seen only during the proliferative phase. They postulated that, since epithelial histodifferentiation in endometrium is known to be influenced by the underlying stroma, the ectopic stroma of endometriosis may be abnormal in itself, thus inducing the differentiation of an epithelium that is different from that of uterine endometrium.

POSSIBLE ENVIRONMENTAL FACTORS INFLUENCING THE RECEPTOR LEVELS

Cyclical changes mimicking hormonal-responsive endometrium has been suggested by morphological and histopathological studies. However, all comparative studies on endometriotic tissue and uterine endometrium obtained simultaneously from the same woman have shown dissimilarities of one kind or another, indicating a defective response in endometriotic tissue to hormonal stimuli. Assuming that endometriotic tissue is ectopic endometrium, it is difficult to explain the sparsity of secretory histological changes in this tissue, especially in view of the fact that PRc level is high in relation to ERc. The question then is whether these dissimilarities are due to differences in the tissues themselves or to differences in the surroundings. Factors such as the anatomical localization of the lesion may influence the behaviour of endometriosis as well as affect alterations in a putative paracrine response that might influence growth and differentiation. Poor vascularity, surrounding fibrosis or exposure to inflammatory cells may also be responsible. A basal membrane is missing in endometriotic lesions. The normal architecture of the endometrium, lacking in endometriotic tissue, and the relative differences in the amount of stroma among implants might contribute to the observed differences. It appears, however, that in certain, but not all, implants, a functional integrity exists[51].

An aberrant vascular pattern close to the endometriotic lesions has been observed. Cornellie and collaborators[60] found that secretory differentiation of endometriotic epithelial cells was only present when the ectopic stroma had a well-developed microvasculature with blood capillaries being present near the glandular epithelium. This might depend on an inflammatory reaction aroused by the endometriotic tissue. The myometrium is usually better vascularized than the structures surrounding the endometriotic lesions. Some locations, such as the ovary, may offer a very different paracrine environment, including increased exposure to steroids. There are numerous studies to support interactions between epithelial and stromal cells that affect growth and differentiation of the reproductive tract. Sometimes endometriotic tissue displays a clear dys-synchrony between glandular cell and stroma[53].

In order to study the two tissue types in the same environment, we transplanted to nude mice endometriotic tissue and uterine endometrium obtained simultaneously from the same woman[34]. Endometriotic samples were implanted subcutaneously to one side of a mouse and the endometrium from the same woman to the other side of the same mouse. Tissue samples from one woman were transplanted to four mice, of which one was treated with oestrogen, one with progesterone, one with danazol and one mouse remained untreated as a control. The success rate of graft acceptance was 50% higher for endometrium than for endometriotic tissue. All grafts became surrounded by a capsule of fibrous tissue, and the fibrosis extended into the grafts to varying degrees. The fibrosis was very thick and rich in collagen in the oestrogen-treated grafts, but less compact in the danazol-treated and gestagen-treated grafts. In this respect there was no difference between endometrial and endometriotic grafts. The grafts seemed to be resolved gradually and replaced by fibrous tissue. In no case was the graft histologically identical to the original tissue after the treatment or observation period. The histological changes in the endometriotic grafts closely resembled those found in the endometrial grafts, i.e. proliferative epithelium was observed in the oestrogen-treated grafts and an inactive pattern in the gestagen-treated and danazol-treated grafts. After 10 weeks in the same environment the untreated grafts of the two tissue types had developed a similar histological expression to the hormonal influence. This experiment indicates that the two tissue types, when localized to the same milieu, develop a similar histological appearance and respond in similar ways to steroidal influences. These findings suggest that the histological and functional discrepancies seen under natural conditions between human uterine endometrium and endometriotic lesions may, at least in part, be the result of environmental differences.

The influence of the anatomical localization of the endometriotic lesions has been studied by two groups. Vierikko and co-workers[43] did not find any differences in receptor level between superficial lesions and ovarian cysts. When monoclonal antibodies were used for receptor assays, we did not find any differences in receptor level in lesions with different localizations. However, Brosens and collaborators[61] found that ovarian lesions appeared to show less histological response than the peritoneal lesions to hormonal influence.

THE EFFECT OF EXOGENOUS HORMONES ON STEROID RECEPTOR LEVELS

During the influence of exogenous hormones such as medroxyprogesterone acetate, danazol and gestrinone, the ERc and PRc levels in uterine endometrium decrease[43]. However, in endometriotic issue, neither short-term nor long-term treatment changed the receptor levels. Neither did the 17β-HSD activity increase in endometriotic tissue as it did in endometrium. However, the immunohistochemical bindings to ER and PR were reduced in endometriotic tissue from the four patients on medical suppression studied by Lessey and collaborators[51]. It is possible that the influence of hormones would be different in fresh compared to that in older endometriotic lesions. This subject remains to be studied. These data might imply that endometriotic tissue is unpredictable in its response to the cyclic hormonal milieu in terms of ER and PR but may retain the ability to respond to hormonal suppression over a prolonged period. Up to now no studies on steroid receptors during GnRH agonist treatment have been published.

CONCLUSION

ER, PR and AR are measurable in endometriotic tissue, ER in a lower level than in endometrium and AR in the same range as in endometrium. The ER level does not change during the menstrual cycle in as pronounced a manner as in endometrium. The ER are obviously biologically active, but the response to hormonal influence is different compared to that in endometrium, indicating a different regulation of the steroid receptor mechanisms.

The studies on PR have shown interesting differences between binding techniques and immunoassays. The monoclonal antibodies detect a similar level of PR in tissue homogenates of endometriotic tissue to that in endometrium and sometimes also histochemically. On the other side, binding techniques measure lower PR level in endometriotic tissue compared to that in endometrium. These findings indicate that there is a high level of biologically inactive PR in endometriotic tissue. As this difference is not found regarding ER and AR, it indicates a different PR regulation in endometriotic tissue. If there is a defect in PR function in endometriotic tissue, it might explain the sometimes weak or absent secretory phase development as well as clinical response of endometriotic tissue to gestagen therapy. Whether the level of biologically active PR is extremely low in endometriotic tissue in the poor responders remains to be studied.

The lack of cyclic variation in the concentrations of ERc and PRc is additional evidence that the hormonal control of endometriotic tissue is different from that in uterine endometrium. The lack of response of 17β-HSD in endometriotic tissue to elevated progesterone concentrations in the latter part of the menstrual cycle, and to the administration of MPA, danazol and gestrinone, confirmed the unresponsive state of endometriotic tissue. As it has been shown that MPA, danazol and gestrinone all induce 17β-HSD in the endometrium, these data suggest that mechanisms other than those mediated via female steroid hormone receptors are involved in the transmission of the therapeutic actions of these drugs in endometriotic tissue.

Further study of the importance of the stroma and of the surrounding tissue is needed. Until now we have no convincing evidence that the steroid receptor levels differ in endometriotic lesions of different localizations or in primary versus recurrent disease, but further, more detailed work is needed.

REFERENCES

1. Jensen, E.V. and Jacobson, H.I. (1962). Basic guides to the mechanism of estrogen action. *Rec. Prog. Horm. Res.*, **18**, 387–395
2. Toft, D. and Gorski, J. (1966). A receptor molecule for estrogens; Isolation from the rat uterus and preliminary characterization. *Proc. Natl. Acad. Sci. USA*, **55**, 1574–1581
3. Edwards, D.P., Chamness, G.C. and McGuire, W.L. (1979). Estrogen and progesterone receptor proteins in breast cancer. *Biochim. Biophys. Acta*, **560**, 457–486
4. King, W.J. and Greene, G.L. (1984). Monoclonal antibodies localize oestrogen receptor in the nuclei of target cells. *Nature*, **307**, 745–747
5. Press, M.F., Holt, J.A., Herbst, A.L. and Greene, G.L. (1985). Immunocytochemical identification of estrogen receptor in ovarian carcinomas. Localization with monoclonal estrophilin antibodies compared with biochemical assays. *Lab. Invest.*, **53**, 349–361
6. Schrader, W.T. (1984). New model for steroid hormone receptors? *Nature*, **308**, 17–18

7. Pertschuk, L.P., Feldman, J.G., Eisenberg, K.B., Carter, A.C., Thelmo, W.L., Cruz, W.P., Thorpe, S.M., Christensen, J., Rasmussen, B.B., Rose, C. and Greene, G.L. (1988). Immunocytochemical detection of progesterone receptor in breast cancer with monoclonal antibody. *Cancer*, **62**, 342–349

8. Korenman, S.G. (1968). Radio-ligand binding assay of specific estrogens using a soluble uterine macromolecule. *J. Clin. Endocrinol. Metab.*, **28**, 127–130

9. Daehnfeldt, J.L. and Briand, P. (1977). Determinations of high-affinity gestagen receptors in hormone-responsive and hormone-independent GR mouse mammary tumours by an exchange assay. In McGuire, W.L. *et al.* (eds.) *Progesterone Receptors in Normal and Neoplastic Tissues*, pp. 59–69. (New York: Raven Press)

10. Scatchard, G. (1949). The attractions of proteins for small molecules and ions. *Ann. N.Y. Acad. Sci.*, **51**, 660–672

11. Gustafsson, J.-Å. Gustafsson, S.A., Nordenskjöld, B., Okret, S., Silfverswärd, C. and Wrange, Ö. (1978). Estradiol receptor analysis in human breast cancer tissue by isoelectric focusing in polyacrylamide gel. *Cancer Res.*, **38**, 4225–4228

12. Auer, G.U., Caspersson, T.O., Gustafsson, S.A., Humla, S.A., Ljung, B.-M., Nordenskjöld, B.A., Silfverswärd, C. and Wallgren, A.S. (1980). Relationship between nuclear DNA distribution and estrogen receptors in human mammary carcinomas. *Anal. Quant. Cytol.*, **2**, 280–284

13. Hasson, J., Luhan, P.A. and Kohl, M.W. (1981). Comparison of estrogen receptor levels in breast cancer samples from mastectomy and frozen section specimens. *Cancer*, **47**, 138–139

14. Peck, E.J. and Clark, J.H. (1977). Effect of ionic strength on charcoal adsorption assays of receptor-estradiol complexes. *Endocrinology*, **101**, 1034–1043

15. Skovgaard Poulsen, H. (1981). Oestrogen receptor assay — limitation of the method. *Eur. J. Cancer*, **17**, 495–501

16. Wittliff, J.L. (1984). Steroid-hormone receptors in breast cancer. *Cancer*, **53**, 630–643

17. Zava, D.T., Landrum, B., Horwitz, K.B. and McGuire, W.L. (1979). Androgen receptor assay with [³H]methyltrienolone (R1881) in the presence of progesterone receptors. *Endocrinology*, **104**, 1007–1012

18. Braunsberg, H. and Hammond, K.D. (1979). Methods of steroid receptor calculation: An interlaboratory study. *J. Steroid Biochem.*, **11**, 1561–1565

19. King, R.J.B., Barnes, D.M., Hawkins, R.A., Leake, R.E., Maynard, P.V., Millis, R.M. and Roberts, M.M. (1979). Measurement of oestrogen receptors by five institutions on common tissue samples. In King, R.J.B. (ed.) *Steroid Receptor Assays in Human Breast Tumours; Methodological and Clinical Aspects*, pp. 7–15. (Cardiff: Alpha Omega Publishing Ltd)

20. Oxley, D.K. (1984). Hormone receptors in breast cancer. Analytic accuracy of contemporary assays. *Arch. Pathol. Lab. Med.*, **108**, 20–23

21. Greene, G.L., Closs, L.E., Fleming, H., DeSombre, E.R. and Jensen, E.V. (1977). Antibodies to estrogen receptor: Immunochemical similarity of estrophilin from various mammalian species. *Proc. Natl Acad. Sci. USA.*, **74**, 3681–3685

22. Greene, G.L. and Jensen, E.V. (1982). Monoclonal antibodies as probes for estrogen receptor detection and characterization. *J. Steroid Biochem.*, **16**, 353–359

23. Fernö, M., Borg, Å. and Sellberg, G. (1986). Enzyme immuno assay of the estrogen receptor in breast cancer biopsy samples. *Acta Radiol. Oncol.*, **25**, 171–175

24. Press, M.F. and Greene, G.L. (1984). Methods in laboratory investigation. An immuno-cytochemical method for demonstrating estrogen receptor in human uterus using monoclonal antibodies to human estrophilin. *Lab. Invest.*, **50**, 480–486

25. Charpin, C., Jacquemier, J., Andrac, L., Vacheret, H., Habib, M.C., Devictor, B., Lavaut, M.N. and Toga, M. (1988). Multiparameteric analysis (SAMBA 200) of the progesterone receptor immunocytochemical assay in nonmalignant and malignant breast disorders. *Am. J. Pathol.*, **132**, 199–211

26. Jänne, O., Kauppila, A., Kontula, K., Syrjälä, P. and Vihko, R. (1979). Female sex steroid receptors in normal, hyperplastic and carcinomatous endometrium. The relationship to serum steroid hormones and gonadotropins and changes during medroxyprogesterone acetate administration. *Int. J. Cancer*, **24**, 545–554

27. Martin, P.M., Rolland, P.H., Gammerre, M., Serment, H. and Toga, M. (1979). Estradiol

and progesterone receptors in normal and neoplastic endometrium: Correlations between receptors, histopathological examinations and clinical responses under progestin therapy. *Int. J. Cancer*, **23**, 321–329

28. Spona, J., Ulm, R., Bieglmayer, C. and Husslein, P. (1979). Hormone serum levels and hormone receptor contents of endometria in women with normal menstrual cycles and patients bearing endometrial carcinoma. *Gynecol. Obstet. Invest.*, **10**, 71–80
29. Levy, C., Robel, P., Gautray, J.P., De Brux, J., Verma, U., Descomps, B., Baulieu, E.E. and Eychenne, B. (1980). Estradiol and progesterone receptors in human endometrium: Normal and abnormal menstrual cycles and early pregnancy. *Am. J. Obstet. Gynecol.*, **136**, 646–651
30. Neumannova, M., Kauppila, A. and Vihko, R. (1983). Cytosol and nuclear estrogen and progestin receptors and 17 beta-hydroxysteroid dehydrogenase activity in normal and carcinomatous endometrium. *Obstet. Gynecol.*, **61**, 181–188
31. Cao, Z.-Y., Eppenberger, U., Roos, W., Torhorst, J. and Almendral, A. (1983). Cytosol estrogen and progesterone receptor levels measured in normal and pathological tissue of endometrium, endocervical mucosa and cervical vaginal portion. *Arch. Gynecol.*, **233**, 109–119
32. Tsibris, J.C.M., Fort, F.L., Cazenave, C.R., Cantor, B., Bardawil, W.A., Notelovitz, M. and Spellacy, W.N. (1981). The uneven distribution of estrogen and progesterone receptors in human endometrium. *J. Steroid Biochem.*, **14**, 997–1003
33. Dizerga, G.S., Barber, D.L. and Hodgen, G.D. (1980). Endometriosis: role of ovarian steroids in initiation, maintenance, and suppression. *Fertil. Steril.*, **33**, 649–653
34. Bergqvist, A., Jeppsson, S., Kullander, S. and Ljungberg, O. (1985). Human uterine endometrium and endometriotic tissue transplanted into nude mice. *Am. J. Pathol.*, **121**, 337–341
35. Schweppe, K.-W., Wynn, R.M. and Beller, F.K. (1984). Ultrastructural comparison of endometriotic implants and eutopic endometrium. *Am. J. Obstet. Gynecol.*, **148**, 1024–1039
36. Bergqvist, A., Ljungberg, O. and Myhre, E. (1984). Human endometrium and endometriotic tissue obtained simultaneously: A comparative histological study. *Int. J. Gynecol. Pathol.*, **3**, 135–145
37. Vasquez, G., Cornillie, F. and Brosens, I.A. (1984). Peritoneal endometriosis: scanning electron microscopy and histology of minimal pelvic endometriotic lesions. *Fertil. Steril.*, **42**, 696–703
38. Tamaya, T., Motoyama, T., Ohono, Y., Ide, N., Tsurusaki, T. and Okada, H. (1979). Steroid receptor levels and histology of endometriosis and adenomyosis. *Fertil. Steril.*, **31**, 396–400
39. Bergqvist, A., Rannevik, G. and Thorell, J. (1980). Estrogen (ER) and progesterone (PR) receptors in endometriosis and intrauterine endometrium. *Acta Obstet. Gynecol. Scand. Suppl.*, **93**, 67
40. Bergqvist, A., Rannevik, G. and Thorell, J. (1981). Estrogen and progesterone cytosol receptor concentrations in endometriotic tissue and intrauterine endometrium. *Acta Obstet. Gynecol. Scand. Suppl.*, **101**, 53–58
41. Jänne, O., Kauppila, A., Syrjälä, P. and Vihko, R. (1980). Comparison of cytosol estrogen and progestin receptor status in malignant and benign tumors and tumor-like lesions of human ovary. *Int. J. Cancer*, **25**, 175–179
42. Jänne, O., Kauppila, A., Kokko, E., Lantto, T., Rönnberg, L. and Vihko, R. (1981). Estrogen and progestin receptors in endometriosis lesions: Comparison with endometrial tissue. *Am. J. Obstet. Gynecol.*, **141**, 562–566
43. Vierikko, P., Kauppila, A., Rönnberg, L. and Vihko, R. (1985). Steroidal regulation of endometriosis tissue: lack of induction of 17β-hydroxysteroid dehydrogenase activity by progesterone, medroxyprogesterone acetate, or danazol. *Fertil. Steril.*, **43**, 218–224
44. Lyndrup, J., Thorpe, S., Glenthøj, A., Obel, E. and Sele, V. (1987). Altered progesterone/estrogen receptor ratios in endometriosis. A comparative study of steroid receptors and morphology in endometriosis and endometrium. *Acta Obstet. Gynecol. Scand.*, **66**, 625–629
45. Gould, S.F., Shannon, J.M. and Cunha, G.R. (1983). Nuclear estrogen binding sites in human endometriosis. *Fertil. Steril.*, **39**, 520–524

46. Eisenfeld, A.J., Gardner, W.U. and van Wagenen, G. (1971). Radioactive estradiol accumulation in endometriosis of the rhesus monkey. *Am. J. Obstet. Gynecol.*, **109**, 124–130

47. Bergqvist, A., Jeppsson, S. and Ljungberg, O. (1985). Histochemical demonstration of estrogen and progesterone binding in endometriotic tissue and in uterine endometrium. A comparative study. *J. Histochem. Cytochem.*, **33**, 155–161

48. Bergqvist, A., Carlström, K. and Ljungberg, O. (1984). Histochemical localization of estrogen and progesterone receptors. Evaluation of a method. *J. Histochem. Cytochem.*, **32**, 493–500

49. Bergqvist, A. and Fernö, M. (1988). Steroid receptors in endometriotic tissue and endometrium assayed with monoclonal antibodies. In Genazzani, A.R., Petraglia, F., Volpe, A. and Facchinetti, F. (eds.) *Recent Research in Gynecological Endocrinology*, vol. 1, pp. 394–399. (Casterton Hall, Carnforth: Parthenon Publ. Group)

50. Bur, M.E., Greene, G.L. and Press, M.F. (1987). Estrogen receptor localization in formalin-fixed, paraffin-embedded endometrium and endometriotic tissues. *Int. J. Gynecol. Pathol.*, **6**, 140–151

51. Lessey, B.A., Metzger, D.A., Haney, A.F. and McCarty, K.S. Jr. (1989). Immunohistochemical analysis of estrogen and progesterone receptors in endometriosis: comparison with normal endometrium during the menstrual cycle and the effect of medical therapy. *Fertil. Steril.*, **51**, 409–415

52. Bergqvist, A., Ljungberg, O. and Fernö, M. (1989). Histochemical localization of estrogen (ER) and progesterone (PR) receptors in endometriotic tissue and endometrium using monoclonal antibodies. Presented at *The Second International Symposium on Endometriosis*, May 1–3, Houston, Texas

53. Sternfeld, M.D., West, N.B. and Brenner, R. M. (1988). Immunocytochemistry of the estrogen receptor in spontaneous endometriosis in rhesus macaques. *Fertil. Steril.*, **49**, 342–348

54. Punnonen, R., Pettersson, K., Vanharanta, R. and Lukola, A. (1985). Androgen, estrogen and progestin binding in cytosols of benign gynecologic tumours and tumour-like lesions. *Horm. Metab. Res.*, **17**, 607–609

55. Carlström, K., Bergqvist, A. and Ljungberg, O. (1988). Metabolism of estrone sulfate in endometriotic tissue and in uterine endometrium in proliferative and secretory cycle phase. *Fertil. Steril.*, **49**, 229–233

56. Bergqvist, A. and Myhre, E. (1986). Glycogen and acid and neutral polysaccharides in endometriotic tissue and in uterine endometrium: a comparative histochemical study. *Int. J. Gynecol. Pathol.*, **5**, 338–344

57. Prakash, S., Ulfelder, H. and Cohen, R.B. (1965). Enzyme-histochemical observations on endometriosis. *Am. J. Obstet. Gynecol.*, **91**, 990–997

58. Vernon, M.W., Beard, J.S., Graves, K. and Wilson, E.A. (1986). Classification of endometriotic implants by morphologic appearance and capacity to synthesize prostaglandin F. *Fertil. Steril.*, **46**, 801–806

59. King, R.J.B., Townsend, P.T., Siddle, N., Whitehead, M.I. and Taylor, R.W. (1982). Regulation of estrogen and progesterone receptor levels in epithelium and stroma from pre- and postmenopausal endometria. *J. Steroid Biochem.*, **16**, 21–30

60. Cornillie, F.J., Brosens, I.A., Vasquez, G. and Riphagen, I. (1986). Histologic and ultrastructural changes in human endometriotic implants treated with the antiprogesterone steroid ethylnorgestrienone (gestrinone) during 2 months. *Int. J. Gynecol. Pathol.*, **5**, 95–109

61. Brosens, I.A., Cornillie, F.J. and Vasquez, G. (1986). Etiology and pathophysiology of endometriosis. In Roland, R., Chadha, D.R. and Willemsen, W.N.P. (eds.) *Gonadotrophin Down-Regulation in Gynecological Practice*, pp. 81–102. (New York: Alan R. Liss)

4
The endometrium and endometriosis

S. K. Smith

INTRODUCTION

Endometriosis represents one of the most intriguing and difficult conditions facing reproductive medicine. The condition is characterized by the finding of tissue with histological similarities to endometrium, outside of the uterine cavity. The controversy surrounding the aetiology of this condition must centre on the endocrine, paracrine and autocrine factors that regulate endometrial differentiation and proliferation. The first description of endometriosis as a discrete entity was made in the 1920s[1] by Sampson, and as most of the disease was found in the pelvis this led to the initial hypothesis of simple implantation[2], which would be dependent on the retrograde passage of endometrium at menstruation. This hypothesis has gained credence more recently, as Halme et al.[3] showed blood in the peritoneal cavity of 90% of 52 women with patent fallopian tubes having sterilization in the premenstrual period. The presence of blood in peritoneal fluid was significantly reduced in women with occluded tubes. The presence of endometrial glands in peritoneal fluid was confirmed by several other authors[4-6] though the endometrial cells constitute less than 20% of the cells, the rest being macrophages and lymphocytes[7,8]. Thus it is likely that most women experience retrograde menstruation. If the implantation hypothesis is correct, then women with endometriosis must differ from normal women either because their endometrium has a greater capacity to implant and grow or because the environment of their peritoneal cavity favours the nurture of the endometrium.

Alternatively, endometrium could be deposited in ectopic sites by haematogenous or lymphatic spread[9], whilst Novak[10] proposed the mesothelial metaplasia hypothesis in which endometrial detritus induces mesothelial changes. It is possible that endometriosis may involve *all* or part of these hypotheses but it is the one of retrograde menstruation that is still considered the most likely cause, at least in women with superficial pelvic endometriosis. The finding of ectopic endometrium obviously raises the question of whether ectopic endometrium is similar to eutopic endometrium.

ECTOPIC AND EUTOPIC ENDOMETRIUM

Histology and ultrastructure

Sampson[1] described endometriotic glands and stroma as being morphologically identical to uterine endometrium and cyclical histological changes have been described by more recent authors[11]. Enzyme-histochemical assessment of endometriotic endometrium in which staining for alkaline phosphatase, acid phosphatase, lactic dehydrogenase, glucose-6-phosphate dehydrogenase, isocitric dehydrogenase and succinic dehydrogenase similarly demonstrated little difference between eutopic and ectopic endometrium[12].

More detailed analysis of endometriotic foci suggests subtle differences between eutopic and ectopic endometrium. Schweppe and Wynn[13] described the ultrastructural changes in 14 endometriotic foci removed from ovary (10 cases), broad ligament (2), cul-de-sac (1) and episiotomy scar (1). The presence of giant mitochondria and nuclear channel systems was absent from ectopic endometrium but in general it was possible to date the endometrium using standard criteria for uterine endometrium, e.g. increases in Golgi complexes, mitochondria, rough endoplasmic reticulum and secretory vesicles during the proliferative phase of the cycle and increases in secretory vesicles and intraluminal secretion during the secretory phase. Further analysis of 77 cases of endometriotic tissue suggested a delay in the development of proliferative changes when compared to uterine endometrium and precise dating of ectopic endometrium in the secretory stage of the cycle was not possible because of the wide variability of endometrial response and the absence of giant mitochondria and nuclear channels[14]. Scanning electron and light microscopy of 36 patients confirmed the diagnosis of endometriosis in a further study but further indicated three types of peritoneal endometriotic lesion[15]. Firstly, endometrial polyps were present covered by predominantly non-ciliated cells, and glandular openings were absent. Secondly, stromal foci were present containing gland openings and covered by non-ciliated glandular cells. Finally, retroperitoneal glandular structures were present in some lesions in which the endometriotic tissue was found beneath the peritoneal surface.

The consistent findings of these studies suggest that endometriotic endometrium has many similarities with uterine endometrium but that development is delayed in the proliferative phase of the cycle and there is

---

Figure 4.1 (opposite) (i) Scanning electron microscopy of endometriotic polyp obtained from the peritoneal cavity at (a) × 125 and (b) × 2500 magnification. Note the reduction of ciliated cells. (ii) Scanning electron microscopy of second type of ectopic endometrium demonstrating the presence of glandular openings and numerous ciliated cells. (iii) Third type of ectopic endometrium demonstrating mesothelial cells covered with microvilli which are flattened and elongated. Published by kind permission of Dr. Vasquez, and *Fertility and Sterility*.

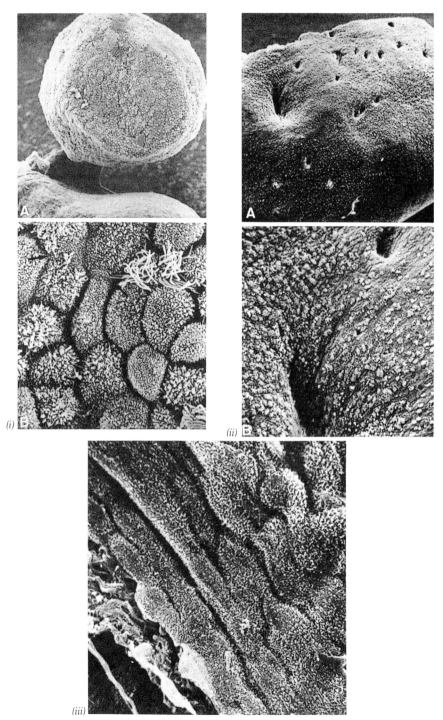

an incomplete progestational response. These observations may suggest an inadequate response to the ovarian steroids mediated by differences in receptor levels.

Steroid receptors and oestrogen metabolism in endometriotic lesions

Studies of nuclear oestrogen receptor content of rhesus and human endometriotic lesions reveal remarkable intraspecies similarities. In both species, cyclical changes of receptor levels do not occur in endometriotic implants. In the rhesus monkey, Sternfeld et al.[16] used monoclonal anti-oestrophilins to demonstrate nuclear oestrogen receptors. In uterine endometrium, glandular cells had the highest content of receptor and both glandular and stromal cell receptor levels fell in the secretory phase. Endometriotic implants had lower levels of receptors that did not change during the cycle. Gould et al.[17] used autoradiography to demonstrate oestrogen receptors in human endometrium and showed consistent staining of stromal cells in endometriotic lesions throughout the cycle whilst staining declined in these cells in the luteal phase. Glandular cells of endometriotic lesions were patchily stained throughout the cycle yet their staining in uterine endometrium was profuse in the proliferative phase and absent in the secretory phase of the cycle.

Uterine and endometriotic tissue also differs with respect to oestrogen metabolism as both 17β-hydroxysteroid dehydrogenase[18] and oestrone sulphatase activity[19] are depressed in endometriotic tissue compared to uterine endometrium.

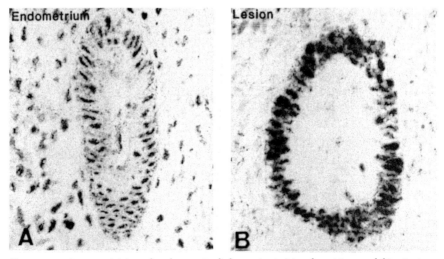

Figure 4.2 Immunostaining of nuclear oestradiol receptor in (a) endometrium, and (b) ectopic endometrium. Published by kind permission of Dr. M. D. Sternfeld, and *Fertility and Sterility*.

ENDOMETRIAL GROWTH

Regulation of cellular proliferation

Despite these subtle differences between uterine endometrium and ectopic endometrium, the tissue is still essentially endometrium and is capable of implanting and proliferating. Based on this fact, present therapy attempts to suppress endometrial growth by the induction of pseudopregnancy (oral contraceptives and gestagens) or pseudomenopause (danazol and LHRH agonists)[20,21]. All of these treatments cause regression of the explants and alleviation of symptoms[22–25]. However, treatment is often associated with unpleasant side-effects[22,23,26], the disease recurs in between 16 and 52% of women[23,27,28], and subsequent conception rates even with mild endometriosis are not improved by medication[25,29–31]. The failure of hormone therapy

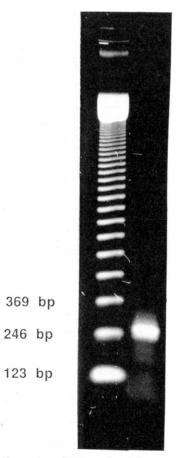

369 bp

246 bp

123 bp

Figure 4.3 Ethidium bromide staining of PCR product following agarose gel electrophoresis of predicted size approximately 257 bp for EGF. Reproduced by kind permission of *Clinics in Obstetrics and Gynaecology.*

probably arises from incomplete suppression of endometriotic foci[32] but clearly it does not alter the underlying pathology of this disorder.

These strategies are inadequate for the treatment of endometriosis and reflect the paucity of knowledge concerning the factors that regulate normal and abnormal endometrial growth. The mammalian cell cycle is a complex mechanism and full discussion of its regulation is beyond the scope of this chapter. Interpretation of such findings in endometriotic implants will be ambiguous because of the likely heterogeneity of the cell population. Nevertheless, little is known of the stages of the cell cycle that endometriotic cells are in and this is likely to be an important area in which a greater understanding of the pathophysiology of endometriosis will arise. Cells arrested in G_0 require competence factors that permit them to be stimulated to proceed through G_1 to DNA synthesis and mitosis. These stimulatory factors are as yet poorly defined but are present in serum[33]. The detailed knowledge of cell cycle regulatory factors has been best outlined in fibroblasts and it is not known whether this is reflected in the regulation of glandular or stromal proliferation in endometriotic explants. However, there is increasing evidence to suggest that peptide growth factors are expressed in mammalian endometrium and that they play an important role in permitting cells to enter the cell cycle.

Growth factors and endometrium

In view of the considerable interest in the role of growth factors in cell growth it is surprising that little is known of their function in the normal endometrium, which undergoes such prolific regeneration every month, nor is there much information about the expression, secretion or effects of growth factors in endometriosis.

Epidermal growth factor
In the light of the obvious identification of endometrial epithelial cells in endometriotic explants it is appropriate to consider the possible role of epidermal growth factor (EGF) in endometrial proliferation as EGF is known to be a potent stimulator of proliferation particularly of fibroblasts, keratinocytes and epithelial cells[34,35]. EGF is a 53-amino-acid peptide that is derived from a larger 1168-amino-acid precursor[36,37]. This large precursor contains at least seven similar repeats and the mature peptide is the unit at the 3' end of the gene coding sequence[38]. Highest levels of EGF are present in the male submaxillary gland of the mouse[39] with significantly lower amounts being present in the female SMG and kidney. Gonzalez et al.[40] detected low amounts of EGF in mouse uterus but found that levels were increased 7-fold by oestradiol. Immunoreactive EGF is present in mouse epithelial cells[41] but was shown only after proteolytic preparation of the tissue. This observation could indicate that prepro-EGF exists as a transmembrane peptide with an α-helical transmembrane scanning peptide[34].

Presence of the message for prepro-EGF has been demonstrated in the mouse uterus. DiAugustine et al.[41] showed the presence of a 4.7 kb prepro-

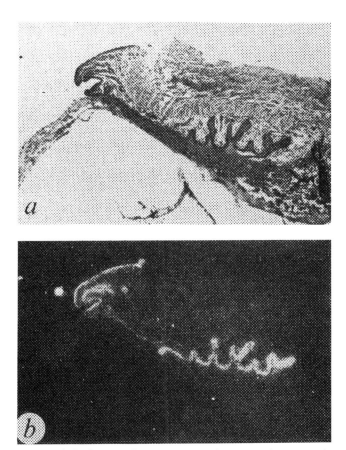

Figure 4.4 *In situ* hybridization of tissue sections of mouse endometrium demonstrating immunofluorescence with a CSF-1 antisense RNA probe. Published by kind permission of Dr. J. W. Pollard, and *Nature*.

EGF mRNA in the uteri of immature mice using a cDNA probe. However, the SMG prepro-EGF mRNA is present in very low copy number and was not demonstrated in human endometrium using radioimmunoassay (RIA)[42]. Recently, application of the gene amplification technique, the polymerase chain reaction (PCR) suggests that human endometrium contains the message for prepro-EGF[43]. Endometrium from women obtained in the proliferative and secretory phases of the cycle were found to have a PCR product of predicted size following synthesis of cDNA by reverse transcriptase[44] and this product was not present in peripheral nucleated white cells. It is possible that oestradiol stimulates EGF synthesis, as Imai[45] demonstrated increased levels in uterine fluid following oestrogen administration and DiAugustine *et al.*[41] showed a rise in prepro-EGF levels in endometrium after similar treatment.

Endometrium is likely to be a target for EGF since EGF receptors are present. EGF receptors are present in rat[46] and human[47] endometrium and appear to be evenly distributed between glandular and stromal cells[48,49]. In the rat, oestradiol stimulates increased binding of EGF[50] and promotes the synthesis of two transcripts of EGF receptor mRNA of sizes 9.5 and 6.6 kb[51], which are similar in size to reported values for EGF receptor mRNA from A431 cells[48] and human placenta[52].

The EGF receptor is a 170-kDa glycosylated transmembrane peptide[53] that contains a 621-amino-acid extracellular domain and a 23-amino-acid transmembrane scanning sequence. Two cysteine-rich regions between residues 134 to 313 and 446 to 612 cooperate to form the high-affinity EGF receptor site[38]. The intracellular domain contains the protein-tyrosine kinase and three autophosphorylation sites all situated towards the C-terminus[54]. The mechanisms of ligand binding and signal transduction are reviewed by Westmark and Heldin[55]. The mechanism whereby EGF activates the protein-tyrosine kinase is not clear, though a process of receptor dimerization appears to be involved[56].

The cellular responses induced by growth factors are complex but include ion fluxes, phospholipid hydrolysis and proto-oncogene activation[57]. The EGF receptor contains a regulatory phosphorylation site at Thr-654 that is phosphorylated by protein kinase C (PKC). Protein kinase C activity is most likely to be involved in proliferation but the exact relationship between PKC and the EGF receptor has not been established, though the potential remains for intracellular autoregulation of receptor function. The activity of the protein tyrosine kinase is central to signal transduction and mitogenesis induced by ligands of the EGF receptor (reported in Westmark and Heldin[55]). Point directed mutagenesis of the adenosine triphosphate- (ATP-) binding site of the EGF receptor abolishes kinase activity and prevents inositol phosphate accumulation, Ca^{2+} influx, c-*fos* and c-*myc* expression and DNA synthesis. As will be discussed later in this chapter, of particular interest is the potential interaction between EGF receptor activation, eicosanoid synthesis and mitogenesis. Several reports suggest that phospholipase C-mediated hydrolysis of phospholipids is involved in the regulation of mitogensis[57], as for example the observation that microinjection of antibodies to PIP2 inhibits platelet derived growth factor- (PDGF-) activated mitogenesis[58]. This evidence for this interaction and its possible significance to the aetiology of endometriosis will be considered in the section on eicosanoids and endometrium.

In the mouse, EGF stimulates proliferation of uterine epithelial cells maintained in serum-free medium supplemented with insulin and hydrocortisone[59]. More recently, Haining *et al.*[60] showed that EGF in combination with oestradiol produced a slight increase in cell numbers of human epithelial but not stromal cells cultured in serum-free medium. It is not known whether endometriotic epithelial cells would respond in the same way, but differences in peritoneal fluid levels of EGF between normal and endometriotic women were not found by DeLeon *et al.*[61]. Of course this does not mean that endometriotic cells do not have greater numbers of receptors than uterine endometrium nor that signal induction arising from these receptors is not different from uterine endometrium. The situation is further complicated because the response of cells to the growth factor is dependent on the concentration of the peptide, the receptivity of the cell and even the presence of other growth-promoting agents like bombesin, PDGF, TGF_α or TGF_β[35]. Furthermore, other agents, including retinoic acid and EGF itself[62], appear to be capable of stimulating expression of the EGF receptor, indicating complicated autoregulatory mechanisms of growth control. There are no data concerning these factors with regard to normal uterine endometrium, still less data concerning endometriotic cells. Nevertheless, a disorder of endometrial growth does arise in women with endometriosis and it is likely to be necessary to obtain this information before rational improvements in therapy can be applied.

Transforming growth factor alpha
Transforming growth factor alpha (TGF_α) is a 50-amino-acid secreted peptide that is derived in the human from a 160-amino-acid precursor[63]. Multiple species of TGF_α exist but the smallest 50-amino-acid form has 30% structural homology to EGF, and conservation of the six cysteine residues with the presumed formation of three disulphide bridges provides a molecular explanation of the ability of both EGF and TGF_α to bind to the EGF receptor[64]. The mRNA for TGF_α is between 4.5 and 4.8 kb long and contains 6 exons from chromosome 2[65]. The precursor peptide consists of a 100-amino-acid extracellular domain containing the mature TGF_α, a hydrophobic transmembrane domain and a 35-residue intracellular domain[66,67]. The peptide is derived by proteolytic cleavage of the extracellular peptide[68]. However, it is possible that cleavage does not occur and that the precursor peptide remains as an extracellular agonist that can bind to EGF receptors, thus exerting a mechanism of cell-to-cell mediated mitogenesis.

TGF$_\alpha$ is expressed by skin keratinocytes[69] and activated macrophages[70]. Using Northern blot and *in situ* hybridization, Han *et al.*[71] were able to demonstrate expression of TGF_α in the stroma of rat decidua but were unable to demonstrate its presence in non-pregnant tissue. It is not known whether human endometrium expresses TGF_α, but human peripheral leukocytes do express the message for TGF_α (Schofield, Jones, Rajput-Williams and Smith, 1990, unpublished data). Alterations in TGF_α expression may confer on cells a proliferative advantage. Although TGF_α has less receptor binding capacity than EGF, both growth factors appear equally potent in their ability to stimulate DNA synthesis in several cell lines[72].

The expression of EGF and TGF_α by normal endometrium is just being evaluated in women, but the factors regulating this expression are unknown. The fact that the message for these peptides is only present in low copy number significantly hinders further advances in this area. The small amount of endometriotic tissue obtained at operation further complicates the study of endometriosis in humans. However, it is most likely that differences do occur in expression of the peptides or the receptor between uterine and endometriotic endometrium, which is complicated by differences in signal transduction. Detailed knowledge is likely to be needed in this field to gain further light on the role of growth factors in ectopic endometrial proliferation.

Colony-stimulating factor
Colony-stimulating factor 1 (CSF-1) is a glycosylated polypeptide homodimer initially thought to be a haemopoietic growth factor but which is now known

to be expressed in endometrium and decidua[73]. Human CSF-1 is the product of a single gene situated on chromosome 5 and arises from three transcripts produced by alternate splicing of the primary RNA. The larger 4-kb message encodes a transmembrane peptide that is rapidly cleaved and released in its glycosylated form as a soluble growth factor[74,75]. Two smaller RNA species are present in the human, a 1.9-kb and a 1.6-kb species, the former lacking 116 amino acids and the latter lacking 298 amino acids compaired to the product of the 4-kb species[76,77]. The product of the smaller RNA species is processed like that of the 4-kb RNA but the product of the 1.9-kb species lacks the endoplasmic reticulum proteolytic cleavage site and is only slowly cleaved by extracellular proteolysis[78].

In situ hybridization studies in the mouse indicate that CSF-1 is expressed in the luminal and glandular cells of the endometrium and that expression is enhanced by the effect of progesterone on an oestradiol-primed endometrium. A role for CSF-1 in trophoblast proliferation is suggested by the finding of the 165-kDa transmembrane tyrosine kinase receptor, which is the product of the c-*fms* proto-oncogene but this receptor has not been demonstrated in endometrium. It is unlikely that CSF-1 exerts an autocrine role in this case, though it might be involved in the well-described activation of peritoneal macrophages that is found in women with endometriosis.

Fibroblast growth factors
As described, endometriosis is characterized by the ability of endometrium to maintain itself in the alien environment of the peritoneal cavity. In addition it seems to stimulate activation not only of peritoneal macrophages but also fibroblasts, as moderate to severe endometriosis is associated with increased fibrosis and vascular proliferation at and around the site of implantation. This latter mechanism, angiogenesis, is mediated in part by an increasing group of polypeptides including TGF_α, TGF_β, angiogenin, tumour necrosis factor and the two 'original' fibroblast growth factors, acidic and basic FGF[79].

Bovine pituitary basic FGF (bFGF) was originally described as a 146-amino-acid peptide[80] that binds to a 145-kDa cell surface receptor[81]. However, it now appears that there are several microheterogeneous forms. Florkiewicz and Sommer[82] recently demonstrated four species of bFGF expressed by the human cell line SK-HEP-1. The smallest mRNA codes for a 17.8-kDa, 155-amino-acid peptide with a putative initiator ATG (methionine) codon. In addition, three further mRNA species 22.5, 23.1 and 24.2-kDa code for peptides that are collinear NH_2-terminal extensions of the original 17.8-kDa bFGF.

Acidic FGF (aFGF) was originally presumed to be found only in neural tissue[83], but was subsequently demonstrated in human prostate[84], bovine kidney[85], and human brain and kidney, including that of the fetus[86]. It was not detected in placenta or fetal liver, though in this latter paper the polymerase chain reaction was not used. Of particular interest to the aetiology of endometriosis, though, is the finding of both FGFs in pig endometrium and uterine flushings[87]. It is now clear that the FGFs are a larger family of peptides that includes *int-2, hst*/KS3 and FGF-5[88]. These peptides contain a common central sequence of about 150 amino acids with N- and C-terminal extensions. The latter three 'FGFs', but not acidic and basic FGF, contain amino-terminal hydrophobic leader sequences that facilitate secretion. It is not clear how these FGFs are released from the cell to exert autocrine effects on cells through binding to cell surface receptors. FGF-5 has been demonstrated in human endometrial carcinoma cells[89], but it is not clear whether it is expressed in non-malignant human endometrium.

FGFs bind to heparin[90,91], which is a significant constituent of the glycosaminoglycans of the extracellular matrix (ECM). Release of FGFs from the ECM is facilitated by heparin sulphatase[92], which probably releases the growth factors to induce endothelial proliferation[93] and angiogenesis[79]. The role of FGF expression from endometriotic explants remains to be elucidated.

Growth factors and angiogenesis

The classic description of moderate or severe endometriosis includes the increased vascularity of peritoneum surrounding the endometriotic implant. This increased vascularity is localized to the implant and is not the result of generalized peritoneal angiogenesis. Angiogenesis is associated with the inflammatory response that appears to be a characteristic of the cells of the peritoneal cavity. The potential role of some better-known growth factors has been outlined above but there are several other peptides that may be involved and the potential of altered growth factor expression for initiating or perpetuating endometriosis is being pursued.

EICOSANOIDS, ENDOMETRIUM AND ENDOMETRIOSIS

Introduction

There is considerable controversy concerning the role of prostaglandins in the aetiology of endometriosis. In this section, the evidence for disturbances of PG synthesis in endometriosis is reviewed, the factors regulating PG synthesis are considered and the potential mechanisms whereby these disturbances may be involved in endometriosis are discussed.

Prostaglandins and endometriosis

New Zealand White rabbits with induced endometriosis have elevated levels of $PGF_{2\alpha}$ in peritoneal fluid[94], whilst elevated concentrations of $PGF_{2\alpha}$ but not PGE_2 were found in the peritoneal fluid of monkeys with autotransplanted endometrium[95]. Levels of various PGs in peritoneal fluid of patients with endometriosis have recently been reviewed by Syrop and Halme[96].

They reviewed 12 communications that had measured PG concentrations. Rock *et al.*[97], Dawood *et al.*[98], DeLeon *et al.*[61], and Chacho *et al.*[99] failed to demonstrate differences in $PGF_{2\alpha}$ levels in peritoneal fluid between women with and without endometriosis when the fluid was removed in the proliferative phase of the cycle. Similarly, Halme *et al.*[100] failed to demonstrate elevated levels of $PGF_{2\alpha}$ in peritoneal fluid of 16 women with endometriosis compared to 24 fertile women. However, Badawy *et al.*[101] found elevated levels of $PGF_{2\alpha}$ in peritoneal fluid throughout the menstrual cycle, whilst DeLeon *et al.*[61] found higher levels only in the secretory part of the cycle when comparing 8 women without endometriosis to 23 women with the disease. PGE_2 levels were also increased in these latter studies but were not elevated in the former studies.

More consistent findings were obtained when levels of the metabolites of thromboxane A_2 and prostacyclin (i.e. 6-keto-$PGF_{1\alpha}$) were measured in peritoneal fluid. Drake *et al.*[102,103], Dawood *et al.*[98], Koskimies *et al.*[104], Ylikorkala *et al.*[105], and DeLeon *et al.*[61] all demonstrated elevated levels of 6-keto-$PGF_{1\alpha}$ in women with endometriosis. The largest differences were found in the study by Drake *et al.*[102] in which 6-keto-$PGF_{1\alpha}$ levels were 44.5 + 13.7 ng/ml in 14 women with endometriosis compared to 3.85 + 2.5 ng/ml in 15 control women. Such a large difference was not found by Dawood *et al.*[98], in whose study peritoneal fluid levels of 6-keto-$PGF_{1\alpha}$ were 3.32 + 0.7 ng/ml in 16 women with endometriosis compared to 0.48 + 0.19 ng/ml in 10 women without the disease. These findings were not confirmed by the studies of Sgarlata *et al.*[106], Badawy *et al.*[101] and Mudge *et al.*[107], who failed to demonstrate differences in 6-keto-$PGF_{1\alpha}$ levels in women with endometriosis; but although DeLeon *et al.*[61] also failed to show differences in these levels in the proliferative phase of the cycle, they did find significant increases in the secretory phase of the cycle.

The findings with respect to 6-keto-$PGF_{1\alpha}$ levels were mirrored in most studies by similar observations for TXB_2 concentrations in which levels were elevated in peritoneal fluid of women with endometriosis.

Prostaglandin synthesis and the origin of peritoneal prostaglandins

Site of prostaglandin release

There are many potential sources of the PGs found in peritoneal fluid of women. These could include passive diffusion from any of the principal organs situated in the peritoneal cavity. Alternatively, they may be derived directly from the peritoneum[108] or from activated peritoneal macrophages[109]. Finally, they may be released from the ovary either by passive diffusion or by release at the time of rupture of the follicle[110].

Thromboxanes are predominantly synthesized by platelets[111] but also by peritoneal macrophages[112]. Prostacyclin is synthesized predominantly by endothelial cells[111], but could also be derived from peritoneum[112] or by diffusion from myometrium[113]. Neither of these PGs is synthesized in large amounts by endometrium[113], from which $PGF_{2\alpha}$ is the principal PG released. Before considering the factors possibly responsible for the elevated levels of PGs present in peritoneal fluid, it is perhaps relevant briefly to consider the mechanisms of PG synthesis since they broadly appear universal to most cell types.

Prostaglandin synthesis

In considering the site of PG synthesis it is important to remember the mechanism whereby PGs are synthesized and metabolized since they have a very short half-life and usually reflect *de novo* synthesis[114]. It is not the remit of this book to consider in detail the synthesis of eicosanoids but it will be considered briefly as it could be relevant to the aetiology of endometriosis and could be involved in the cause of the infertility and symptomatology of this disorder.

The primary PGs like $PGF_{2\alpha}$, PGE_2, PGI_2 and TXA_2 are all derived from the same precursors, i.e. the PG endoperoxides, which are themselves derived from free arachidonic acid (AA)[115]. Free AA in the cytosol (accounting for approximately only 5% of AA) is the substrate for metabolism to PGs. Arachidonic acid is bound to cell-membrane phospholipids and is released by the action of at least two families of phospholipases, A and C[116,117]. Phospholipase A_2 results in the cleavage of AA from the c-2 position of phosphatidylethanolamine and phosphatidylcholine. However, PLC activity results in the formation of two compounds. Although PLCs will use phosphatidylserine and choline as substrate, it is the phosphatidylinositol-PLCs (PI-PLCs) that have raised most interest because they play a central role in transmembrane cell signalling and are integrally involved in cell differentiation and proliferation[118]. The PI-PLCs cleave diacylglycerol (DAG) from phosphatidyl 4,5-bisphosphate (PIP_2). DAG, in conjunction with Ca^{2+} and phosphatidylserine activate protein kinase C[119]. In addition, DAG is a substrate for diacyl and monoacyl glycerol lipases that release free AA into the cytosol[116]. The other products derived from the hydrolysis of PIP_2 are the inositol phosphates[120]. Inositol 1,4,5-trisphosphate ($InsP_3$) promotes the release of Ca^{2+} from endoplasmic reticulum[121] (for a review see Rana and Hokin[122]) which results in oscillatory changes[123] of intracellular Ca^{2+}. Human endometrium contains both PLA2 and PLC activities[124,125] but it is not known which enzymes are present in endometriotic foci. The mechanisms whereby disturbances in PG synthesis may be involved in the aetiology of endometriosis or in the infertility and symptomatology associated with endometriosis will now be considered. Regrettably, there is little direct evidence and many of these views will inevitably be speculative.

Prostaglandin synthesis and the aetiology of endometriosis
Proliferation of endometriotic foci. There is evidence that prostaglandins may function to regulate cellular proliferation and/or differentiation, particularly in endometrium. Prostaglandin $F_{2\alpha}$ induces decidualization in the rat[126], inhibitors of PG synthesis impair decidual change[127,128], and this inhibition may be partially reversed by the administration of exogenous PGs[129,130]. More specifically, $PGF_{2\alpha}$ stimulates DNA synthesis and increased cell numbers of rabbit endometrial cells[131]. This action is antagonized by PGE_2 and PGE_1. Furthermore, $PGF_{2\alpha}$ appears to be required for oestradiol-mediated stimulation of endometrial proliferation[132].

The role of phosphoinositides in cell proliferation has been extensively studied over the past five years and there are many extensive reviews[118,133]. The PG and phosphoinositide pathways are integrally linked and feedback mechanisms exist. Phospholipase A_2 has a greater affinity for Ca^{2+} than PLCs[134] and the rise of intracellular Ca^{2+} induced by $InsP_3$ may stimulate PLA2 activity. In addition, PGs stimulate inositol phosphate accumulation in fibroblasts[135] and endometrium[131]. More recently this simplistic relationship has been questioned[136], but nevertheless PG and inositol phosphate accumulation are integral parts of the second-messenger system of cells that do seem to be involved in the process of proliferation and differentiation.

Endometriotic implants contain and release less $PGF_{2\alpha}$ than endometrium obtained from the uterine cavity[137]. Highest amounts of PGs were released from implants described as being reddened petechial, with the lowest amounts being present in powder-burn foci. These findings suggest that in the active phase of endometrial growth there is an increased release of $PGF_{2\alpha}$. Indeed, in endometriotic implants taken from women with severe or extensive endometriosis, the release and content of PG was low. These findings indicate that endometriotic foci are dissimilar to eutopic endometrium not only in their morphological characteristics but also in their capacity to synthesize PGs. However, where the tissue appears active and is presumably proliferating, PG levels increase, consistent with the requirement for PGs in endometrial proliferation.

Interaction between endometriotic foci and peritoneal fibroblasts. Drake *et al.*[102] suggested that the raised levels of PGs found in peritoneal fluid of women with endometriosis were derived from the stimulation of a peritoneal reaction by the endometrium. This requires either that the endometrium of women with endometriosis is different from normal women or that the peritoneal response is altered in these women. Such mechanisms exist. Firstly, AA is capable of stimulating fibroblast proliferation, a mechanism that may involve the generation of the superoxide radical[138] O_2^-. The activation of peritoneal macrophages has been described and the fibrosis of endometriosis is well recognized. Alternatively, the activated macrophages may stimulate PG synthesis and could influence endometrial proliferation. Interleukin-1β is a potent stimulator of PG synthesis from human amnion[139], though its effect on endometrium is poorly defined.

Endometrium and the infertility and symptomatology of endometriosis
The cause of the profound infertility associated even with mild endometriosis remains obscure. Disturbances of PG synthesis in the peritoneal cavity could influence ovum pick-up, tubal transport and even embryonic development. Hahn *et al.*[140] suggest that failure of implantation is part of the mechanism of infertility in rabbits with ectopically implanted endometrium, and in rodents a strong correlation exists between PG synthesis, decidualization and successful implantation. It is not clear whether this relationship exists in the uteri of women. Disorders of PG synthesis by the endometrium of women with endometriosis could result in abnormal implantation or placentation. There is no evidence to substantiate these hypotheses at present. Similarly, the cause of the characteristic symptoms of abdominal pain, dysmenorrhoea and dyspareunia is obscure. There is considerable evidence to link excessive release of PGs by endometrium with the aetiology of dysmenorrhoea[141], which may arise in women with endometriosis since Willman[142] showed increased synthesis of PGs in endometrium of women with the disease. The mechanism whereby endometriotic explants induce pain is not known but in some ways mirrors the pain of chronic pelvic infection, with a peritoneal cavity containing

activated macrophages and enhanced fibroblast activity.

The expression of growth factors by human endometrium is poorly understood and is only now being elucidated. It is highly likely that this is an important factor in the regulation of normal endometrial proliferation and differentiation and clearly the role of growth factors in abnormal proliferation needs to be investigated. The importance of the role of endometrial-derived growth factors and embryonic development and subsequently placental growth is being increasingly understood[143] and this could provide a further mechanism of endometriosis-derived infertility.

Conclusion

The differences between eutopic and ectopic endometrium have been considered in this chapter and possible mechanisms for the cause of endometriosis have been suggested. However, the basic question of the aetiology of this disorder remains unanswered. Does it arise because of abnormal endometrium being deposited in the peritoneal cavity, or is the environment of the endometrial cavity different in women who develop endometriosis?

Endometriosis is the cause of extensive pain and suffering to women, whether because of unpleasant symptoms or because of the pain of infertility. The cause of this syndrome has remained obscure for too long. Extensive research is required to elucidate its cause and to lead to effective means of treatment that will bring relief to many thousands of women.

REFERENCES

1. Sampson, J.A. (1927). Peritoneal endometriosis due to the menstrual dissemination of endometrial tissue into the peritoneal cavity. *Am. J. Obstet. Gynecol.,* **14**, 422–429
2. Sampson, J.A. (1940). The development of the implantation theory for the origin of peritoneal endometriosis. *Am. J. Obstet. Gynecol.,* **40**, 549–557
3. Halme, J., Hammond, M.G., Hulka, J.F., Raj, S.G. and Talbert, L.M. (1984). Retrograde menstruation in healthy women and in patients with endometriosis. *Obstet. Gynecol.,* **64**, 151–154
4. Beyth, Y., Yaffe, H., Levij, I. and Sadovsky, E. (1975). Retrograde seeding of endometrium: a sequela of tubal flushing. *Fertil. Steril.,* **26**, 1094–1097
5. Portuondo, J.A., Herran, C., Echanojauregui, A.D. and Riego, A.G. (1982). Peritoneal flushing and biopsy in laparoscopically diagnosed endometriosis. *Fertil. Steril.,* **38**, 538–541
6. Bartosik, D., Jacobs, S.L. and Kelly, L.J. (1986). Endometrial tissue in peritoneal fluid. *Fertil. Steril.,* **46**, 796–999
7. Halme, J., Becker, S. and Wing, R. (1984). Accentuated cyclic activation of peritoneal macrophages in patients with endometriosis. *Am. J. Obstet. Gynecol.,* **148**, 85–90
8. Haney, A.F., Muscato, J.J. and Weinberg, J.B. (1981). Peritoneal fluid cell populations in infertile patients. *Fertil. Steril.,* **35**, 696–704
9. Halban, J. (1924). Hysteroadenosis Metastica; Die lymphogene Genese der sog Adeno-fibromatosis heterotopica. *Dien. Klin. Wochenschr.,* **37**, 1205–1205
10. Novak, E. (1926). The significance of uterine mucosa in the fallopian tubes with a discussion of the origin of the aberrant endometrium. *Am. J. Obstet. Gynecol.,* **12**, 484–526
11. Roddick, J.W., Conkey, G. and Jacobs, E.J. (1960). The hormonal response of endometrium in endometriotic implants and its relationship to symptomatology. *Am. J. Obstet. Gynecol.,* **79**, 1173–1177

12. Prakash, S., Ulfeder, H. and Cohen, R.B. (1965). Enzyme-histochemical observations on endometriosis. *Am. J. Obstet. Gynecol.*, **91**, 990–997
13. Schweppe, K.W. and Wynn, R.M. (1981). Ultrastructural changes in endometriotic implants during the menstrual cycle. *Obstet. Gynecol.*, **58**, 465–473
14. Schweppe, K.W., Wynn, R.M. and Beller, F.K. (1984). Ultrastructural comparison of endometriotic implants and eutopic endometrium. *Am. J. Obstet. Gynecol.*, **148**, 1024–1039
15. Vasquez, G., Cornillie, F. and Brosens, I.A. (1984). Peritoneal endometriosis: scanning electron microscopy and histology of minimal pelvic endometriotic lesions. *Fertil. Steril.*, **42**, 696–703
16. Sternfeld, M.D., West, N.B. and Brenner, R.M. (1988). Immunocytochemistry of the estrogen receptor in spontaneous endometriosis in rhesus macaques. *Fertil. Steril.*, **49**, 342–348
17. Gould, S.F., Shannon, J.M. and Cunha, G.R. (1983). Nuclear estrogen binding sites in human endometrium. *Fertil. Steril.*, **39**, 520–524
18. Vierikko, P., Kauppila, A., Ronnberg, L. and Vihko, R. (1985). Steroidal regulation of endometriosis tissue: lack of induction of 17β-hydroxysteroid dehydrogenase activity by progesterone, medroxyprogesterone acetate, or danazol. *Fertil. Steril.*, **43**, 218–224
19. Carlstrom, K., Berqvist, A. and Ljunberg, O. (1988). Metabolism of estrone sulfate in endometriotic tissue and in uterine endometrium in proliferative and secretory cycle phase. *Fertil. Steril.*, **49**, 229–233
20. Schmidt, C.L. (1985). Endometriosis: a reappraisal of pathogenesis and treatment. *Fertil. Steril.*, **44**, 157–173
21. Olive, D.L. and Haney, A.F. (1985). Endometriosis-associated infertility: a critical review of therapeutic approaches. *Obstet. Gynecol. Rev.*, **41**, 538–555
22. Moghissi, K.S. and Boyce, C.R. (1976). Management of endometriosis with oral medroxyprogesterone acetate. *Obstet. Gynecol.*, **47**, 265–267
23. Barbieri, R.L., Evans, S. and Kistner, R.W. (1982). Danazol in the treatment of endometriosis: analysis of 100 cases with a 4-year follow-up. *Fertil. Steril.*, **37**, 737–746
24. Shaw, R.W., Fraser, H.M. and Boyle, H. (1983). Intranasal LHRH in the treatment of women with endometriosis. *Br. Med. J.*, **287**, 1667
25. Thomas, E.J. and Cooke, I.D. (1986). Successful treatment of asymptomatic endometriosis; does it benefit infertile women? *Br. Med. J.*, **294**, 1117–1119
26. Meldrum, D.R., Chang, R.J., Lu, J.H.K., Vale, W., Rivier, J. and Judd, H.L. (1982). 'Medical oophorectomy' using a long-acting GN-RH agonist — a possible new approach to the treatment of endometriosis. *J. Clin. Endocrinol. Metab.*, **54**, 1081–1085
27. Kistner, R.W. (1962). Infertility with endometriosis: a plan of therapy. *Fertil. Steril.*, **13**, 237–245
28. Moore, E.E., Harger, J.H., Rock, J.A. and Archer, D.F. (1981). Management of pelvic endometriosis with low-dose danazol. *Fertil. Steril.*, **36**, 15–19
29. Seibel, M.M., Berger, M.J., Weinstein, F.G. and Taymor, M.L. (1982). The effectiveness of danazol on subsequent fertility in minimal endometriosis. *Fertil. Steril.*, **38**, 534–540
30. Portuondo, J.A., Echanojauregui, A.D., Herran, C. and Alijarte, I. (1983). Early conception in patients with untreated mild endometriosis. *Fertil. Steril.*, **39**, 22–25
31. Buttram, V.C., Reiter, R.C. and Ward, S. (1985). Treatment of endometriosis with danazol: report of a 6-year prospective study. *Fertil. Steril.*, **43**, 353–360
32. Nisolle-Pochet, M., Casanas-Roux, F. and Donnez, J. (1988). Histologic study of ovarian endometriosis after hormonal therapy. *Fertil. Steril.*, **49**, 423–426
33. Russell, W.E., VanWyk, J.J. and Pledger, W.J. (1984). Inhibition of the mitogenic effects of plasma by a monoclonal antibody to somatomedin C. *Proc. Natl. Acad. Sci. USA*, **81**, 2389–2392
34. Carpenter, G. and Cohen, S. (1979). Epidermal growth factor. *Annu. Rev. Biochem.*, **48**, 193–216
35. Burgess, A.W. (1989). Epidermal growth factor and transforming growth factor a. *Br. Med. Bull.*, **45**, 401–424
36. Gray, A., Dull, T.J. and Ullrich, A. (1983). Nucleotide sequence of epidermal growth factor cDNA predicts a 128,000-molecular weight protein precursor. *Nature*, **303**, 722–725

37. Scott, J., Urdea, M., Quirigo, M., Sanchez-Pescador, R., Fong, N., Selby, M., Rutter, W.J. and Bell, G.I. (1983). Structure of a mouse submaxillary gland messenger RNA encoding epidermal growth factor and seven related proteins. *Science*, **221**, 236–240

38. Gill, G.N., Bertics, P.J. and Santon, J.B. (1987). Epidermal growth factor and its receptor. *Mol. Cell. Endocrinol.*, **51**, 169–186

39. Rall, L.B., Scott, J. and Bell, G.I. (1985). Mouse preproepidermal growth factor synthesis by the kidney and other tissues. *Nature*, **313**, 228–231

40. Gonzalez, F., Lakshmanan, J., Hoath, S. and Fisher, D.A. (1984). Effect of oestradiol-17beta on uterine epidermal growth factor concentration in immature mice. *Acta Endocrinol. Copenh.*, **105**, 425–428

41. DiAugustine, R.P., Petrusz, P., Bell, G.I., Brown, C.F., Korach, K.S., McLachlan, J.A. and Teng, C.T. (1988). Influence of estrogens on mouse uterine epidermal growth factor precursor protein and messenger ribonucleic acid. *Endocrinology*, **122**, 2355–2363

42. Hirata, Y. and Orth, D.N. (1979). Epidermal growth factor (urogastrone) in human tissue. *J. Clin. Endocrinol. Metab.*, **48**, 667–673

43. Smith, S.K. (1989). Prostaglandins and growth factors in the endometrium. In Drife, J.O. (ed.), *Clinical Obstetrics and Gynecology*, Ch. 3, pp. 249–270 (London: Baillière Tindall)

44. Ehrlich, H.A. (1989). *PCR Technology. Principles and Applications for DNA Amplification.* (New York: Stockton Press)

45. Imai, Y. (1982). Epidermal growth factor in rat luminal fluid. *Endocrinol. Abstr.*, **110**, 331

46. Mukku, V.R. and Stancel, G.M. (1985). Receptors for epidermal growth factor in the rat uterus. *Endocrinology*, **117**, 149–154

47. Hofmann, G.E., Rao, C.V., Barrows, G.H., Schultz, G.S. and Sanfilippo, J.S. (1984). Binding sites for epidermal growth factor in human uterine tissues and leiomyomas. *J. Clin. Endocrinol. Metab.*, **58**, 880–884

48. Lin, T.H., Mukku, V.R., Verner, G., Kirkland, J.L. and Stancel, G.M. (1988). Autoradiographic localization of epidermal growth factor receptors to all major uterine cell types. *Biol. Reprod.*, **38**, 403–411

49. Chegini, N., Rao, C.H., Wakim, N. and Sanfilippo, J. (1986). Binding of ^{125}I-epidermal growth factor in human uterus. *Cell Tissue Res.*, **246**, 543–548

50. Mukku, V.R. and Stancel, G.M. (1985). Regulation of epidermal growth factor receptor by estrogen. *J. Biol. Chem.*, **260**, 9820–9824

51. Lingham, R.B., Stancel, G.M. and Loose-Mitchell, D.S. (1988). Estrogen regulation of epidermal growth factor receptor messenger ribonucleic acid. *Mol. Endocrinol.*, **2**, 230–235

52. Ullrich, A., Coussens, L., Hayflick, J.S., Dull, J.J., Gray, A., Tam, A.W., Lee, J., Yarden, Y., Libermann, T.A., Schlessinger, J., Downward, J., Mayes, E.L.V., Whittle, N., Waterfield, M.D. and Seeburg, P.H. (1984). Human epidermal growth factor receptor cDNA sequence and aberrant expression of the amplified gene in A431 epidermoid carcinoma cells. *Nature*, **309**, 418–425

53. Cohen, S., Ushiro, H., Stoschek, C. and Chinkers, M. (1982). A native 170000 Da epidermal growth factor receptor-kinase complex from shed plasma membrane vesicles. *J. Biol. Chem.*, **257**, 1523–1531

54. Carpenter, G. (1987). Receptors for epidermal growth factor and other polypeptide mitogens. *Ann. Rev. Biochem.*, **56**, 881–914

55. Westmark, B. and Heldin, C.H. (1989). Growth factors and their receptors. *Curr. Opin. Cell Biol.*, **1**, 279–285

56. Schlessinger, J. (1988). The epidermal growth factor receptor as a multifunctional allosteric protein. *Biochemistry*, **27**, 3119–3123

57. Rozengurt, E. (1986). Early signals in the mitogenic response. *Science*, **234**, 161–166

58. Matuoka, K., Fukami, K., Nakashishi, O., Kawai, S. and Takenawa, T. (1988). Mitogenesis in response to PDGF and bombesin abolished by microinjection of antibody to PIP2. *Science*, **239**, 640–642

59. Tomooka, Y., DiAugustine, R.P. and McLachlan, J.A. (1986). Proliferation of mouse uterine epithelial cells in vitro. *Endocrinology*, **118**, 1011–1018

60. Haining, R.E.B., Fraser, H.M. and Smith, S.K. (1990). The effect of epidermal growth factor and estrogen on the proliferation of separated cells of human endometrium. *Fertil. Steril.* (submitted)

61. DeLeon, F.D., Vijayakumar, R., Brown, M., Rao, V., Yussman, M.A. and Schulz, G. (1986). Peritoneal fluid volume, estrogen, progesterone, prostaglandin, and epidermal growth factor concentrations in patients with and without endometriosis. *Obstet. Gynecol.*, **68**, 189−194

62. Thompson, K.L. and Rosner, M.R. (1989). Regulation of epidermal growth factor receptor gene expression by retinoic acid and epidermal growth factor. *J. Biol. Chem.*, **264**, 3230−3234

63. Derynck, R., Roberts, A.B., Winkler, M.E., Chen, E.Y. and Goeddel, D.V. (1984). Human transforming growth factor-α: precursor structure and expression in *E. coli*. *Cell*, **38**, 287−297

64. Massague, J. (1983). Epidermal growth factor-like transforming growth factor. II. Interaction with epidermal growth factor receptors in human placenta membranes and A431 cells. *J. Biol. Chem.*, **258**, 13614−13620

65. Derynck, R. (1988). Transforming growth factor α. *Cell*, **54**, 593−595

66. Brachmann, R., Lindquist, P.B., Nagashima, M., Kohr, W., Lipari, T., Napier, M. and Derynck, R. (1989). Transmembrane TGF-alpha precursors activate EGF/TGF-alpha receptors. *Cell*, **56**, 691−700

67. Gentry, L.E., Twardzik, D.R., Lim, G.J., Ranchalis, J.E. and Lee, D.C. (1987). Expression and characterisation of transforming growth factor α precursor protein in transfected mammalian cells. *Mol. Cell. Biol.*, **7**, 1585−1591

68. Teixido, J., Gilmore, R., Lee, D.C. and Massague, J. (1987). Integral membrane glycoprotein properties of the prohormone pro-transforming growth factor-a. *Nature*, **326**, 883−885

69. Coffey, R.J., Derynck, R., Wilcox, J.N., Bringman, T.S., Goustin, A.S., Moses, H.L. and Pittelkow, M.R. (1987). Production and auto-induction of transforming growth factor α in human keratinocytes. *Nature*, **328**, 817−820

70. Rappolee, D.A., Mark, D., Banda, M.J. and Werb, Z. (1988). Wound macrophages express TGF-alpha and other growth factors in vivo: analysis by mRNA phenotyping. *Science*, **241**, 708−711

71. Han, V.K.M., Hunter, E.S., Pratt, R.M., Zendegui, J.G. and Lee, D.C. (1987). Expression of rat transforming growth factor alpha mRNA during development occurs predominantly in maternal decidua. *Mol. Cell Biol.*, **7**, 2335−2343

72. Schreiber, A.B., Winkler, M.E. and Derynck, R. (1986). Transforming growth factor-alpha: a more potent angiogenic mediator than epidermal growth factor. *Science*, **232**, 1250−1253

73. Pollard, J.W., Bartocci, A., Arceci, R., Orlofsky, A., Ladner, M.B. and Stanley, E.R. (1987). Apparent role of the macrophage growth factor, CSF-1, in placental development. *Nature*, **330**, 484−486

74. Manos, M.M. (1988). Expression and processing of a recombinant human macrophage colony stimulating factor in mouse cells. *Mol. Cell. Biol.*, **8**, 5035−5039

75. Rettenmier, C.W., Roussel, M.F. and Sherr, C.J. (1988). The colony-stimulating factor 1 (CSF-1) receptor (c-fms proto-oncogene product) and its ligand. *J. Cell Sci. Suppl.*, **9**, 27−44

76. Kawasaki, E.S., Ladner, M.B., Wang, A.M., van Arsdell, J., Warren, M.K., Coyne, M.Y., Schweickart, V.L., Lee, M.T., Wilson, K.J., Boosman, A., Stanley, E.R., Ralph, P. and Mark, D.F. (1985). Molecular cloning of a complementary DNA encoding human macrophage-specific colony-stimulating factor (CSF-1). *Science*, **230**, 291−296

77. Cerretti, D.P., Wignall, J., Anderson, D., Tushinski, R.J., Gallis, B.M., Stya, M., Gillis, S., Urdal, D.L. and Cosman, D. (1988). Human macrophage-colony stimulating factor: alternative RNA and protein processing from a single gene. *Mol. Immunol.*, **25**, 761−770

78. Rettenmier, C.W., Roussel, M.F., Ashmun, R.A., Ralph, P., Price, K. and Sherr, C.J. (1987). Synthesis of membrane-bound colony-stimulating factor-1 (CSF-1) and down-modulation of CSF-1 receptors in NIH 3T3 cells transformed by cotransfection of the human CSF-1 and c-fms (CSF-1 receptor) genes. *Mol. Cell. Biol.*, **7**, 2378−2387

79. Folkman, J. and Klagsbrun, M. (1987). Angiogenic factors. *Science*, **235**, 442−447

80. Esch, F.A., Baird, N., Ling, N., Ueno, F., Hill, L., Denoroy, R., Klepper, D., Gospodarowicz, P., Bohlen, P. and Guillemin, R. (1985). Primary structure of bovine pituitary basic fibroblast growth factor (FGF) and comparison with the amino-acid terminal sequence

of bovine brain acidic FGF. *Proc. Natl. Acad. Sci. USA*, **82**, 6507–6511
81. Gospodarowicz, D., Baird, A., Cheng, J., Lui, G.M., Esch, F. and Bohlen, P. (1986). Isolation of fibroblast growth factor from bovine adrenal gland: physico-chemical and biological characterisation. *Endocrinology*, **118**, 82–90
82. Florkiewicz, R.Z. and Sommer, A. (1989). Human basic fibroblast growth factor gene encodes four polypeptides: three initiate translation from non-AUG codons. *Proc. Natl Acad. Sci. USA*, **86**, 3978–3981
83. Lobb, R.R., Harper, J.W. and Fett, J.W. (1986). Purification of heparin-binding growth factors. *Ann. Biochem.*, **154**, 1–14
84. Crabb, J.W., Armes, L.G., Carr, S.A., Johnson, C.M., Roberts, G.D., Bordoli, R.S. and McKeehan, W.L. (1986). Complete primary structure of prostatropin, a prostate epithelial cell growth factor. *Biochemistry*, **25**, 4988–4993
85. Gautschi-Sova, P., Jiang, Z.P., Frater-Schroder, M. and Bohlen, P. (1987). Acidic fibroblast growth factor is present in nonneural tissue: isolation and chemical characterization from bovine kidney. *Biochemistry*, **26**, 5844–5847
86. Wang, W.P., Lehtoma, K., Lee Varban, M., Krishnan, I. and Chiu, I.M. (1989). Cloning of the gene coding for human class 1 heparin-binding growth factor and its expression in fetal tissues. *Mol. Cell. Biol.*, **9**, 2387–2395
87. Brigstock, D.R., Heap, R.B. and Brown, K.D. (1989). Polypeptide growth factors in uterine tissues and secretions. *J. Reprod. Fertil.*, **85**, 747–758
88. Thomas, K.A. (1988). Transforming potential of fibroblast growth factor genes. *Trends Biochem. Sci.*, **13**, 327–328
89. Zhan, X., Bates, B., Hu, X. and Goldfarb, M. (1988). The human FGF-5 oncogene encodes a novel protein related to fibroblast growth factors. *Molec. Cell. Biol.*, **8**, 3480–3495
90. Bohlen, P.A.A., Baird, A., Esch, F., Ling, N. and Gospodarowicz, D. (1984). Isolation of brain fibroblast growth factor by heparin Sepharose affinity chromatography: identity with pituitary fibroblast growth factor. *Proc. Natl Acad. Sci. USA*, **81**, 6963–6967
91. Shing, Y., Folkman, J., Sullivan, R., Butterfield, C., Murray, J. and Klagsbrun, M. (1984). Heparin affinity: purification of a tumour-derived capillary endothelial cell growth factor. *Science*, **223**, 1296–1299
92. Baird, A. and Ling, N. (1987). Fibroblast growth factors are present in the extracellular matrix produced by endothelial cells *in vitro*: implications for a role of heparinase-like enzymes in the neovascular response. *Biochem. Biophys. Res. Comm.*, **142**, 428–435
93. Thomas, K.A. and Gimenez-Gallego, G. (1986). Fibroblast growth factors; broad spectrum mitogens with potent angiogenic activity. *Trends Biochem. Sci.*, **11**, 81–84
94. Schenken, R.S. and Asch, R.H. (1980). Surgical induction of endometriosis in the rabbit: Effect on fertility and concentrations of peritoneal fluid prostaglandins. *Fertil. Steril.*, **34**, 581–587
95. Schenken, R.S., Asch, R.H., Williams, R.F. and Hodgen, G.D. (1984). Etiology of infertility in monkeys with endometriosis: measurement of peritoneal fluid prostaglandins. *Am. J. Obstet. Gynecol.*, **150**, 349–355
96. Syrop, C.H. and Halme, J. (1987). Peritoneal fluid environment and infertility. *Fertil. Steril.*, **48**, 1–9
97. Rock, J.A., Dubin, N.H., Ghodgaonkar, R.B., Bergquist, C.A., Erozan, Y.S. and Kimball, A.W. (1982). Cul-de-sac fluid in women with endometriosis: fluid volume and prostanoid concentration during the proliferative phase of the cycle–days 8 to 12. *Fertil. Steril.*, **37**, 747–750
98. Dawood, M.Y., Khan-Dawood, F.S. and Wilson, L. (1984). Peritoneal fluid prostaglandins and prostanoids in women with endometriosis, chronic pelvic inflammatory disease, and pelvic pain. *Obstet. Gynecol.*, **148**, 391–395
99. Chacho, K.J., Stronkowski Chacho, M., Andresen, P.J. and Scommegna, A. (1986). Peritoneal fluid in patients with and without endometriosis: Prostanoids and macrophages and their effect on the spermatozoa penetration assay. *Am. J. Obstet. Gynecol.*, **154**, 1290–1296
100. Halme, J., Becker, S., Hammond, M.G., Raj, M.H.G. and Raj, S. (1983). Increased activation of pelvic macrophages in infertile women with mild endometriosis. *Am. J. Obstet. Gynecol.*, **145**, 333–337
101. Badawy, S.Z.A., Marshall, L. and Cuenca, V. (1985). Peritoneal fluid prostaglandins in

various stages of the menstrual cycle: role in infertile patients with endometriosis. *Int. J. Fertil.*, **30**, 48–53

102. Drake, T.S., O'Brien, W.F., Ramwell, P.W. and Metz, S.A. (1981). Peritoneal fluid thromboxane B2 and 6-keto-prostaglandin F1α in endometriosis. *Am. J. Obstet. Gynecol.*, **140**, 401–404

103. Drake, T.S., O'Brien, W.F. and Ramwell, P.W. (1983). Peritoneal fluid prostanoids in unexplained infertility. *Am. J. Obstet. Gynecol.*, **147**, 63–64

104. Koskimies, A.I., Tenhunen, A. and Ylikorkala, O. (1984). Peritoneal fluid 6-keto-prostaglandin F1α, thromboxane B2 in endometriosis and unexplained infertility. *Acta Obstet. Gynecol. Scand. Suppl.*, **123**, 19–21

105. Ylikorkala, O., Koskimies, A., Laatkainen, T., Tenhunen, A. and Viinikka, L. (1984). Peritoneal fluid prostaglandins in endometriosis, tubal disorders and unexplained infertility. *Obstet. Gynecol.*, **63**, 616–620

106. Sgarlata, C.S., Hertelendy, F. and Mikhail, G. (1983). The prostanoid content in peritoneal fluid and plasma of women with endometriosis. *Am. J. Obstet. Gynecol.*, **147**, 563–565

107. Mudge, T.J., James, M.J., Jones, W.R. and Walsh, J.A. (1985). Peritoneal fluid 6-keto-prostaglandin F1α levels in women with endometriosis. *Am. J. Obstet. Gynecol.*, **152**, 901–904

108. Herman, A., Claeys, M., Moncada, S. and Vane, J.R. (1979). Biosynthesis of prostacyclin PG12 and 12-HETE by pericardium, pleura, peritoneum, and aorta of the rabbit. *Prostaglandins*, **18**, 439–446

109. Halme, J., Becker, S. and Haskill, S. (1987). Altered maturation and function of peritoneal macrophages: Possible role in pathogenesis of endometriosis. *Am. J. Obstet. Gynecol.*, **156**, 783–789

110. Lenton, E.A., King, H., Thomas, E.J., Smith, S.K., McLachlan, R.I., MacNeil, S. and Cooke, I.D. (1988). The endocrine environment of the human oocyte. *J. Reprod. Fertil.*, **82**, 827–841

111. Moncada, J. and Vane, J.R. (1980). Prostacyclin in the cardiovascular system. *Adv. Prostaglandin Thomboxane Res.*, **6**, 43–60

112. Sun, G.Y. and Su, K.L. (1979). Metabolism of arachidonyl phosphoglycerides in mouse-brain subcellular fractions. *J. Neurochem.*, **32**, 1053–1059

113. Smith, S.K., Abel, M.H., Kelly, R.W. and Baird, D.T. (1981). A role for prostacyclin (PG12) in excessive menstrual bleeding. *Lancet*, **1**, 522–524

114. Bito, L.Z. (1975). Are prostaglandins intracellular, transcellular or extracellular autocoids? *Prostaglandins*, **9**, 51–55

115. Samuelsson, B., Goldyne, M., Granstrom, E., Hamberg, M., Hammarstrom, S. and Malmstem, C. (1978). Prostaglandins and thromboxanes. *Annu. Rev. Biochem.*, **47**, 997–1029

116. Lapetina, E.G. (1982). Regulation of arachidonic acid production: Role of phospholipase C and A2. *Trends Pharmacol. Sci.*, **3**, 115–118

117. Little, C. (1989). Phospholipase C. *Biochem. Soc. Trans.*, **17**, 271–273

118. Berridge, M.J. (1987). Inositol trisphosphate and diacylglycerol: Two interacting second messengers. *Annu. Rev. Biochem.*, **56**, 159–179

119. Nishizuka, Y. (1986). Studies and perspectives of protein kinase C. *Science*, **233**, 305–312

120. Berridge, M.J. and Irvine, R.F. (1984). Inositol trisphosphate, a novel second messenger in cellular signal transduction. *Nature*, **312**, 315–321

121. Streb, H., Irvine, R.F., Berridge, M.J. and Schulz, I. (1983). Release of Ca^{2+} from a nonmitochondrial intracellular store in pancreatic acinar cells by inositol-1,4,5-trisphosphate. *Nature*, **306**, 67–69

122. Rana, R.S. and Hokin, L.E. (1990). Role of phosphoinositides in transmembrane signalling. *Physiol. Rev.*, **70**, 115–164

123. Berridge, M.J., Cobbold, P.H. and Cuthbertson, K.S.R. (1988). Spatial and temporal aspects of cell signalling. *Philos. Trans. R. Soc. Lond. (Biol.)*, **320**, 325–343

124. Bonney, R.C. (1985). Measurement of phospholipase A2 activity in human endometrium during the menstrual cycle. *J. Endocrinol.*, **107**, 183–189

125. Bonney, R.C. and Franks, S. (1987). Phospholipase C activity in human endometrium: its significance in endometrial pathology. *Clin. Endocrinol.*, **27**, 307–320

76

126. Miller, M.M. and O'Morchoe, C.C.C. (1982). Decidual cell reaction induced by prostaglandin F2α in the mature oophorectomised rat. *Cell Tissue Res.*, **255**, 189–199

127. Hoffman, L.H., DePietro, D.L. and McKenna, T.J. (1978). Effects of indomethacin on uterine capillary permeability and blastocyst development in rabbits. *Prostaglandins*, **15**, 823–828

128. Phillips, C.A. and Poyser, N.L. (1981). Studies on the involvement of prostaglandins in implantation in the rat. *J. Reprod. Fertil.*, **62**, 73–81

129. Sananes, N., Baulieu, E.E. and Le Goascogne, C. (1976). Prostaglandins as inductive factor of decidualisation in the rat uterus. *Mol. Cell. Endocrinol.*, **6**, 153–158

130. Kennedy, T.G. and Lukich, L.A. (1982). Induction of decidualization in rats by the intrauterine infusions of prostaglandins. *Biol. Reprod.*, **27**, 253–260

131. Orlicky, D.J., Silio, M., Williams, C., Gordon, J. and Gerschenson, L.E. (1986). Regulation of inositol phosphate levels by prostaglandins in cultured endometrial cells. *J. Cell Physiol.*, **128**, 105–112

132. Orlicky, D.J., Lieberman, R., Williams, C. and Gerschenson, L.E. (1987). Requirement for prostaglandin F2 in 17β-estradiol stimulation of DNA synthesis in rabbit endometrial cultures. *J. Cell Physiol.*, **130**, 292–300

133. Whitman, M., Fleischman, L., Chahwala, S.B., Cantley, L. and Rosoff, P. (1986). Phosphoinositides, mitogenesis, and oncogenesis. In Putney, J.R. (ed.) *Phosphoinositides and Receptor Mechanisms*, vol. 7, pp. 197–217. (New York: Alan R. Liss)

134. Billah, M.M., Lapetina, E.G. and Cuatrecasas, P. (1980). Phospholipase A2 and phospholipase C activities of platelets. Differential substrate specificity, Ca^{2+} requirement, pH dependence, and cellular localization. *J. Biol. Chem.*, **255**, 10227–10231

135. Black, F.M. and Wakelam, J.O. (1990). Activation of inositol phospholipid breakdown by prostaglandin F2α without any stimulation of proliferation in quiescent NIH-3T3 fibroblasts. *Biochem. J.*, **266**, 661–667

136. Crouch, M.F. and Lapetina, E.G. (1988). No direct correlation between Ca^{2+} mobilisation and dissociation of G during platelet phospholipase A activation. *Biochem. Biophys. Res. Commun.*, **153**, 21–30

137. Vernon, M.W., Beard, J.S., Graves, K. and Wilson, E.A. (1986). Classification of endometriotic implants by morphologic appearance and capacity to synthesize prostaglandin F. *Fertil. Steril.*, **46**, 801–806

138. Murrell, G.A.C., Francis, M.J.O. and Bromley, L. (1989). Cyclo-oxygenase and oxygen free radical-stimulated fibroblast proliferation. *Biochem. Soc. Trans.*, **17**, 482–483

139. Romero, R., Durum, S., Dinarello, C., Oyarzun, E., Hobbins, J.C. and Mitchell, M. D. (1989). Interleukin-1 stimulates prostaglandin biosynthesis by human amnion. *Prostaglandins*, **37**, 13–22

140. Hahn, D.W., Carraher, R.P., Foldsey, R.G. and McGuire, J.L. (1986). Experimental evidence for failure to implant as a mechanism of infertility associated with endometriosis. *Am. J. Obstet. Gynecol.*, **155**, 1109–113

141. Smith, S.K. (1990). The role of eicosanoids in menstruation and disorders of menstruation. In Mitchell, M.D. (ed.) *Eicosanoids in Reproduction*, pp. 87–102. (Baton Rouge, Fla.: CRC Press Inc.)

142. Willman, E.A., Collins, W.D. and Clayton, S.L. (1976). Studies on the involvement in prostaglandins in uterine symptomatology and pathology. *Br. J. Obstet. Gynaecol.*, **83**, 337–341

143. Pollard, J.W. (1990). Regulation of polypeptide growth factors synthesis and growth factor-related gene expression in the rat and mouse uterus before and after implantation. *J. Reprod. Fertil.*, **88**, 721–731

5
The peritoneal environment in endometriosis

B. S. Hurst and J. A. Rock

Endometriosis is frequently found in patients with infertility and pelvic pain. It is estimated that 30% to 40% of women with infertility have endometriosis[1]. Dysmenorrhoea, dyspareunia, back and rectal pain are common complaints in women with endometriosis[2]. The relationship of endometriosis to pelvic pain and infertility is clearly evident, with disease resulting in extensive scarring and fixation of the adnexa, or with extensive distortion of ovarian anatomy by endometriomas. Infertility may occur when endometriosis on the ovarian capsule interferes with the ovulatory process and ovum pick-up.

However, symptoms do not directly correspond with the extent of visible endometriosis. There is no universally accepted hypothesis that explains how endometriosis can cause these symptoms, especially in the case of minimal and mild endometriosis. Investigators have attempted to identify factors present in patients with endometriosis that would explain the symptoms of pain and infertility. Many investigators have proposed that patients with endometriosis have an altered pelvic environment that interferes with fertility and provides the mechanism for pain. The mesothelium may directly produce toxic factors or may serve as a site of accumulation of toxic substances with endometriosis.

To understand the role of the mesothelium in endometriosis, a basic understanding of the anatomy and physiology of the mesothelium is helpful. The mesothelium is composed of a single layer of flattened cells forming an epithelium that lines serous cavities including the peritoneum, pericardium and pleura. The peritoneum is a completely enclosed sac with the exception of the openings of the fallopian tubes. The peritoneum is highly permeable. Water, electrolytes, urea and other small molecules and toxins are freely transported across the peritoneal membrane[3].

Microscopically, the peritoneum consists of a simple squamous cell layer of mesothelium and a deeper loose connective-tissue layer that contains collagen, elastic fibres, fat cells, reticulum and macrophages. With peritoneal irritation or inflammation, the squamous cells may become cuboidal and develop small spaces[3].

The peritoneal cavity normally contains 20 ml or less of straw-coloured fluid. Normal peritoneal fluid contains approximately 1 000 000 cells/ml[4]. Ninety per cent of these cells are macrophages. The remainder are mostly composed of desquamated mesothelial cells and lymphocytes. Granulocytes, normally present in small numbers, are greatly increased with pelvic inflammation.

Because of the uncertain aetiology of infertility and pelvic pain in patients with minimal and mild endometriosis, many authors have evaluated specific alterations in the pelvic environment. Endometriosis may cause peritoneal fluid volume changes by changing mesothelial permeability or altering peritoneal fluid volume by other mechanisms. Alterations in macrophage numbers, concentration or activation may occur in patients with endometriosis. Prostanoids may be produced directly by peritoneal surfaces, by endometriosis implants, or as a result of menstrual debris. The peritoneum may also be a site of abnormal production or accumulation of toxic substances in patients with endometriosis (Figure 5.1). These alterations in the pelvic environment may provide insight to the association of endometriosis and pain and infertility.

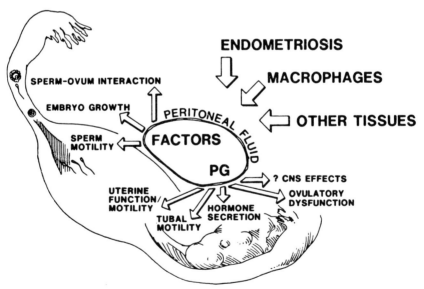

Figure 5.1 Prostaglandin and peritoneal fluid alterations that may contribute to infertility in endometriosis. Prostaglandins secreted directly by implants or by 'activated' macrophages may induce ovarian dysfunction or altered tubal or uterine motility. Unknown peritoneal fluid components may adversely affect sperm function, fertilization, or early embryo growth. (From Muse[5] with permission of the publisher)

ROLE OF MESOTHELIUM IN THE PATHOPHYSIOLOGY OF ENDOMETRIOSIS

Peritoneal fluid is an ultrafiltrate of plasma. In normally cycling women, the peritoneal fluid volumes are low. As the cycle progresses, peritoneal fluid volume gradually increases to its maximum volume of approximately 20 ml during the third week of the cycle. Peritoneal fluid volume then decreases following the mid-luteal phase[6,7].

The source of the peritoneal fluid is debated in the literature. Some investigators have suggested that oestradiol may cause accumulation of fluid within the peritoneal cavity[6]. Others believe that the volume changes are a direct result of ovarian exudative fluid, with an additional contribution from follicular rupture[7]. The fallopian tube contribution to peritoneal fluid is minimal in most conditions[8]. Endometriosis may alter peritoneal fluid volumes by the following mechanisms: increased fluid production by the ovaries, altered mesothelial permeability, or increases in the colloid osmotic pressure as a result of altered protein content.

The alterations in peritoneal fluid volume may play a direct physiological role in normal reproduction, although this role is not certain. Peritoneal fluid may affect ovulation by providing substances necessary for breakdown of the follicle wall, ovum pick-up by the fallopian tube, ovum maturation, sperm capacitation, tubal motility, and transport of the fertilized ovum. Dramatic increases or decreases in peritoneal fluid volume could result in infertility by altering ovum pick-up at the time of ovulation or by altering tubal transport. A more likely role of peritoneal fluid in infertility is by serving as a reservoir of toxic cells or substances.

Many studies have been performed to look at specific peritoneal factors that interfere with fertilization by evaluating peritoneal fluid from women with and without endometriosis. Muse *et al.* found no difference in sperm motility in peritoneal fluid from women with endometriosis when compared to peritoneal fluid from women with endometriosis[9]. No difference was found in the penetration of zona-free hamster oocytes by human sperm when cultured in heat-treated peritoneal fluid from women with and without endometriosis[10]. Other studies have observed a detrimental mouse sperm–ova interaction in peritoneal fluid of women with endometriosis[11]. Peritoneal fluid from women with endometriosis is toxic to growth and development of mouse embryos[12].

If peritoneal fluid volume itself causes infertility in women with endometriosis, there should be a measurable difference in peritoneal fluid volumes. There is a considerable amount of data in the literature regarding peritoneal fluid volume in women with endometriosis (Table 5.1). In 1980, Drake[13] published data that showed an increase in peritoneal fluid throughout the cycle in patients with endometriosis. Peritoneal fluid volumes were highest in patients with severe disease. Koninckx[7] found significantly higher peritoneal volume in patients with mild and moderate endometriosis during cycle days 1 to 5. Peritoneal fluid volumes were comparable to controls in the remainder of the follicular phase. Patients with severe endometriosis had reduced volumes in the early luteal phase. Oak[29] found increased peritoneal fluid in the early luteal phase in patients with endometriosis. Other investigators have found

Table 5.1 Studies of peritoneal fluid volume in women with endometriosis

Author/date	No. of patients		Cycle timing	Volume changes with endometriosis
	Endometriosis	Controls		
Drake, 1980[13]	32	34	Throughout	↑
Koninckx, 1980[7]	72	74	Days 1–5	↑
			Proliferative	↔
			luteal phase	↓
Drake, 1981[14]	14	15	Throughout	↑
Haney, 1981[15]	10	22	Days 11–19	↑
Rock, 1982[16]	45	17	Days 8–12	↔
Sgarlatta, 1983[17]	25	10	Days 8–12	↔
Crain, 1983[18]	21	37	Throughout	↔
Dawood, 1984[19]	49	10	Throughout	↔
Mudge, 1985[20]	42	71	Luteal phase	↔
Olive, 1985[21]	42	61	Throughout	↔
Badawy, 1985[22]	39	45	Throughout	↔
DeLeon, 1986[23]	31	14	Throughout	↔
Chaco, 1986[24]	24	31	Proliferative	↔
			luteal phase	↑
Rezai, 1987[25]	45	28	Days 13–18	↔
Awadalla, 1987[26]	49	73	Throughout	↔
Syrop, 1987[27]	119	134	Throughout	↑
Hill, 1988[28]	33	8	Throughout	↑

elevated peritoneal fluid volume in patients with endometriosis[15,27,28].

Some investigators have failed to show an alteration in peritoneal fluid volume in women with endometriosis. Rock studied patients during cycle days 8 to 12, and found no difference in fluid volumes in patients with endometriosis compared to controls[16]. The severity of disease did not affect the measured quantities. In a similar study, Rezai et al. found no difference in fluid volumes when evaluating patients with and without endometriosis during days 13 to 18[25]. Olive et al. found no difference in peritoneal fluid volume of infertile patients with or without endometriosis without reference to cycle day[21]. Other investigators have failed to show an association of peritoneal fluid volume and endometriosis[17,19,20,23,26].

There are many explanations for the discrepancies in the data regarding peritoneal fluid volumes. Cycle day variations have a significant effect on peritoneal fluid volumes. Control groups not properly selected may include infertile patients with microscopic endometriosis and thus diminish the differences between patients and controls. Techniques used in obtaining follicular fluid may vary. Furthermore, patients who are receiving hormonal therapies such as oral contraceptives that suppress ovulatory function will have lower cul-de-sac fluid volumes[6,7].

It is unlikely that fluid volume alone plays a role in the aetiology of endometriosis. Most investigators have looked at toxic substances that may be contained in the peritoneal fluid. Indeed, some investigators have shown alterations in macrophages, prostanoids, interleukins, peritoneal fluid proteins, and other substances.

MACROPHAGES

Normal peritoneal fluid contains approximately 10^6 cells/ml. Eighty-five per cent of these cells are macrophages, with the remainder composed of desquamated mesothelial cells and lymphocytes[4]. Macrophages are derived from bone marrow stem cells. Monocytes, the product of stem cells, circulate in the vascular system. Monocytes cross blood vessel walls by diapedesis in response to a local inflammatory process. Macrophages, once activated, differentiate to larger, enzymatically active macrophages with increased phagocytic abilities. Macrophages produce a great number of products that can serve as mediators of the inflammatory response such as prostanoids, interleukins, and other substances that may be harmful to reproduction. Macrophages have receptors for the Fc portion immunoglobulins, and receptors for complement C3. Macrophages produce complement[30]. The major physiological role of macrophages is as phagocytic scavenger cells for cellular debris, including red blood cells and sperm.

Many authors have suggested that macrophages are the mediator of infertility in patients with minimal and mild endometriosis. Macrophages may interefere with the reproductive process by sperm phagocytosis. Ovulation and corpus luteum function may be influenced by macrophages. Macrophages and factors produced by macrophages may interefere with sperm motility, oocyte pick-up, and early embryo survival.

Sperm phagocytosis by macrophages has been demonstrated in animals[31]. Phagocytosis of human sperm by human macrophages has been shown to occur *in vitro*[32]. An elevated number, concentration, or activation of macrophages could therefore interfere with sperm transport or survival.

Studies evaluating sperm survival in the peritoneal fluid from women with endometriosis are limited. Two studies have examined sperm recovery from peritoneal fluid in women following artificial insemination. Hoxsey *et al.* supported the macrophage hypothesis, with sperm recovered in peritoneal fluid from 18% of patients with endometriosis compared to 78% of controls[33]. Others have obtained conflicting data, with sperm recovered in 45% of patients with endometriosis compared to 35% of the control group[34]. These studies are limited by low patient numbers involved. Control groups included patients with infertility, which may bias results.

Other investigators have shown an inhibition of sperm phagocytosis *in vitro* with ethiodol. Ethiodol, a lipid-based contrast agent formerly used with hysterosalpingograms, is associated with a temporary increase in fertility after its use. This increase in fertility may be due to inhibition of sperm phagocytosis[35].

Macrophages may interefere with ovulation or corpus luteum function in patients with endometriosis. Macrophages are found within the developing follicles. Macrophages may decrease granulosa cell progesterone production[36]. It is unlikely that direct macrophage alteration of ovulatory function and corpus luteum function plays a role in the pathophysiology of endometriosis, although it is possible that this mechanism plays a minor role in endometriosis-associated infertility.

To have a pathological effect, macrophages would be expected to be present in higher numbers, higher concentrations, or at higher activation states in patients with endometriosis. Macrophages may be present as a result of local inflammation produced by endometrial implants or by retrotubal menstruation. Peritoneal fluid from patients with minimal and mild endometriosis increases macrophage proliferation *in vitro*[37]. The mitogens involved are unknown, although interleukins may play a role.

The currently favoured hypothesis states that macrophages are present due to retrograde menstruation. Approximately 90% of normal women experience retrotubal menstruation. Women with endometriosis may have more macrophages as a result of a larger tubal reflux. Patients with endometriosis may have a higher number of tubal macrophages. Macrophage populations are elevated in the ampullary portion of the fallopian tubes in patients with endometriosis[38]. Patients with tubal occlusion have lower numbers of macrophages when compared to women with infertility due to endometriosis, pelvic adhesions, or unexplained infertility[39]. The alteration of peritoneal macrophages, if real, appears to be a local effect. No alterations in circulating white blood cell population characteristics have been identified in endometriosis patients[40].

If the pathological effect of endometriosis is mediated through macrophages, one should be able to demonstrate alterations in macrophage numbers, concentrations, or activation. The peritoneal fluid has been examined by investigators to determine changes in macrophage characteristics with endometriosis. Haney *et al.* in 1981 showed an increase in the total macrophage number in patients with endometriosis[15]. Many other investigators have confirmed an increase in macrophages in the peritoneal fluid with endometriosis[21,24,27,28,38,41,44-46] (Table 5.2). There are no studies that show a decrease in macrophage number with endometriosis. Two studies, however, failed to show an increase in patients with endometriosis[26,47]. There are criticisms of studies that look only at the total macrophage numbers. A higher total number of macrophages may occur if volume is raised without affecting concentration. Thus, for those who propose that endometriosis is associated with higher total peritoneal fluid volumes, the change in macrophage numbers may be an associated process and not an indicator of pathology. With this in mind, many investigators have examined macrophage concentration in the peritoneal fluid from patients with endometriosis.

Haney *et al.* showed an increase in macrophage concentration in peritoneal fluid in women with endometriosis[15]. The increase in macrophage concentration was supported by Haney and Halme[38,41]. Later studies from Halme showed an insignificant increase in macrophage concentration in women with endometriosis[39,42]. Other investigators have been unable to demonstrate altered macrophage concentrations with endometriosis[24,38,41,42,44,46,47] (Table 5.2).

Macrophage number and concentration may be less important than macrophage activation. A macrophage is activated before it becomes a phagocytic scavenger. Activation is manifest by several changes, including

THE PERITONEAL ENVIRONMENT IN ENDOMETRIOSIS

Table 5.2 Studies of peritoneal fluid macrophages in women with endometriosis

Author/date	No. of patients Endometriosis	Controls	Cycle timing	Macrophage number	Macrophage concentration	Macrophage 'activation'	Method to determine activation
Haney, 1981[15]	10	22	Days 11–19	↑	↑		
Halme, 1982[41]	46	34	Days 13–21	↑	↑		
Muscatto, 1982[32]	10	22	Days 11–20			↑	Sperm phagocytosis
Haney, 1983[36]	12	28	Days 11–19	↑	↑		
Halme, 1983[42]	18	36	Throughout		↑	↑	Myeloperoxidase and acid phosphatase staining
Becker, 1983[43]	(not defined)		Days 10–20			↑	Leucine amino-peptidase, acid phosphatase, and phagocytosis
Halme, 1984[39]	29	78	Throughout		↔	↑	Acid phosphatase, leucine aminopeptidase, macrophage size
Badawy, 1984[44]	45	57	Throughout	↑	↑	↑	Acid phosphatase
Olive, 1985[21]	42	61	Throughout	↑	↔		
Chaco, 1986[24]	35	34	Throughout	↑	↑	↑	Acid phosphatase
Syrop, 1987[27]	119	134	Throughout	↑	↔		
Awadalla, 1987[26]	49	73	Throughout	↔	↔	↕	Sperm phagocytosis, macrophage size, capping
Dunselman, 1988[46]	13	12	Throughout	↑	↑	↑	Chemiluminescence, erythrophagocytosis
Hill, 1988[28]	33	17	Throughout	↑	↑		

85

cellular enlargement. Capping, or segregation of ligand-specific cell membrane receptors at one pole of the cell, also indicates activation. Increases in enzymes such as acid phosphatase, myeloperoxidase, leucine aminopeptidase, and chemiluminescence are other measurable indicators of macrophage activation. Macrophage activation can be evaluated *in vitro* by the observation of phagocytic ability. Investigators who have evaluated macrophage activation have used at least one of the above criteria to determine activity. Halme's group has demonstrated macrophage activation in several studies[39,42,45]. Each study demonstrated macrophage activation using different techniques including myeloperoxidase staining, acid phosphatase, leucine aminopeptidase and macrophage size, and macrophage size and cellular capping[42,45]. Muscatto *et al.* reported improved macrophage phagocytosis of sperm when macrophages were recovered from peritoneal fluid from endometriosis patients[32]. Others have shown macrophage activation with endometriosis[24,46]. While most investigators have shown activation of macrophages with endometriosis, not all studies have demonstrated this effect. Awadalla was unable to demonstrate improved sperm phagocytosis in patients with endometriosis[26].

Studies evaluating peritoneal macrophages have limitations, as do studies evaluating peritoneal fluid volumes. Cycle day at the time of recovery is rarely controlled, and variation in the cycle day may have a profound effect. Increased peritoneal fluid during the third week of the cycle may result in a lower macrophage concentration. A relative increase in concentration during the early follicular phase may occur when fluid volume is low. Furthermore, total macrophage number may be influenced by menstrual reflux before, during, or after menses, owing to inflammation, menstrual debris, or tubal macrophages. Macrophage number or activation may vary with cyclic hormonal changes of the menstrual cycle, although there are no data to confirm this hypothesis. Further criticism is directed at the lack of validation of collection techniques. Collection techniques require consistency. Minimal variations may bias results. Selection of control groups has been a major source of criticism. Most studies include infertility patients with no visible evidence of endometriosis at the time of laparoscopy. Patients with unexplained infertility may indeed have active microscopic or atypical endometriosis. Patients with tubal occlusion have fewer macrophages present in peritoneal fluid than patients with patent tubes. Patients with pelvic infections are likely to have higher macrophage counts.

While many investigators have suggested that gamete phagocytosis by macrophages mediates endometriosis-associated infertility, many others believe that toxic factors in the pelvis are the explanation for symptoms associated with endometriosis. The source of the toxic factors may be macrophages, endometrial implants, or retrotubal reflux. Prostaglandins, interleukins, proteins, growth factors, protein hormones, and plasminogen activators have been proposed as mediators of the symptoms of pain and infertility in endometriosis. Of these factors, prostanoids have received the greatest attention.

PROSTANOIDS

Prostanoids are physiologically active compounds derived from arachidonate or other 20-carbon fatty acids. They form the active prostaglandins (PG), thromboxane (Tx), prostacycline (PGI_2), and leukotrienes. Prostaglandin formation is initiated when arachodonate is liberated from phospholipids in the plasma membrane as a result of phospholipase A_2 activation. The stimuli include angiotensin II, bradykinin, epinephrine, and thrombin. Glucocorticoids and local anaesthetics inhibit prostanoid production by inhibiting phospholipase A_2.

Arachodonate, once formed, is rapidly catalysed to prostaglandin G (PGG_2), then to prostaglandin H_2 (PGH_2). PGH_2 is then converted to prostaglandin D (PGD_2), F (PGF_2), thromboxane (TxA_2) or prostacycline (PGI_2) depending on cell type. Each cell type produces only one type of prostanoid. Thromboxane synthetase, present in platelets, spleen and lung, catalyses the formation of thromboxane. Thromboxane causes vasoconstriction and platelet aggregation. Prostacyclines, on the other hand, are produced by blood vessel walls and the peritoneum via prostacycline synthetase. Prostacycline is a potent inhibitor of platelet aggregation. Prostaglandins D, E and F produce smooth-muscle contraction. Prostaglandins increase cyclic AMP in platelets, corpus luteum, thyroid, fetal bone, pituitary and lung. Cyclic AMP is lowered in the renal tubules and adipose tissue by prostaglandins[48].

Leukotrienes are formed by hydroxylation of arichodonate at carbon 12. The leukotrienes are formed in leukocytes, platelets and macrophages in response to immunological and non-immunological stimuli. Leukotrienes have potent chemotactic activity. Leukotrienes form the slow-reacting substance of anaphylaxis, which results in constriction of bronchial musculature. Leukotrienes also cause vascular permeability and are involved in immediate hypersensitivity reactions[48].

Prostaglandins are rapidly metabolized by a number of enzymes, and have a very short half-life. Ninety-five per cent of prostaglandins are removed in one circulation through the lung and 80% are removed passing through the liver. Thromboxane A_2 is converted to thomboxane B_2 (TxB_2), an inactive metabolite. Prostacycline is converted to the inactive 6-keto-prostaglandin $F_{1\alpha}$ (6-k-$PGF_{1\alpha}$). $PGF_{2\alpha}$ is metabolized to 13,14-dihydro-15-keto-$PGF_{2\alpha}$ (PGFM). PGDM and PGEM are the inactive metabolites of PGD and PGE, respectively. These metabolites have a longer half-life and are more stable than active precursors and are usually the substances measured in peritoneal fluid.

Prostaglandins play many roles in the normal reproductive physiological process. Prostaglandins affect ovulation, tubal motility, luteolysis, implantation and uterine contractility. Prostanoids also appear to play a role in embryogenesis. Because of the profound influences of prostanoids in reproductive physiology, prostanoids have been proposed as a mechanism of endometriosis-associated infertility. It is widely accepted that prostaglandins play a role in the ovulatory process. Inhibition of prostaglandin formation by non-steroidal anti-inflammatory agents has been shown to increase the incidence of luteinized unruptured follicle syndrome in animals[49]. Prostaglandins as a result of endometriosis may interfere with oocyte release by desensitization of the follicle to prostaglandins[50] There are no studies to our knowledge, however, that would suggest that increased prostaglandins due to endometriosis interfere with ovulation *in vivo*.

Many investigators have proposed that tubal motility is altered due to prostaglandins in patients with endometriosis. 15-Methyl $PGF_{2\alpha}$ accelerates ovum transfer and reduces fertility when administered intravaginally in the rabbit[51]. Eddy demonstrated accelerated ovum transport in the fallopian tube of rhesus monkeys with prostaglandins[52]. Altered tubal ovum transport could cause early arrival of the embryo into the uterus, which would result in suboptimal timing for implantation. Studies in humans have been unable to show altered transport of tubal oocytes with prostaglandins[53].

Prostaglandins appear to play a role in luteolysis. Injection of prostaglandin synthetase inhibitor into the corpus luteum causes premature luteolysis in the rhesus monkey[54]. Administration of pharmacological levels of $PGF_{2\alpha}$ results in premature luteolysis when injected directly into the rhesus monkey ovary[55]. Treatment of humans in the luteal phase with high doses of PGF is associated with decreased levels of progesterone and premature menstrual bleeding[56]. The physiological role of prostaglandins for the initiation of luteolysis is controversial in humans, however[57]. Prostaglandins are present in endometrial tissue. Increased metabolites have been found in women with dysmenorrhoea[58]. Prostaglandin synthetase inhibitors effectively relieve dysmenorrhoea in patients with endometriosis. Prostaglandins may cause strong uterine contractions and cervical dilatation, which may result in explusion of an early pregnancy. Furthermore, a pathological level of prostaglandins may interfere with early embryo development. Endometriosis may be associated with higher rates of preclinical or clinical spontaneous abortions due to elevated prostaglandins.

Abnormal levels of prostaglandins may occur directly from endometrial implants, macrophages, the peritoneum, menstrual reflux, or from the ovaries. Drake *et al.* proposed that endometriosis implants cause a peritoneal reaction[14]. This reaction leads to an increase in macrophage number. Macrophage activation occurs with a subsequent release of thromboxane A_2. The peritoneal reaction results in increased prostacycline. Altered levels of prostanoids then interfere with the normal reproductive physiology. Peritoneal implants produce increased levels of prostaglandins[59,60]. The endometrium and the fallopian tube are other possible sources of peritoneal fluid prostaglandins. Prostaglandin production or accumulation as a result of retrograde tubal menstruation is possible but has not been established. The ovaries may be a source of peritoneal fluid prostaglandins. Follicular fluid $PGF_{2\alpha}$ increases in follicles before ovulation[61]. There are no convincing data that show that the production of prostaglandins from the follicle is abnormal with endometriosis.

In an attempt to evaluate the role of prostaglandins in peritoneal fluid in patients with endometriosis, many investigators have measured prostanoids directly from peritoneal fluid (Table 5.3). The studies of peritoneal fluid prostaglandins have the same limitations stated for peritoneal fluid volume and peritoneal fluid macrophages. Cycle timing, control group selection, and collection techniques have varied from one study to another, making it difficult to interpret the data. Studies of peritoneal fluid prostaglandins are limited by the ubiquitous nature of prostaglandins and their short half-lives of seconds or minutes. Because of the short half-life, prostaglandin metabolites have been measured instead of their physiologically active precursors. PGEM, PGFM, 6-keto-$PGF_{1\alpha}$, and TxB_2 have been measured as representatives of their active precursors PGE, $PGF_{2\alpha}$, PGI_2 and TxA_2, respectively. Another

Table 5.3 Studies of peritoneal fluid prostaglandins in women with endometriosis

Author/date	No. of patients		Prostaglandins				
	Endometriosis	Controls	$F_{2\alpha}$	E_2	FM	$6\text{-}k\text{-}F_{1\alpha}$	TXB_2
Drake, 1981[14]	14	15				↑	↑
Badawy, 1982[62]	15	5	↔	↑			
Rock, 1982[16]	45	17	↔	↔	↔		↔
Sondheimer, 1982[63]	10	4	↔				
Halme, 1983[42]	16	24	↔	↔			
Sgarlatta, 1983[17]	21	6	↔	↔	↔	↔	↔
Badawy, 1984[44]	26	24	↑	↑			
Dawood, 1984[19]	16	10	↔	↔		↑	↔
Ylikorkla, 1984[60]	29	25				↑	↑
Badawy, 1985[22]	39	45	↑	↑			
Mudge, 1985[20]	42	81				↔	
Chacho, 1986[24]	5	5		↔	↔	↔	↔
DeLeon, 1986[23]	31	14	↑	↑		↑	↑
Rezai, 1987[25]	45	28	↔	↔	↔		↔

shortcoming of these studies arises from the observation that minimal trauma can elicit a large and rapid prostaglandin response. Studies measuring gross changes in prostaglandin metabolites may not be adequately sensitive to explain subtle differences in patients with endometriosis.

Drake and associates measured peritoneal fluid thromboxane B_2 and 6-keto-$PGF_{1\alpha}$ and noted a 10-fold increase in the patient with endometriosis[14]. Ylikorkla and Viinikka supported the observation from Drake et al., although the degree of increase of 6-keto-$PGF_{1\alpha}$ and TxB_2 in patients with endometriosis was less than twice the controls[60]. Sondheimer and Flickinger measured $PGF_{2\alpha}$ from patients in the follicular phase[63]. Elevated prostaglandins were seen in this study when there was blood-tinged fluid. The highest levels were found in patients with moderate and severe endometriosis in the presence of blood or 'chocolate' fluid. However, other patients with a similar extent of disease had undetectable levels, while some patients with no endometriosis had high $PGF_{2\alpha}$ levels.

When cycle stage is controlled, Rock and Rezai failed to demonstrate a significant change in prostaglandin levels in peritoneal fluid from patients with endometriosis compared to controls[16,25]. Sgarlatta[17] et al., Dawood[19] et al., Chacho[24] et al., and Halme[42] were unable to show an alteration of prostaglandins with endometriosis. Dawood et al., however, noted an elevated concentration of the prostacycline metabolite with endometriosis[19]. The explanation for contradictions in these studies evaluating peritoneal fluid is uncertain. These differences may in part be explained by the differences in collection techniques, selection of controls, and cycle day. Vernon et al., proposes that prostaglandin production may be altered with the histology of the endometrial implants[64]. Active petechial implants, which contain endometrial glands and stroma, produce much higher levels of PGF than inactive implants that contain isolated or few endometrial cells in vitro. Although PGF production is much higher in active implants, PGF content is comparable in active and inactive implants. These findings suggest that *in vitro* incubation techniques may be a more useful indication of prostaglandin alterations than direct measurement of prostaglandins.

Prostaglandins play an important role in reproductive physiology, but the role of prostaglandins in endometriosis is uncertain. While prostaglandins may play some role, investigators have actively pursued other explanations for the pain and infertility associated with endometriosis.

INTERLEUKINS/LYMPHOKINES

Lymphokines may play a role in endometriosis-associated infertility. Lymphokines are substances whose function involves regulation of proliferation and differentiation of lymphocytes. Lymphokines are protein products of stimulated macrophages. Of the lymphokines, interleukin-1 has recently received a great deal of attention. Interleukin-1 is produced by macrophages and is a primary mediator of the inflammatory response. It induces prostaglandin synthesis[65]. Interleukin-1 stimulates B-cells to produce immunoglobulins[66].

Although the potential effects of interleukins on reproductive physiology in patients with endometriosis have not been completely defined, interleukin-1 has been found in peritoneal fluid. Levels of peritoneal fluid interleukin are significantly higher with endometriosis than in controls[37,67]. Patients with tubal ligation or tubal occlusion have no detectable interleukin-1 in the peritoneal fluid. Interleukin-1 adversely affects mouse embryo growth *in vitro*[67]. Embryos exposed to interleukins are less likely to develop to the eight-cell stage at 24 hours, and a lower percentage progress to the morula and blastocyst stage at 48 and 72 hours. High levels of interleukin-1 result in embryo degeneration. Interleukin-1 stimulates fibroblast proliferation, collagen deposition, and fibrinogen formation[68]. Fakih *et al.* have proposed that elevated levels of interleukin-1 may explain the occurrence of fibrosis and adhesion formation associated with advanced stages of endometriosis[67].

Clearly, more information is needed. Interleukins may provide an explanation for endometriosis-associated adhesions. Infertility may be partly explained by interleukin-mediated embryo toxicity. Early work is exciting and further investigation should clarify the role of interleukins in endometriosis.

PERITONEAL FLUID PROTEINS

There is potential for other factors, not yet defined, to play a role in endometriosis-associated infertility. Suginami *et al.* examined peritoneal fluid proteins toxic to reproductive function and identified a protein in peritoneal fluid from patients with endometriosis that inhibits the fimbrial capture of ovum *in vitro*[69]. This substance is a water-soluble protein with a molecular weight greater than 100 000. A mechanism by which this protein interferes with ovum pick-up is not clear, however[70].

Joshi *et al.* have identified a progestogen-associated endometrial protein (PEP) that is elevated in peritoneal fluid in the secretory phase of the menstrual cycle from women with moderate to severe endometriosis compared to patients with mild endometriosis and disease-free controls[71]. PEP is a major secretory protein of the human endometrium and rises rapidly during the late luteal phase of the menstrual cycle[72]. The tissue origin of peritoneal fluid PEP has not been determined but may result from retrograde flow or secretion of endometriosis implants. Serum concentrations of this protein are elevated on days 5–20 in patients with severe endometriosis compared to controls[73]. Serum levels of PEP are lowered by conservative surgery or medical therapy in patients with endometriosis[73]. Further confirming studies are necessary before PEP may be used as a clinical marker for endometriosis, although early reports are encouraging. The physiological role of PEP in endometriosis has not been established.

Other investigators have looked at the association of growth factors in peritoneal fluid of patients with endometriosis. Epidermal growth factor is increased in peritoneal fluid during the secretory phase of the cycle, but there is no difference between patients with endometriosis and controls[23]. Macrophage-derived growth factor, on the other hand, is produced in higher amounts from macrophages from patients with endometriosis[74]. Halme has proposed that macrophage-derived growth factor enhances the ectopic growth of endometrial cells in the peritoneal cavity[74]. Tumour necrosis factor is elevated in patients with moderate or severe endometriosis[75]. Although tumour necrosis factor is elevated with advanced endometriosis, elevated levels have been found in women with pelvic inflammatory disease. Further investigation is necessary to define the role of growth factors with endo-metriosis.

Other proteins in peritoneal fluid have been examined. Acid phosphatase is elevated in peritoneal fluid from patients with endometriosis, although the significance of this finding is not clear[42]. Plasminogen activator is a trypsin-like proteinase that is present in high concentrations of many extracellular fluids. When plasminogen activator is reduced by 50% or more, fibrin cannot be cleared and permanent adhesions may subsequently form[76]. Malick has proposed that a deficiency in plasminogen activation activity in patients with endometriosis may explain adhesion formation with endometriosis[77]. Plasminogen activator activity, however, is unchanged in peritoneal fluid from endometriosis patients[78]. The severity of endometriosis does not affect plasminogen activator activity levels[79]. Although prolactin is a secretory product of normal endometrium, peritoneal fluid prolactin levels are unchanged with endometriosis[80].

CA-125 is a cell surface antigen expressed in derivatives of coelomic epithelium, peritoneum, and the endocervix. CA-125 is elevated in peritoneal fluid of women with moderate and severe endometriosis, although other investigators have found that serum CA-125 levels are a more sensitive indicator of endometriosis than peritoneal fluid levels[81,82]. CA-125 is not likely to play a direct role in the pathophysiology of endometriosis, but serum levels may provide a useful indicator of the extent of disease or responses to therapy. In addition, radiolabelled monoclonal antibodies to CA-125 have been used to image ovarian endometriosis with immunoscintigraphy. In an early study, two women with severe endometriosis had positive immunoscintigraphy[83]. These results are preliminary and the technique experimental. However, if further studies confirm the initial report, immunoscintigraphy may be useful in the diagnosis or management of endometriosis.

CONCLUSION

There remains no universally accepted explanation for the symptoms that occur in patients with endometriosis. Local peritoneal factors provide at least a partial explanation for the pathophysiological changes that occur with endometriosis. Data continue to accumulate supporting the role of macrophages in endometriosis. Macrophages present in higher numbers, concentrations, or activation states may cause infertility by gamete phagocytosis. Activated macrophages may release factors that interfere with reproduction such as lymphokines. A role for prostaglandins in endometriosis, once a popular notion, has fallen into disfavour. Studies measuring prostaglandins have been inconclusive, contradictory, and limited by the ubiquitous nature of prostaglandins and their rapid half-lives. Peritoneal fluid proteins or growth factors may be altered with endometriosis. These substances may interfere with reproduction. More studies are needed to confirm preliminary reports of endometriosis-associated peritoneal proteins.

Much insight has been gained by measurements of suspected toxins in peritoneal fluid. Inferences based on these observations, although helpful, need support. New models are necessary to establish the pathophysiology of endometriosis. Controlled, randomized clinical studies are critical to clarify the conflicts present in the literature.

REFERENCES

1. Kistner, R.W. (1979). Endometriosis in infertility. *Clin. Obstet. Gynecol.*, **22**, 101
2. Stevenson, C.S. and Campbell, C.G. (1960). The symptoms, physical findings, and clinical diagnosis of pelvic endometriosis. *Clin. Obstet. Gynecol.*, **3**, 441
3. Rohr, M.S. and McDonald, J.C. (1986). Abdominal wall, umbilicus, peritoneum, mesenteries, omentum, and retroperitoneum. In Sabiston, D.C., Jr. (ed.) *Textbook of Surgery*, 13th edn, p. 774 (Philadelphia: W.B. Saunders)
4. van Furth, R., Raeburn, J.A. and van Zwet, T.L. (1979). Characteristics of human mononuclear phagocytes. *Blood*, **54**, 485
5. Muse, K. (1987). Endometriosis and infertility. In Wilson, E. A. (ed.) *Endometriosis*, p. 94. (New York: Alan R. Liss)
6. Maathuis, J.B., VanLook, P.F.A. and Michie, E.A. (1978). Changes in volume, total protein, and ovarian steroid concentrations of peritoneal fluid throughout the human menstrual cycle. *J. Endocrinol.*, **76**, 123
7. Koninckx, P.R., Renaer, M. and Brosens, I.A. (1980). Origin of peritoneal fluid in women: An ovarian exudation product. *Br. J. Obstet. Gynaecol.*, **87**, 177
8. Lippes, J., Enders, R.G., Pragay, D.A. and Bartholomew, W.R. (1972). The collection and analysis of human follicular tubal fluid. *Contraception*, **5**, 85
9. Muse, K.N., Estes, S., Vernon, M., Zavos, P. and Wilson, E.A. (1986). Effect of endometriosis on sperm motility in peritoneal fluid in vitro. *Fertil. Steril.* (suppl.), **46**, 99
10. Halme, J. and Hall, J.L. (1982). Effect of pelvic fluid from endometriosis patients on human sperm penetration of zona-free hamster ova. *Fertil. Steril.*, **37**, 573
11. Sueldo, C.E., Lambert, H., Steinleitner, A.J. and Swanson, J.A. (1986). Effect of peritoneal fluid on murine sperm ova interaction. *Fertil. Steril.* (suppl.), **46**, 8

12. Morcos, R.N., Gibbons, W.E. and Findley, W.E. (1985). Effect of peritoneal fluid on in vitro cleavage of 2-cell mouse embryos: Possible role in infertility associated endometriosis. *Fertil. Steril.*, **44**, 678

13. Drake, T.S., Metz, S.A., Grunert, G.M. and O'Brien, W.F. (1980). Peritoneal fluid volume in endometriosis. *Fertil. Steril.*, **34**, 280

14. Drake, T.S., O'Brien, W.F., Ramwell, P.W. and Metz, S.A. (1981). Peritoneal fluid thromboxane B_2 and 6-keto-prostaglandin $F_{1\alpha}$ in endometriosis. *Am. J. Obstet. Gynecol.*, **140**, 401

15. Haney, A.F., Muscato, J.J. and Weinberg, J.B. (1981). Peritoneal fluid cell populations in infertility patients. *Fertil. Steril.*, **35**, 696

16. Rock, J.A., Dubin, N.H., Ghodgaonkar, R.B., Bergquist, C.A., Erozan, Y.S. and Kimball, A.W. (1982). Cul-de-sac fluid in women with endometriosis: Fluid volume and prostanoid concentration during the proliferative phase of the cycle — days 8 to 12. *Fertil. Steril.*, **37**, 747

17. Sgarlatta, C.S., Hertelendy, F. and Mikhail, G. (1983). The prostanoid content in peritoneal fluid and plasma of women with endometriosis. *Am. J. Obstet. Gynecol.*, **147**, 563

18. Crain, J.L. and Luciano, A.A. (1983). Peritoneal fluid evaluation in infertility. *Obstet. Gynecol.*, **61**, 159

19. Dawood, M.Y., Kahn-Dawood, F.S. and Wilson, L. Jr. (1984). Peritoneal fluid prostaglandins and prostanoids in women with endometriosis, chronic pelvic inflammatory disease, and pelvic pain. *Am. J. Obstet. Gynecol.*, **148**, 391

20. Mudge, T.J., James, M.J., Jones, W.R. and Walsh, J.A. (1985). Peritoneal fluid 6-keto prostaglandin $F_{1\alpha}$ levels in women with endometriosis. *Am. J. Obstet. Gynecol.*, **152**, 901

21. Olive, D.L., Weinberg, J.B. and Haney, A.F. (1985). Peritoneal macrophages and infertility: The association between cell number and pelvic pathology. *Fertil. Steril.*, **44**, 772

22. Badawy, S.Z., Marshall, L. and Cuenca, V. (1985). Peritoneal fluid prostaglandins in various stages of the menstrual cycle: Role in infertile patients with endometriosis. *Int. J. Fertil.*, **30**, 48

23. DeLeon, F.D., Vijayakumar, R., Brown, M., Rao, C.V., Yussman, M.A. and Schultz, G. (1986). Peritoneal fluid volume, estrogen, progesterone, prostaglandin, and epidermal growth factor concentrations in patients with and without endometriosis. *Obstet. Gynecol.*, **68**, 189

24. Chacho, K.J., Chacho, M.S., Andresen, P.J. and Scommegna, A. (1986). Peritoneal fluid in patients with and without endometriosis: Prostanoids and macrophages and their effects on the spermatozoa penetration assay. *Am. J. Obstet. Gynecol.*, **154**, 1290

25. Rezai, N., Ghodgaonkar, R.B., Zacur, H.A., Rock, J.A. and Dubin, N.H. (1987). Cul-de-sac fluid in women with endometriosis: Fluid volume, protein and prostanoid concentrations during the periovulatory period — days 13 to 18. *Fertil. Steril.*, **48**, 29

26. Awadalla, S.G., Friedman, C.I., Haq, A.U., Roh, S.I., Chin, N.W. and Kim, M.W. (1987). Local peritoneal factors: Their role in infertility associated with endometriosis. *Am. J. Obstet. Gynecol.*, **157**, 1207

27. Syrop, C.H. and Halme, J. (1987). Cyclic changes of peritoneal fluid parameters in normal and infertile patients. *Obstet. Gynecol.*, **69**, 416

28. Hill, J.A., Faris, H.M.P., Schiff, I. and Anderson, D.J. (1988) Characterization of leukocyte subpopulations in the peritoneal fluid of women with endometriosis. *Fertil. Steril.*, **50**, 216

29. Oak, M.K., Chantler, E.N., Williams, C.A.V. and Elstein, M. (1985). Sperm survival studies in peritoneal fluid from infertile women with endometriosis and unexplained infertility. *Clin. Reprod. Fertil.*, **3**, 297

30. Werb, Z. (1987). Macrophages. In Stites, D.P., Stobo, J.D. and Wells, J.V. (eds.) *Basic and Clinical Immunology*, 6th edn, p. 96. (Norwalk, Conn.: Appleton and Lange)

31. Ball, R.Y., Scott, N. and Mitchinson, M.J. (1984). Further observations on spermiphagy by murine peritoneal macrophages in vitro. *J. Reprod. Fertil.*, **71**, 221

32. Muscato, J.J., Haney, A.F. and Weinberg, J.B. (1982). Sperm phagocytosis by human peritoneal macrophages: A possible cause of infertility in endometriosis. *Am. J. Obstet. Gynecol.*, **144**, 503

33. Hoxsey, R.J., Rao, R. and Scommegna, A. (1984). Sperm recovery in peritoneal fluid of endometriosis versus 'normal' infertile patients. *Fertil. Steril.*, **41**, 395 [abstract]

34. Stone, S.C. and Himsl, K. (1986). Peritoneal recovery of motile and nonmotile sperm in

the presence of endometriosis. *Fertil. Steril.*, **46**, 338

35. Boyer, P., Territo, M.C., deZiegler, D. and Meldrum, D.R. (1986). Ethiodol inhibits phagocytosis by pelvic peritoneal macrophages. *Fertil. Steril.*, **46**, 715
36. Halme, J., Hammond, M.G., Syrop, C.H. and Talbert, L.M. (1985). Peritoneal macrophages modulate human granulosa luteal cell progesterone production. *J. Clin. Endocrinol. Metab.*, **16**, 912
37. Hill, J.A. and Anderson, D.J. (1989). Lymphocyte activity in the presence of peritoneal fluid from fertile women and infertile women with and without endometriosis. *Am. J. Obstet. Gynecol.*, **161**, 861
38. Haney, A.F., Misukonis, M.A. and Weinberg, J.B. (1983). Macrophages and infertility: Oviductal macrophages as potential mediators of infertility. *Fertil. Steril.*, **39**, 310
39. Halme, J., Becker, S. and Wing, R. (1984). Accentuated cyclic activation of peritoneal macrophages in patients with endometriosis. *Am. J. Obstet. Gynecol.*, **148**, 85
40. Gleicher, N., Dmowski, W.P., Siegel, I., Lin, T.L., Friberg, J., Radwanska, E. and Toder, V. (1984). Lymphocyte subsets in endometriosis. *Obstet. Gynecol.*, **63**, 463
41. Halme, J., Becker, S., Hammond, M.G. and Raj, S. (1982). Pelvic macrophages in normal and infertile women: The role of patent tubes. *Am. J. Obstet. Gynecol.*, **142**, 890
42. Halme, J., Becker, S., Hammond, M.G., Raj, M.H.G. and Raj, S. (1983). Increased activation of pelvic macrophages in infertile women with mild endometriosis. *Am. J. Obstet. Gynecol.*, **145**, 333
43. Becker, S., Halme, J. and Haskill, S. (1983). Heterogeneity of human peritoneal macrophages: Cytochemical and flow cytometric studies. *J. Reticuloendothelial Soc.*, **33**, 127
44. Badawy, S.Z., Cuenca, V., Marshall, L., Munchback, R., Rinas, A.C. and Coble, D.A. (1984). Cellular components in peritoneal fluid in infertile patients with and without endometriosis. *Fertil. Steril.*, **42**, 704
45. Halme, J., Becker, S. and Haskill, S. (1987). Altered maturation and function of peritoneal macrophages: Possible role of pathogenesis of endometriosis. *Am. J. Obstet. Gynecol.*, **156**, 783
46. Dunselman, G.A., Hendrix, M.G., Bouckaert, P.X. and Evers, J.L. (1988). Functional aspects of peritoneal macrophages in endometriosis of women. *J. Reprod. Fertil.*, **82**, 707
47. Zeller, J.M., Hening, I., Radwanska, E. and Dmowski, W.P. (1987). Enchancement of human monocyte and peritoneal macrophage chemiluminescence activities in women with endometriosis. *Am. J. Reprod. Immunol. Microbiol.*, **13**, 78
48. Mayes, P.A. (1988). Metabolism of unsaturated fatty acids and eicosanoids. In Murry, R.K., Granner, D.K., Mayes, P.A. and Rodwell, V.W. (eds.) (1988). *Harper's Biochemistry*, 21st edn, p. 210. (Norwalk, Conn.: Appleton and Lange)
49. Schenken, R.S., Asch, R.H., Williams, R.F. and Hodgen, G.D. (1984). Etiology of infertility in monkeys with endometriosis: Luteinized unruptured follicles, luteal phase defects, pelvic adhesions and spontaneous abortions. *Fertil. Steril.*, **41**, 122
50. Burns, W.N. and Schenken, R.S. (1989). Pathophysiology. In Schenken, R.S. (ed.) (1989). *Endometriosis: Contemporary Concepts in Clinic Management*, p. 83. (Philadelphia: J.P. Lippincott)
51. Spillman, C.H., Beubing, D.C., Roseman, T.J. and Larion, L.J. (1976). Effect of vaginally administered 15(S)-15-methyl $PGF_{2\alpha}$ on egg transport and fertility in rabbits. *Proc. Soc. Exp. Biol. Med.*, **151**, 575
52. Eddy, C.A. (1980). Ovum transport in the Rhesus monkey following postovulatory intravaginal 15(S)-15-methyl prostaglandin $F_{2\alpha}$ methyl ester administration. *Am. J. Obstet. Gynecol.*, **137**, 966
53. Croxatto, H.B., Ortiz, M.E., Guiloff, E. and Ibarra, A. (1978). Effect of 15(S)-15-methyl prostaglandin $F_{2\alpha}$ on human oviductal motility and ovum transport. *Fertil. Steril.*, **30**, 408
54. Sargent, E.L. and Stouffer, R.L. (1987). An obligatory luteotrophic role for prostaglandins in the Rhesus monkey. Presented at the 20th Annual Meeting for the Society of a Study of Reproduction, Urbana, Ill., July 20–23 [abstract 171]
55. Auletta, F.J., Kamps, D.L., Pories, S., Bisset, J. and Gibson, M. (1984). An intracorpus luteum site for the luteolytic action of prostaglandin $F_{2\alpha}$ in the Rhesus monkey. *Prostaglandins*, **27**, 285
56. Wentz, A.C. and Jones, G.S. (1973). Transient luteolytic effect of prostaglandin $F_{2\alpha}$ in the human. *Obstet. Gynecol.*, **42**, 172

57. Stouffer, R.L. (1988). Perspectives on the corpus luteum of the menstrual cycle and early pregnancy. *Semin. Reprod. Endocrinol.*, **6**, 103
58. Lundstrom, V. and Green, K. (1978). Endogenous levels of prostaglandin $F_{2\alpha}$ and its main metabolites in plasma and endometrium of normal and dysmenorrheic women. *Am. J. Obstet. Gynecol.*, **130**, 640
59. Moon, Y.S., Jeung, P.C.S., Yuen, B.H. and Gomel, V. (1981). Prostaglandin F in human endometriotic tissue. *Am. J. Obstet. Gynecol.*, **141**, 344
60. Ylikorkla, O. and Viinikka, C. (1983). Prostaglandins in endometriosis. *Acta Obstet. Gynecol. Scand.* [suppl.], **113**, 105
61. Marsh, J.M. and Le Maire, W.J. (1974). Cyclic AMP accumulation and steroidogenesis in the human corpus luteum: Effect of gonadotropins and prostaglandins. *J. Clin. Endocrinol. Metab.*, **38**, 99
62. Badawy, S.Z., Marshall, L., Gabal, A.A. and Nusbaum, M.L. (1982). The concentration of 13,14-dihydro-15-keto prostaglandin $F_{2\alpha}$ and prostaglandin E_2 in peritoneal fluid of infertile patients with and without endometriosis. *Fertil. Steril.*, **38**, 166
63. Sondheimer, S.J. and Flickinger, G. (1982). Prostaglandin $F_{2\alpha}$ in the peritoneal fluid of patients with endometriosis. *Int. J. Fertil.*, **27**, 73
64. Vernon, M.S., Beard, J.S., Graves, K. and Wilson, E.A. (1986). Classification of endometriotic implants by morphologic appearance and capacity to synthesize prostaglandin F. *Fertil. Steril.*, **46**, 801
65. Rossi, V., Breviario, F., Ghezzi, P., Dejana, E. and Montovani, A. (1985). Interleukin-1 induces prostacyclin in vascular cells. *Science*, **229**, 174
66. Falkoff, R.J., Muraguchi, A., Hong, J.X., Butler, J.L., Dinarello, C.A. and Fauci, A.S. (1983). The effects of interleukin-1 on human B-cell activation and proliferation. *J. Immunol.*, **131**, 801
67. Fakih, H., Baggett, B., Holtz, G., Tsang, K.Y., Lee, J.C. and Williamson, H.O. (1987). Interleukin-1: A possible role in the infertility associated with endometriosis. *Fertil. Steril.*, **47**, 213
68. Postlethwaite, A.E., Lachman, L.B. and Kang, A.H. (1984). Induction of fibroblast proliferation by interleukin-1 derived from human monocytic leukemic cells. *Arthritis Rheum.*, **27**, 995
69. Suginami, H., Yano, K., Watanabe, K. and Matsuura, S. (1986). A factor inhibiting ovum capture by the oviductal fimbriae present in endometriosis peritoneal fluid. *Fertil. Steril.*, **46**, 1140
70. Mahi-Brown, C.A. and Yanagimachi, R. (1983). Parameters influencing ovum pickup by oviductal fimbria in the golden hamster. *Gamete Res.*, **8**, 1
71. Joshi, S.G., Zamah, N.M., Raikar, R.S., Buttram, V.C., Jr., Henriques, E.S. and Gordon, M. (1986). Serum and peritoneal fluid proteins in women with and without endometriosis. *Fertil. Steril.*, **46**, 1077
72. Joshi, S.G., Bank, J.F., Henriques, E.S., Makarachi, A. and Malties, G. (1982). Serum levels of progestagen-associated endometrial protein during menstrual cycle and pregnancy. *J. Clin. Endocrinol. Metab.*, **55**, 642
73. Telimaa, S., Kauppila, A., Ronnberg, L., Suikkari, A.M. and Seppala, M. (1989). Elevated serum levels of endometrial secretory protein PP14 in patients with advanced endometriosis. *Am. J. Obstet. Gynecol.*, **161**, 866
74. Halme, J., White, C., Kauma, S., Estes, J. and Haskill, S. (1988). Peritoneal macrophages from patients with endometriosis release growth factor activity in vitro. *J. Clin. Endocrinol. Metab.*, **66**, 1044
75. Eiserman, J., Gast, M.J., Pineda, J., Odem, R.R. and Collins, J.L. (1988). Tumour necrosis factor in peritoneal fluid of women undergoing laparoscopic surgery. *Fertil. Steril.*, **50**, 573
76. Buckman, R.F., Woods, M., Sargent, L. and Gervin, A.S. (1976). A unifying pathogenetic mechanism in the etiology of intraperitoneal adhesions. *J. Surg. Res.*, **20**, 1
77. Malick, J.E. (1982). The etiology of endometriosis. *J. Am. Osteopath. Assoc.*, **81**, 407
78. Batzofin, J.H., Holmes, S.D., Gibbons, W.E. and Buttram, V.C. Jr. (1985). Peritoneal fluid plasminogen activator activity in endometriosis and pelvic adhesive disease. *Fertil. Steril.*, **44**, 277
79. Olive, D.L., Hobbs, M.M., Misukonis, M.A., Weinberg, J.B. and Haney, A.F. (1986). Macrophages and infertility: The association between lysozyme activity and cell number.

Fertil. Steril., **46**(5), 110

80. Haney, A.F., Handwerger, S. and Weinberg, J.B. (1984). Peritoneal fluid prolactin in infertile women with endometriosis: Lack of evidence of secretory activity by endometrial implants. *Fertil. Steril.*, **42**, 935
81. Williams, R.S., Rao, Ch.V. and Yussman, M.A. (1988). Interference in the measurement of CA-125 in peritoneal fluid. *Fertil. Steril.*, **49**, 547
82. Moretuzzo, R.W., Di Lauro, S., Jenison, E., Chen, S.L., Reindollar, R.H. and McDonough, P.G. (1988). Serum and peritoneal lavage fluid CA-125 levels in endometriosis. *Fertil. Steril.*, **50**, 430
83. Kennedy, S.H., Soper, N.D., Mojiminiyi, O.A., Sheepstone, B.J. and Barlow, D.H. (1988). Immunoscintigraphy of ovarian endometriosis: A preliminary study. *Br. J. Obstet. Gynaecol.*, **95**, 693

6
The immune system in endometriosis

W. P. Dmowski, D. Braun and H. Gebel

INTRODUCTION

Endometriosis is a poorly understood disease of unknown aetiology and histogenesis. It affects women as well as menstruating female primates of other species. The disease is characterized by ectopic growth and function of endometrial cells. Current data indicate that endometriosis begins with retrograde transport through the fallopian tubes into the peritoneal cavity of endometrial cells or fragments desquamated during the menstrual period. These cells (or tissue fragments) then implant, proliferate and develop into characteristic endometriotic lesions. Under cyclic stimulation of the ovarian hormones, ectopic endometrial cells undergo similar cyclic changes to those of the uterine endometrium. From the peritoneal cavity, endometriosis may spread through lymphatic and vascular channels into distant locations. Alternatively, endometrial cells from the uterus may disseminate systemically into the pelvic cavity and distant locations. It is unclear why, in some women, endometrial cells are transported through lymphatic and vascular channels to various parts of the body, and why they are allowed to implant and function in the ectopic sites. In many respects, this process resembles metastases of neoplastic cells and is the reason why endometriosis in the past has been referred to as 'a benign cancer'.

The concept of retrograde tubal transport and ectopic implantation of the endometrial fragments was proposed more than 60 years ago by Sampson as the 'transplantation theory'[1]. According to this concept, which became generally accepted, retrograde tubal transport is the aetiologic factor in the development of endometriosis. However, retrograde menstrual flow occurs commonly in all menstruating females and endometrial fragments have been identified in the peritoneal cavity of women without, as well as with, endometriosis[2]. It is unknown why endometriotic fragments implant in ectopic locations and develop into endometriosis only in some women.

During the past decade, numerous reports have suggested that endometriosis is associated with changes in the immune system. Alterations in both cell-mediated and humoral immunity in rhesus monkeys, and in women with endometriosis, have been observed by several investigators. Furthermore, systemic radiation or immunotoxicants, both of which are immunosuppressive, have been followed by an increase in the incidence of endometriosis. Rhesus monkeys given total-body exposure to proton irradiation developed endometriosis during subsequent years more frequently than controls[3]. Similarly, monkeys treated with polychlorinated biphenyls (PCBs) which are known immunotoxicants, developed more frequently aggressive forms of endometriosis leading to intestinal obstruction and death[4]. It is possible that suppression of the immune system by systemic irradiation or by PCBs facilitated implantation of the endometrial fragments in ectopic locations and resulted in the development of endometriosis.

It is unclear at this time what is the exact role, if any, of the immune system in the pathogenesis of endometriosis. It is possible, and suggested by some, on the basis of changes in humoral immunity, that endometriosis is a form of autoimmune disease[5]. Alternatively, endometriosis could develop coincidentally with, or as a result of, changes in cell-mediated immunity similar to events that occur in metastatic neoplasia. Which specific cell-mediated mechanisms may be involved is unknown at present. Nevertheless, and regardless of the specific pathogenetic mechanisms, it now appears likely that the development of endometriosis involves an interaction between the immune system and self-antigens. In this chapter we will examine the immune system in endometriosis in the context of recognition and interaction with self-antigens.

IMMUNE SYSTEM: RECOGNITION AND INTERACTION WITH SELF-ANTIGENS

The immune system is usually viewed as a collection of cells distributed at strategic locations throughout the body. However, it probably should be considered as an organ since, collectively, the immune system is as large as the liver and equally crucial for survival. The immune system protects us from a variety of diseases, ranging from viral infections to malignancies. There are four major types of mononuclear cells involved in generating, maintaining and propagating an immune response[6]. These are T lymphocytes, B lymphocytes, monocytes and natural killers, which each have multiple characteristics and functions (Table 6.1). These include the production of cytokines such as interleukins-1 and -2, γ-interferon and tumour necrosis factor. Cytokines, in turn, augment the functional activity of B cells, T cells, monocytes and natural killer (NK) cells.

Cells of the immune system: phenotypes and functions

T lymphocytes
Functionally, T lymphocytes contain multiple subpopulations including helper, suppressor and cytotoxic cells[7–12]. Phenotypically, these T cells are divided

Table 6.1 Mononuclear cells: surface markers and functions

	Monocytes	NK cells	T cells	B cells
Phagocytic	+	−	−	−
Cytotoxic	+	+	+ (subsets)	−
Cytokine production	+	+	+	+
Antibody production	−	−	−	+
Antigenic specificity	−	−	+	+
Surface Ig	−	−	−	+
FcR	+	+	+	+
Histocompatibility antigens:				
Class I	+	+	+	+
Class II	+	±	−[a]	+
E-rosette receptors		+	+	−
(CD2)		(low affinity)	(high affinity)	

[a] Unless activated

into two major groups, CD4 (helper/inducer) and CD8 (suppressor/cytotoxic) which can be subdivided further[7]. One subset of CD4 cells can act as helpers for B cell differentiation[8]; the second subset can function as inducers of suppression[9,10]. Similarly, subsets of CD8 T cells have also been defined[11,12].

B cells
B cells are precursors of plasma cells, the antibody-producing cells of the immune system. Like T cells, there are defined subpopulations of B cells[13]. For example, 10–20% of B cells express CD5, a surface determinant not found on the majority of B cells[14]. It has been suggested that CD5 B cells are responsible for autoantibody production, as these cells are elevated in patients with autoimmune diseases such as systemic lupus erythematosus and rheumatoid arthritis[15].

Monocytes
Monocytes or macrophages are phagocytic cells that ingest, process, and present antigens to lymphocytes, initiating an antigen-specific immune response[16]. In addition, these cells participate in surveillance, protecting the host against neoplastic cells and clearing the system of senescent cells, for example, red blood cells. Monocytes are also protective by directly ingesting and killing invading organisms. The antigen-presenting cell function of monocytes is mediated by class II major histocompatibility complex (MHC) antigens such as HLA-DR[17]. Similar to B and T cells, subpopulations of monocytes have been described. For example, one population of monocytes expresses the class II MHC antigens HLA-DR and HLA-DQ, while a second population expresses only HLA-DR.

NK cells
Natural killer (NK) cells have recently emerged as an important cell type in various disease states, mediating non-MHC-restricted lysis of various malignant cells[18]. NK cells are large granular lymphocytes that appear to be derived from a cell lineage distinct from T cells, B cells or macrophages. Phenotypic

and functional studies indicate that NK cells contain multiple subpopulations. Some NK subsets have functional activity in addition to cytotoxicity[19,20], including cytokine production and immunoregulation of B cells. Recent evidence demonstrates that NK cells are also precursors to lymphokine-activated killer (LAK) cells. LAK cells are now used therapeutically in certain malignant diseases, particularly in renal cell carcinoma and malignant melanoma.

In summary, the cells involved in an immune response have multiple functions and regulatory activities. These cells interact with themselves and one another to protect the host from disease. However, in order to function, there is a fundamental requirement for immune cells to distinguish self from non-self, i.e. to eliminate foreign antigens and ignore autologous antigens. This concept is referred to as tolerance.

Immunological tolerance: induction and maintenance

In simple terms, tolerance is achieved in two ways: cells that react with self-antigens are either physically removed or functionally inactivated[21,22]. The actual mechanisms by which tolerance is maintained are not fully understood and are the subject of intense investigation. Recent studies in mice, utilizing molecular biology techniques, have elucidated several distinct mechanisms whereby tolerance is established and maintained. These include: (1) clonal abortion or deletion; (2) failure of cellular activation due to a missing co-stimulator that is required; (3) active suppression of autoreactive cells[21].

The majority of B cell responses to antigens depend on interaction with T cells. Thus, if T cells are deleted, inactivated or suppressed, tolerance of the B cells is effectively maintained. In mice, it is clear that the expression of self-antigens in the thymic microenvironment plays a prominent role in determining which clones of T cells are destroyed (negative selection) or allowed to mature (positive selection)[23]. Some self-antigens that are not normal thymic constituents may still migrate to the thymus following shedding from other tissues. In either circumstance, expression of self-antigens in the thymic microenvironment selects against autoreactive clones. However, it should be recognized that many self-antigens are not normally expressed or exposed to the thymic microenvironment. In these situations, it is reasonable to assume that tolerance occurs after emigration of mature T cells from the thymus.

Tolerance to self-antigens is proposed to occur during embryogenesis through thymic selection, but can also occur in adults. Not surprisingly, it is much more difficult to promote tolerance in an adult than in a fetus. Until recently, most work on tolerance was performed with antigens foreign to the host immune system and not with autologous constituents. The ability to develop strains of transgenic mice has revolutionized the study of tolerance. Briefly, a foreign gene is introduced into the male pronucleus of a fertilized egg. The fetus develops with this foreign gene being recognized as self[24,25].

Other studies have suggested that some self-antigens are tolerated because they are either not exposed to the immune system (i.e. 'privileged') and/or because they are not immunogenic. A modern approach has been utilized to determine whether tissue normally tolerated can be made immunogenic. For example, beta cells of the islets of Langerhans do not normally express class II MHC antigens[26]. Recently, investigators inserted a class II gene into beta cells, so that they would express those molecules. A destruction, perhaps immunological, of beta cells and diabetes followed. Whether this phenomenon is related to the development of autoimmunity or is simply an aberrant physiology is at this time unclear.

Breakdown of immunological tolerance

Under certain circumstances, tolerance is not maintained. For example, even though autoreactive T cell clones against a specific self-antigen may have been deleted, other T cells, reactive against foreign antigens (e.g. viral proteins) may cross-react with the self-antigens. The effect is an apparent breakdown of self-tolerance. Alternatively, in circumstances where tolerance is maintained by active suppression of autoreactive clones, the loss of suppression could result in the breakdown of tolerance. The loss of tolerance may lead to autoimmune diseases such as rheumatoid arthritis, systemic lupus erythematosus (SLE) and Graves' disease to name but a few. Several factors could contribute to the breakdown of tolerance and the development of autoimmune diseases, including age, heredity and variable exposure to environmental agents involved in the aetiology and pathogenesis of the particular disease.

Autoreactivity as a normal homeostatic mechanism

It is not necessarily true that autoimmune responses are always deleterious to the host. For example, there are numerous circumstances wherein the immune system is likely to be involved in the elimination of self-cells. These are generally cells that are not desirable, such as senescent cells or malignant clones. In these situations, autoreactivity should be considered as beneficial.

Little-understood, yet fascinating, are homeostatic mechanisms through which the host limits autologous tissue growth in ectopic sites. It has been reported that autotransplants such as skin engraft better near donor sites[27] and that testes of dogs when surgically transferred into the peritoneal cavity undergo lymphocytic infiltration and destruction[28].

Several investigators have also described *in vitro* phenomena wherein normal T cells recognize and respond to self components. This response is referred to as the autologous mixed lymphocyte reaction (AMLR) and displays both specificity and memory, two hallmarks of an immune response[29]. The AMLR is severely impaired when lymphocytes are obtained from patients with Hodgkin's disease[30] and active SLE[31]. There is no direct evidence to suggest a corresponding *in vivo* role for the AMLR. Some investigators have suggested that the AMLR is involved in self-regulation of an immune response in neoplasia.

101

ALTERATIONS IN HUMORAL IMMUNITY IN ENDOMETRIOSIS

The first report indicating changes in the immune response in endometriosis was published in 1980 in the Russian medical literature. Startseva[32] observed increased B-cell and reduced T-cell reactivity in women with adenomyosis and endometriosis. The possibility of abnormal antigen–antibody reaction was suggested the same year by the studies of Weed and Arguembourg[33]. These authors demonstrated C3 and IgG deposits in the uterine endometrium and a corresponding reduction in the serum total complement levels in women with endometriosis. Two years later, Mathur et al.[34] identified IgG and IgA autoantibodies against endometrial and ovarian tissues in the sera and cervical and vaginal secretions of women with endometriosis. In a subsequent study, these authors[35] demonstrated that both fertile women and those with endometriosis have low levels of circulating and peritoneal fluid antibodies to endometrial antigens of molecular weight (MW) 19, 31, 38 and 42 kd. They postulated that this may be a mechanism for clearing the reproductive tract of the menstrual debris. Women with endometriosis, unlike normal fertile controls, additionally had in their sera and peritoneal fluids antibodies to endometrial antigens of MW 26 kd and 34 kd. Other investigators using different techniques confirmed high frequencies of antiendometrial antibodies in the sera, peritoneal fluids and endometrial tissues in women with endometriosis[36–39].

A different approach to the study of humoral immunity in endometriosis was taken by other investigators who measured autoantibodies against subcellular elements (i.e. antinuclear antibodies) or against chemical substances integral to the cell structure (i.e. anti-DNA, or anti-cardiolipin antibodies). A high frequency of these autoantibodies has been demonstrated in women with autoimmune diseases and with various forms of reproductive failure, such as infertility and recurrent abortions[40,41]. Gleicher and associates[5] reported that among 31 women with endometriosis, 65% had IgG and 45% had IgM autoantibodies to at least one of 16 antigens investigated. Those detected most frequently were autoantibodies to phospholipids, particularly phosphatidyl serine, histones and nucleotides. Such multiple autoantibodies suggest polyclonal B-cell activation. In collaborative studies with Gleicher's laboratory we confirmed these observations[42]. In a group of 20 women with laparoscopically diagnosed and staged endometriosis, 19 (95%) had at least one, and 10 (50%) had more than five autoantibodies against at least one of 45 antigens tested. The most frequent were IgG autoantibodies against phospholipids.

Autoimmune diseases are characterized by increased total immunoglobulin levels and decreased complement, secondary to immune complex formation and complement consumption. Several humoral factors such as serum complement and its components, immunoglobulins and CA-125 antigen levels have been studied in endometriosis but the results are conflicting. Serum complement, C3 and C4 were reported reduced[33,34], unchanged[44] or increased[36]. Similarly, total immunoglobulins were also found to be increased[5], unchanged[44] or decreased[43]. There is a general agreement, however, that CA-125 antigen is elevated in endometriosis, although to a lesser degree than in other pelvic disorders[45]. Serum concentrations range from 10 to 60 U/ml and seem to correlate with the stage of the disease. This is a low range of sensitivity and currently available assays need to be modified to achieve the standard curve between 2 and 50 U/ml. Although at this time CA-125 levels cannot be used for the diagnosis of endometriosis, the test appears to be a good marker to follow the clinical course of the disease and the effect of treatment.

ALTERATIONS IN CELL-MEDIATED IMMUNITY

The possibility that both humoral and cell-mediated immunity are altered in women with endometriosis was first suggested by the already quoted study of Startseva[32], who reported reduced T-cell immunity along with increased B-cell reactivity in women with adenomyosis and endometriosis. Our studies in rhesus monkeys and in women with endometriosis demonstrated alterations in cell-mediated immune mechanisms that are directed against endometrial antigens. In rhesus monkeys with spontaneous endometriosis, we observed a decreased *in vivo* reactivity, measured as intensity of perivascular lymphocytic infiltration compared with normal controls to intradermal injection of autologous endometrial antigens[46]. *In vitro* lymphocyte proliferation in response to the same autologous endometrial antigens was also less pronounced in monkeys with endometriosis. In women with endometriosis, cytotoxicity assays using peripheral lymphocytes and autologous ^{51}Cr-labelled endometrial cells as the target cells demonstrated decreased target cell lysis, with differences between subjects and controls most significant among patients with moderate and severe endometriosis[44]. Tests of non-specific immune function were comparable between subjects and controls, suggesting that both monkeys and women with endometriosis were otherwise immunologically competent.

In order to identify potential changes in the immune cell numbers, peripheral mononuclear leukocyte populations have been quantified by two groups of investigators. However, peripheral blood may not necessarily reflect changes in the peritoneal cavity, where endometriosis develops. Gleicher *et al.*[47] found no significant differences between women with endometriosis and infertile controls. On the other hand, Badawy *et al.*[48] reported an increase in the number of T and B cells and an increase in the T helper to T suppressor ratio in the peripheral blood and peritoneal fluid from women with endometriosis.

In the peritoneal cavity, macrophages are considered to play a major role in maintaining homeostasis. Resident macrophages originating from blood monocytes sequestered in the peritoneal cavity remove red blood cells, damaged tissue fragments, and most likely endometrial cells that gain access to the peritoneal cavity through fallopian tubes. Several studies indicate that in endometriosis the concentration, total number and activational status of peritoneal macrophages are increased[49–51]. They also produce higher levels of IL-1[52] and fibronectin[53], the latter of which may contribute to the development of peritoneal adhesions. In addition to phagocytic activities, peritoneal macrophages may also regulate other events in the peritoneal cavity by release of products such as cytokines, prostaglandins, growth factors, complement components and hydrolytic enzymes. Furthermore, macrophages release low levels of reactive oxygen intermediates, such as superoxide anion, hydrogen peroxide and singlet oxygen.

During stimulation by a phagocytic particle or immune complexes, macrophages increase dramatically the generation of the reactive oxygen intermediates. Although these products are important for degradation of materials within the phagocytic vacuole, they may also damage adjacent normal tissues. The generation of reactive oxygen products, called respiratory burst activity, can be estimated by measuring light emission or chemiluminescence from phagocytic cells stimulated with different chemical or biological activators. We have reported that in endometriosis, resting chemiluminescence of peritoneal macrophages is significantly increased, indicating the increase in their activational status[51]. More interestingly, peripheral blood monocytes stimulated with phorbol myristate acetate or serum-opsonized zymosan showed significantly higher chemiluminescence in patients than in controls. Similarly, peripheral monocytes from women with endometriosis may also produce higher levels of IL-1 *in vitro*, as recently reported[54]. These data indicate that in endometriosis, peripheral blood monocytes are functionally different and suggest that endometriosis may be a systemic rather than a local disorder involving the immune system.

Alterations in the activational characteristics and morphological appearance of peritoneal macrophages in endometriosis were the basis for an interesting hypothesis on the pathophysiology of endometriosis postulated by Halme *et al.*[55]. These authors suggested that higher numbers and increased activational status of peritoneal macrophages in endometriosis may lead to secretion of putative growth factors, facilitating implantation and growth of endometrial cells in ectopic locations and giving origin to endometriosis.

EFFECT OF DANAZOL IN ENDOMETRIOSIS

Danazol, a synthetic steroid derivative used commonly in the management of endometriosis, may possess the ability to modulate immunological functions both *in vivo* and *in vitro*.

The effect of danazol in several haematologic and autoimmune disorders is little understood and extremely interesting. In idiopathic thrombocytopenic purpura (ITP), danazol treatment results in clinical improvement, a decrease in antiplatelet antibodies, and normalization of platelet counts[56]. Similarly, in systemic lupus erythematosus (SLE), clinical improvement during danazol treatment is associated with a decrease in abnormal IgG, IgM, and IgA autoantibodies to nDNA and platelets, and in an increase in C1 inhibitor, C4, C5 and CH-50[57]. In hereditary angioneurotic oedema (HAE), clinical improvement during danazol treatment coincides with an increase in genetically deficient α-globulin C1 inhibitor[58]. Similarly, levels of genetically deficient factor VIII in classic haemophilia and of factor IX in Christmas disease increase during danazol treatment, coinciding with clinical improvement[59].

The mechanisms of immunosuppressive effects of danazol in ITP and SLE probably involve several immune cell types. It has been reported recently that in ITP danazol increases the number of T-helper/inducer cells, and the ratio of T-helper/inducer to T-suppressor/cytotoxic cells[60]. This could, in turn, lead to further induction and activation of effector T-suppressor cells, which may then inhibit B-cell proliferation and autoantibody production in ITP and SLE. The mechanism of danazol's effect in HAE, haemophilia and Christmas disease is less clear. It has been suggested that the drug functions at the genetic level, stimulating the normal allele to increase production of the deficient protein, thus overcoming the structural defect of the other allele.

In vitro, danazol in concentrations of 10^{-6} M (equivalent to therapeutically effective plasma levels) displays an immunosuppressive effect on macrophage-dependent T-lymphocyte proliferation[61]. This effect was comparable to that of glucocorticoids, whereas similar concentrations of oestradiol or testosterone were not immunosuppressive. In the same concentration (10^{-6} M), danazol did not significantly suppress macrophage-dependent T-cell activation of B lymphocytes, although at a higher concentration (10^{-5} M) the suppressive effect was observed. It is unclear whether these effects are at the macrophage or T lymphocyte level, but they seem to be mediated through glucocorticoid receptors.

In a recent prospective, randomized study we compared the effect of danazol and gonadotropin-releasing hormone agonists (GnRH-a) on autoantibody production in women with endometriosis[42]. Ten women treated with danazol and 10 treated with GnRH-a for a period of 6 months were studied. Clinical and endocrine assessments were performed before, during and after treatment, and laparoscopic staging of the disease before and after treatment was also performed. The samples for the autoantibody profile were obtained every 4 weeks, beginning 8 weeks before and ending 8 weeks after treatment. These samples were assayed in a blinded fashion for total immunoglobulins and IgG, IgM and IgA autoantibodies to six phospholipids, five histones and four polynucleotides.

During treatment, amenorrhoea and suppressed ovarian function, as indicated by follicle-stimulating hormone (FSH), luteinizing hormone (LH), oestradiol and progesterone levels were observed in all subjects. The degree of ovarian suppression did not differ between the groups. A significant and comparable degree of resolution of the disease during treatment was observed in both groups. Total IgG, IgM and IgA levels decreased significantly during danazol therapy but not during GnRH-a treatment.

Five patients (50%) in each group initially had more than five autoantibodies elevated. The number and concentration of autoantibodies decreased gradually during danazol but not during GnRH-a treatment. These autoantibodies were predominantly in the phospholipid group and of the IgG isotype. Autoantibodies to phosphatidyl inositol decreased by 94% (IgM) and 86% (IgG); to phosphatidyl ethanolamine by 93% (IgM), 87.5% (IgA) and 85% (IgG); to phosphatidyl serine by 90% (IgG); to cardiolipin by 83% (IgG); to histones H2A by 91% (IgG); and to dsDNA by 66% (IgG). After treatment, autoantibody levels remained suppressed for 8 weeks, although some tendency to a gradual increase was noted. There was no significant change in the concentration of any autoantibodies during treatment with GnRH-a.

During post-treatment follow-up period, five of ten patients in the danazol group conceived. Three of five initially had a significant number of antibodies (9, 16, and 19). Two of five initially had two autoantibodies each. All of these autoantibodies became suppressed during treatment. Four patients were delivered at term and one had a spontaneous, first-trimester abortion. In the GnRH-a group, four patients conceived after treatment. Three of four had fewer than five autoantibodies each (0, 1 and 3), which remained essentially unchanged during treatment. All three were delivered at term of healthy infants. The fourth patient in the GnRH-a group who conceived had 22 autoantibodies, and no change in their number or concentration during treatment. She conceived 28 weeks after treatment but had a spontaneous, first-trimester abortion. She did not conceive again during the subsequent 24 months of follow-up in spite of aggressive treatment with advanced reproductive techniques.

We concluded from this study that both danazol and the GnRH agonists are capable of inducing a comparable degree of ovarian suppression and resolution of endometriosis, but they seem to differ in their effect on the immune system. Suppression of elevated autoantibody concentrations by danazol may suggest another mechanism of action of this steroid in endometriosis and may contribute to the improved reproductive performance after treatment.

POSSIBLE MECHANISMS OF IMMUNE SYSTEM INVOLVEMENT IN ENDOMETRIOSIS

Currently available data seem to indicate that the immune system plays a role in the pathophysiology of endometriosis, although the exact mechanism of this involvement is not clear. It is possible that endometriosis is an autoimmune disease, not unlike SLE, with which it seems to be frequently associated[62]. Increased immunoglobulin levels and high frequency of auto-antibodies indicate polyclonal activation of B cells. Other characteristics of autoimmune diseases, such as female preponderance, familial occurrence, tissue damage, and multiorgan involvement are also present. Furthermore, treatment with danazol inhibits autoantibody production and brings about clinical improvement in several autoimmune disorders as well as in endometriosis.

Alternatively, it is possible that changes in humoral immunity in endome-triosis are secondary to deficient cellular mechanisms. According to this concept, endometrial cells or fragments displaced physiologically into the peritoneal cavity of healthy women are 'disposed of' by the local immune system, consisting primarily of the peritoneal macrophages. Endometriosis may develop when the peritoneal 'disposal system' is defective and permits implantation of the endometrial cells or fragments. It is also possible that endometriosis may develop if the peritoneal 'disposal system' is overwhelmed by the increased retrograde transport due to obstructed menstrual flow, as in cervical stenosis. Ectopic endometrial cells implanted in the peritoneal cavity are then processed by activated macrophages and presented to the T cells. Under the influence of macrophage-released cytokines, T cells proliferate and differentiate into functional subsets with different properties. A host of T cell-derived factors then play a critical role in the activation and differentiation of B cells. The activated B cells then produce autoantibodies against endometrial cells or against endometrial cell-derived phospholipids, histones, or nucleotides. Autoantibodies may in turn reduce fertility by interfering with ovum capture or implantation as well as by increasing the frequency of abortions.

Recently, we have tested the functional capacity of macrophages from women with endometriosis to mediate cytotoxic activities. We compared normal, fertile and infertile controls with women having stages I–IV endometriosis. Peritoneal macrophages recovered during laparoscopy were stimulated with various macrophage-activating cytokines, particularly γ-interferon (γIFN) and endotoxin, and subsequently tested for their capacity to kill a reference target cell, the Chang hepatoma cell line[63].

In normal, fertile controls, peritoneal macrophages could be activated to a cytocidal state by the combination of γIFN and endotoxin. In infertile controls peritoneal macrophages were significantly more active in their response to γIFN and endotoxin. This level of hyperactivity was also observed in women with stage I and II endometriosis. However, in stage III and IV endometriosis, peritoneal macrophage responses to γIFN and endotoxin were significantly reduced to a level that was slightly below that of the normal control group. In order to explore the mechanisms for increasing the responsiveness of peritoneal macrophages, we studied the effect of prostaglandin synthetase inhibitors. In these studies, a prostaglandin antagonist, indomethacin, was introduced into the macrophage activation cultures, together with γIFN and endotoxin; this was done because of the well-known relationship between monocyte prostaglandin metabolism and immune suppression[64]. The results of these studies demonstrated the following. (1) Peritoneal macrophages from fertile controls did not change their response to macrophage activators in the presence of indomethacin. (2) The elevated response of peritoneal macrophages from infertile controls or from women with stage I and II endometriosis was not increased in the presence of indomethacin. (3) The low response of peritoneal macrophages to activating cytokines in women with stage III and IV endometriosis was significantly increased in the presence of indomethacin.

We interpret these data to indicate that the macrophage disposal function in women with extensive endometriosis is impaired; this may be due, at least in part, to prostaglandin metabolism changes in these macrophages. Our future studies will be aimed at further exploration of this phenomenon.

CONCLUSIONS

The emphasis of this review has been concerned with the evidence for a role for the immune response in the development of and the severity of endometriosis. Clearly, the evidence for such a role appears compelling, albeit circumstantial. The possibility that the peritoneal 'disposal system' may function to eliminate misplaced endometrial cells is a hypothesis that has been advanced to explain the development of endometriosis. According to this concept, women with endometriosis have impaired ability of this 'disposal system', which is presumably mediated by either macrophages or peritoneal lymphocytes or both. Alternatively, it is possible that there are differences in the capacity of endometrial tissues to be destroyed even in immunocompetent environments. Whether such differences exist amongst endometrial tissues in women with endometriosis, and what the nature of those differences might be, is at present completely unknown and highly speculative. However, one fundamental aspect of those tissue differences might be a loss of immunogenicity. This could come about through a loss or an alteration of antigenic structures on endometrial tissues. While neither of these mechanisms is mutually exclusive, both are subject to testing. Similarly, the role of humoral responses in endometriosis needs to be further defined. Future studies must determine whether the autoantibodies observed in women with endometriosis are directly involved in the induction, maintenance, or exacerbation of the disease. Furthermore, such studies should determine whether the production of those antibodies is the result of a failure to maintain tolerance to endometrial antigens, or, alternatively, represents a necessary homeostatic mechanism to prevent the disease. Finally, the role of various lymphokines and monokines in facilitating or retarding endometrial tissue implantation or growth must be determined. If the above can be accomplished, then the prospects for better understanding of this enigmatic disease and for manipulating the immune response in favour of clinical disease control are quite good.

REFERENCES

1. Sampson, J.A. (1925). Heterotropic or misplaced endometrial tissue. *Am. J. Obstet. Gynecol.*, **10**, 649
2. Bartosik, D., Jacobs, S.L. and Kelly, L.J. (1986). Endometrial tissue in peritoneal fluid. *Fertil. Steril.*, **46**, 796–800
3. Wood, D.H., Yochmowitz, M.G., Salmon, Y.L., Eason, R.L. and Boster, R.A. (1983). Proton irradiation and endometriosis. *Aviat. Space Environ. Med.*, **54**, 718–724
4. Campbell, J.S., Wong, J., Tryphonas, L., Arnold, D.L., Nera, E., Cross, B. and LaBossiere, E. (1985). Is simian endometriosis an effect of immunotoxicity? Presented at the *Annual Meeting, Ontario Association of Pathology*, October 4, London, Ontario
5. Gleicher, N., El-Roeiy, A., Confino, E. and Friberg, J. (1987). Abnormal autoantibodies in endometriosis: Is endometriosis an autoimmune disease? *Obstet. Gynecol.*, **70**, 115–122
6. Dmowski, W.P., Gebel, H.M. and Rawlins, R.G. (1989). Immunologic aspects of endometriosis. *Obstet. Gynecol. Clin. North Am.*, **16**, 93–103
7. Engleman, E.G., Warnke, R., Fox, R.I., Dilley, S., Benili, C.J. and Levy, R. (1981). Studies of a human T lymphocyte antigen recognized by a monoclonal antibody. *Proc. Natl Acad. Sci., USA*, **78**, 1791–1795
8. Morimoto, C., Letvin, N., Boyd, A., Hagan, M., Brown, H., Kornacki, M. and Schlossman, S.F. (1985). The isolation and characterization of the human helper inducer cell subset. *J. Immunol.*, **134**, 3762–3769
9. Morimoto, C., Letvin, N., Distaso, J., Aldrich, W. and Schlossman, S.F. (1985). The isolation and characterization of the human suppressor inducer T cells subset. *J. Immunol.*, **134**, 1508–1515
10. Sanders, M.E., Makgoba, M.W. and Shaw, S. (1987). Human naive and memory T cells. *Immunol. Today*, **1**, 1–3
11. Damle, N.K. and Engleman, E.G. (1983). Immunoregulatory T cells circuits in man: alloantigen-primed T cells activate alloantigen-specific suppressor T cells in the absence of the initial antigen stimulus. *J. Exp. Med.*, **158**, 159–173
12. Landay, A., Gartland, G.L. and Clemant, L. (1983). Characterization of a phenotypically distinct subpopulation of Leu 2+ cells which suppress T cell proliferation responses. *J. Immunol.*, **131**, 2757–2761
13. Stashenko, P., Nadler, L.M., Hardy, R. and Scholssman, S.F. (1980). Characterization of

human B lymphocyte specific antigen. *J. Immunol.*, **125**, 1678–1685

14. Gadol, N. and Ault, K.A. (1986). Phenotypic and functional characterization of human Leu 1 (CD5) B cells. *Immunol. Rev.*, **93**, 23–24

15. Lydyard, P.M., Youinou, P.Y. and Cooke, A. (1987). CD5-positive B cells in rheumatoid arthritis and chronic lymphocytic leukemia. *Immunol. Today*, **8**, 37–38

16. Johnston, R. (1988). Monocytes and macrophages. *N. Engl. J. Med.*, **318**, 747–752

17. Basham, T., Smith, W., Lanier, L., Morhenn, U. and Merigan, T. (1984). Regulation of expression of class II major histocompatibility antigens on human peripheral blood monocytes and Langerhans cells by interferon. *Human Immunol.*, **10**, 83–93

18. Ades, E. and Lopez, C. (eds.) (1989). *Natural Killer Cells and Host Defense*. (San Francisco: Karger)

19. Cascon, P., Zoumbos, N. and Young, N. (1986). Analysis of natural killer cells in patients with aplastic anemia. *Blood*, **67**, 1349–1355

20. Bray, R.A., Gottschalk, L.R., Landay, A.L. and Gebel, H.M. (1987). Differential surface marker expression in patients with CD16+ lymphoproliferative disorders: In vivo model for NK differentiation. *Human Immunol.*, **19**, 105–115

21. Miller, J.F.A.P., Morahan, G. and Allison, J. (1989). Immunological tolerance; New approaches using transgenic mice. *Immunol. Today*, **10**, 53–57

22. Kappler, J.W., Roehm, N. and Marrack, P. (1987). T cell tolerance by clonal elimination in the thymus. *Cell*, **49**, 273–280

23. Sha, W.C., Nelson, C.S., Newberry, R.D., Kranz, D.M., Russell, J.H. and Loh, D.Y. (1988). Positive and negative selection of an antigen receptor on T cells in transgenic mice. *Nature*, **336**, 73–76

24. Goodnow, C.C., Crosbie, J., Adelstein, S., Lavoie, T.B., Smith-Gill, S.J., Brink, R.A., Pritchard-Briscoe, H., Wotherspoon, J.S., Loblay, R.H., Raphael, K., Trent, R.J. and Basten, A. (1988). Altered immunoglobulin expression and functional silencing of self-reactive B lymphocytes in transgenic mice. *Nature*, **334**, 676–682

25. Kisielow, P., Bluthmann, H., Staerz, U.D., Steinmetz, M. and von Boehmer, H. (1988). Tolerance in T-cell-receptor transgenic mice involves deletion of nonmature CD4+ 8+ thymocytes. *Nature*, **333**, 742–746

26. Arnold, B., Dill, O., Kublbeck, G., Jatsch, L., Simon, M.M., Tucker, J. and Hammerling, G.J. (1988). Alloreactive immune responses of transgenic mice expressing a foreign transplantation antigen in a soluble form. *Proc. Natl Acad. Sci., USA*, **85**, 2269–2273

27. Steele, R.W., Eichberg, J.W., Heberling, R.L., Kalter, S.S. and Kniker, W.T. (1977). Correlation of mixed lymphocyte reactivity and skin graft rejection in nonhuman primates. *J. Med. Primatol.*, **6**, 119–126

28. Shirai, M., Matsushita, S., Kagayama, M., Ichijo, S. and Takeuchi, M. (1966). Histological changes of the scrotal testis in unilateral cryptorchidism. *Tohoku J. Exp. Med.*, **90**, 363–373

29. Weksler, M.E., Moody, C.E. and Kozak, R.W. (1981). The autologous mixed lymphocyte reaction. *Adv. Immunol.*, **31**, 271–312

30. Engleman, E.G., Benike, C.J., Hoppe, R.T., Kaplan, H.S. and Berberich, F.R. (1980). Autologous mixed lymphocyte reaction in patients with Hodgkin's disease. Evidence for a T-cell defect. *J. Clin. Invest.*, **66**, 149–158

31. Sakane, T., Steinberg, A.P. and Green, I. (1978). Failure of autologous mixed lymphocyte reactions between T and non-T cells in patients with systemic lupus erythematosus. *Proc. Natl Acad. Sci., USA*, **75**, 3464

32. Startseva, N.V. (1980). Clinico-immunological aspects of genital endometriosis. *Akush. Ginekol. (Mosk.)*, **3**, 23–26

33. Weed, J.C. and Arguembourg, P.C. (1980). Endometriosis: can it produce an autoimmune response resulting in infertility? *Clin. Obstet. Gynecol.*, **23**, 885–893

34. Mathur, S., Peress, M.R., Williamson, H.O., Youmans, C.D., Maney, S.A., Garvin, A.J., Rust, P.F. and Fudenberg, H.H. (1982). Autoimmunity to endometrium and ovary in endometriosis. *Clin. Exp. Immunol.*, **50**, 259–266

35. Mathur, S., Chihal, H.J., Homm, R.J., Garza, D.E., Rust, P.F. and Williamson, H.O. (1988). Endometrial antigens involved in the autoimmunity of endometriosis. *Fertil. Steril.*, **50**, 860–863

36. Badawy, S.Z., Cuenca, V., Stitzel, A., Jacobs, R.D. and Tomar, R.H. (1984). Autoimmune

phenomena in infertile patients with endometriosis. *Obstet. Gynecol.*, **63**, 271–275
37. Kreiner, D., Fromowitz, F.B., Richardson, D.A. and Kenigsberg, D. (1986). Endometrial immunofluorescence associated with endometriosis and pelvic inflammatory disease. *Fertil. Steril.*, **46**, 243–245
38. Saifuddin, A., Buckley, C.H. and Fox, H. (1983). Immunoglobulin content of the endometrium in women with endometriosis. *Int. J. Gynecol. Pathol.*, **2**, 255–263
39. Wild, R.A. and Shivers, C.A. (1985). Antiendometrial antibodies in patients with endometriosis. *Am. J. Reprod. Immunol. Microbiol.*, **8**, 84–86
40. Cowchock, S., Smith, J.B. and Gocial, B. (1986). Autoantibodies to phospholipids and nuclear antigens in patients with repeated abortions. *Am. J. Obstet. Gynecol.*, **155**, 1002–1010
41. Gleicher, N., El-Roeiy, A., Confino, E. and Friberg, J. (1987). Autoantibodies in patients with unexplained infertility and recurrent pregnancy loss (abstract 249). Presented at the *34th Annual Meeting, Society for Gynecologic Investigation*, March 18–21, Atlanta, p. 153
42. El-Roeiy, A., Dmowski, W.P., Gleicher, N., Radwanska, E., Harlow, L., Binor, Z., Tummon, I. and Rawlins, R.G. (1988). Danazol but not gonadotropin-releasing hormone agonist suppresses autoantibodies in endometriosis. *Fertil. Steril.*, **50**, 864–871
43. Meek, S.C., Hodge, D.D. and Musich, J.R. (1988). Autoimmunity in infertile patients with endometriosis. *Am. J. Obstet. Gynecol.*, **158**, 1365–1373
44. Steele, R.W., Dmowski, W.P. and Marmer, D.J. (1984). Immunologic aspects of human endometriosis. *Am. J. Reprod. Immunol.*, **6**, 33–36
45. Pittaway, D.E. (1989). CA-125 in women with endometriosis. *Obstet. Gynecol. Clin. North Am.*, **16**, 273–252
46. Dmowski, W.P., Steele, R.W. and Baker, G.F. (1981). Deficient cellular immunity in endometriosis. *Am. J. Obstet. Gynecol.*, **141**, 377–383.
47. Gleicher, N., Dmowski, W.P., Siegel, I., Liu, T.L., Friberg, J., Radwanska, E. and Toder, V. (1984). Lymphocyte subsets in endometriosis. *Obstet. Gynecol.*, **63**, 463–466
48. Badawy, S.Z., Cuenca, V., Stitzel, A. and Tice, D. (1987). Immune rosettes of T and B lymphocytes in infertile women with endometriosis. *J. Reprod. Med.*, **32**, 194–197
49. Halme, J., Becker, S. and Wing, R. (1984). Accentuated cyclic activation of peritoneal macrophages in patients with endometriosis. *Am. J. Obstet. Gynecol.*, **148**, 85–90
50. Haney, A.F., Muscato, J.J. and Weinberg, J.B. (1981). Peritoneal fluid cell populations in infertility patients. *Fertil. Steril.*, **35**, 696–698
51. Zeller, J.M., Henig, I., Radwanska, E. and Dmowski, W.P. (1987). Enhancement of human monocyte and peritoneal macrophage chemiluminescence activities in women with endometriosis. *Am. J. Reprod. Immunol. Microbiol.*, **13**, 78–82
52. Fakih, H., Baggett, B., Holtz, G., Tsang, K.Y., Lee, J.C. and Williamson, H.O. (1987). Interleukin-1: a possible role in the infertility associated with endometriosis. *Fertil. Steril.*, **47**, 213–217
53. Kauma, S., Clark, M.R., White, C. and Halme, J. (1988). Production of fibronectin by peritoneal macrophages and concentration of fibronectin in peritoneal fluid from patients with or without endometriosis. *Obstet. Gynecol.*, **72**, 13–18
54. Parvizi, S.T., Jensen, P., DeCherney, A., Polan, M.L. and Comite, F. (1988). Elevated interleukin-1 (IL-1) synthesis by peripheral monocytes in endometriosis (abstract 450). Presented at the *35th Annual Meeting, Society for Gynecologic Investigation*, March 17–20, Baltimore, p. 284.
55. Halme, J., Becker, S. and Haskill, S. (1987). Altered maturation and function of peritoneal macrophages: possible role in pathogenesis of endometriosis. *Am. J. Obstet. Gynecol.*, **156**, 783–789
56. Ahn, Y.S., Harrington, W.J., Simon, S.R., Mylvaganam, R., Pall, L.M. and So, A.G. (1983). Danazol for the treatment of idiopathic thrombocytopenic purpura. *N. Engl. J. Med.*, **308**, 1396–1399
57. Agnello, V., Pariser, K., Gell, J., Gelfand, J. and Turksoy, R.N. (1983). Preliminary observations on danazol therapy of systemic lupus erythematosus: effects on DNA antibodies, thrombocytopenia and complement. *J. Rheumatol.*, **10**, 682–687
58. Gelfand, J.A., Sherins, R.J., Alling, D.W. and Frank, M.M. (1976). Treatment of hereditary angioedema with danazol: Reversal of clinical and biochemical abnormalities. *N. Engl. J. Med.*, **295**, 1444–1448

59. Gralnick, H.R. and Rick, M.E. (1983). Danazol increases Factor VIII and Factor IX in classic hemophilia and Christmas disease. *N. Engl. J. Med.*, **308**, 1393–1395
60. Mylvaganam, R., Ahn, Y.S., Harrington, W.J. and Kim, C.I. (1987). Immune modulation by danazol in autoimmune thrombocytopenia. *Clin. Immunol. Immunopathol.*, **42**, 281–287
61. Hill, J.A., Barbieri, R.L. and Anderson, D.J. (1987). Immunosuppressive effects of danazol in vitro. *Fertil. Steril.*, **48**, 414–418
62. Grimes, D.A., LeBolt, S.A., Grimes, K.R. and Wingo, P.A. (1985). Systemic lupus erythematosus and reproductive function: a case control study. *Am. J. Obstet. Gynecol.*, **153**, 179–186
63. Dmowski, W.P., Braun, D., Gebel, H., Rotman, C. and Madanes, A. Peripheral blood monocyte (PBM) and peritoneal macrophage (PM) cytotoxicity in women with endometriosis and the effect of danazol. 46th Annual Meeting of the American Fertility Society, Washington, D.C., October, 1990
64. Braun, D.P., Harris, J.E. and Rubenstein, M. (1984). Relationship of arachidonic acid metabolism to indomethacin sensitive immunoregulatory function and lymphocyte PGE sensitivity and peripheral blood mononuclear cells of disseminated solid tumor cancer patients. *J. Immunol. Pharmacol.*, **6**(3), 227–236

7
Endometriosis and infertility

E. J. Thomas

INTRODUCTION

It is axiomatic that before treatment of a disease can be justified it must be shown to confer benefit. Since the introduction of the laparoscope, clinicians have been diagnosing endometriosis in the infertile woman with increasing frequency. It is current practice to treat this either medically or surgically and yet perhaps the most controversial clinical problem with endometriosis is whether, if there is no mechanical damage, it has a causal relationship with infertility. The picture is further obscured by recent evidence that pelvic endometriosis is a more ubiquitous phenomenon than previously realized. It is quite possible that the finding of endometriosis is coincidental to the infertility.

This discussion is not academic. Various studies have reported the incidence of endometriosis in infertile women at laparoscopy as between 20% and 50%[1-5]. A population of 400 000 people will yield 472 new infertility referrals each year of which 6% are diagnosed as having endometriosis[6]. This is probably an underestimate as all the patients in this study did not have a laparoscopy. However, if the 6% figure is used, then approximately 4000 new cases of endometriosis will be diagnosed in infertile women in the United Kingdom each year, which increases to between 8000 and 9000 if all women with unexplained infertility have a laparoscopy. The comparable figure for the United States is up to 50 000 women per year. It is important to stress that most of these women will not have symptoms. For example, Thomas and Cooke[7] performed 99 laparoscopies in women with unexplained infertility in which endometriosis was visually diagnosed in 51. In only three women was the disease associated with mechanical damage and no patient was symptomatic. Current medical treatments are potently contraceptive, inappropriate in an infertile population, and all have side-effects. Therefore, to justify their use in infertile women, we must be able to show that they increase

113

fertility, because there is no other possible justification for their use in women without symptoms.

The aim of this chapter is to investigate the role of endometriosis in infertility and to examine critically the evidence that it is an important cause. Firstly, the mechanisms by which the disease may impede fertility mechanically will be described. This will be followed by an analysis of the experimental evidence that endometriosis causes infertility in animals. The hypothesized mechanisms by which endometriosis causes infertility in humans will be analysed. Next, the impact of therapy in benefiting future fertility will be examined. Finally, the current understanding of the natural history of endometriosis will be described. The overall aim is to place the treatment of endometriosis in the infertile woman in context, critically examining whether there is any need for it.

MECHANICAL DAMAGE

Although there may be some debate about the role of filmy peritubal or periovarian adhesions in infertility, there would be unanimous agreement that endometriosis, especially moderate to severe disease, can cause significant damage to the fallopian tubes, ovaries and peritoneal mesothelium. This damage can result in tubal occlusion or fimbrial damage. It can cause dense peritubal adhesions that severely limit the ability of the fimbria to retrieve oocytes. It can cause dense periovarian adhesions that may immobilize completely the ovaries as well as damage ovarian tissue directly by the formation of cysts. It may be that endometriosis causes damage locally by disrupting tissue with its physical presence or by inflammation or by the release of prostaglandins or other factors. Whether it is one or a combination of these mechanisms, the end result is serious compromise of fertility. The treatment of choice in this situation must be surgical. Unlike pelvic infection, endometriosis does not usually cause major damage to the tubal epithelium and good success rates can be expected if the correct surgical techniques are used. These techniques are described elsewhere in this book. Whether adjunctive medical therapy should be prescribed and if so whether before or after surgery and for how long has not been resolved in the literature and appears to be a matter of individual preference. This is addressed in more detail by Barbieri elsewhere in this book.

EXPERIMENTAL ANIMAL EVIDENCE

Before analysing data in the human, I would briefly like to discuss the evidence showing that experimental endometriosis adversely affects fertility in animals. There is good evidence to show that experimental endometriosis will cause periovarian and peritubal adhesions that will mechanically impede fertility[8]. Schenken et al. reported abnormalities in the concentrations of peritoneal fluid prostaglandins in monkeys with experimental endometriosis[9]. Abnormalities of ovulation including the luteinized unruptured follicle syndrome (LUF), have been described in both monkeys[10] and rabbits[11]. Recent evidence has shown less ovulation points in rabbits with experimental ovarian endometriosis[12] that was not related to mechanical damage. Autoimmune abnormalities have been described in monkeys[13]. An embryotoxic effect has been reported in rabbits, both in those with the experimental disease and in normal animals injected with the peritoneal fluid from the experimental animals[14]. There is, however, conflicting evidence that shows no change in the previously described mechanisms in rabbits with experimental endometriosis[15]. The same authors could also find no effect of the presence of endometriosis on subsequent embryonic cleavage[16] and concluded that the likely impact of the disease was on implantation.

Although there is some conflict, good evidence exists that the disease will affect fertility when experimentally induced in animals. This would appear to provide a firm basis from which to hypothesize that similar consequences of the disease can be expected in humans. However, care should be taken before concluding too much from these data. It is important to remember that experimental endometriosis in animals is created by placing normal endometrium in extrauterine locations. There is increasing evidence in humans that endometriosis differs greatly from endometrium in morphology[17-19], in oestrogen and progesterone receptor expression[20,21] and in endocrine function[22]. It cannot, therefore, be considered as just ectopic endometrium. It is logical that the converse of this must also hold true, namely that normal endometrium placed in ectopic locations cannot be considered to behave in the same manner as endometriosis. I believe that this, taken in combination with the fact that these are animal models, means that care should be taken before extrapolating the data to the human. The observations are further compromised by the fact that spontaneous endometriosis has only been reported in the monkey and then at a low incidence[23]. It has not been reported in any of the other animals, especially the rabbit or the mouse, which undermines the relevance of these as models.

MECHANISMS BY WHICH ENDOMETRIOSIS MAY CAUSE INFERTILITY

In this next part of the chapter I shall review individually those mechanisms through which endometriosis has been postulated to cause infertility. I shall analyse the data that support and negate them and also address the biological plausibility of the mechanism. I shall only investigate those mechanisms that do not cause mechanical impediment to fertility because, as I have already discussed, there is little debate that this is a cause of infertility.

The following have been promoted as possible mechanisms:

- genetic predisposition;
- abnormalities of reproductive hormones;
- adverse factors in the peritoneal fluid;
- immune abnormalities;
- abnormal oocytes;
- increased spontaneous abortions.

GENETIC PREDISPOSITION

It has been shown that endometriosis is significantly ($p < 0.05$) more common in the first-degree relatives of patients with the disease[24,25]. A polygenic or multifactorial mode of inheritance is postulated. Although good evidence about a genetic predisposition to infertility has not been reported, it can be hypothesized that there is a link between those genes that control fertility and those that are involved in the phenotypic expression we recognize as endometriosis. In this case we would expect to see endometriosis more commonly in infertile women without the relationship being causal. In line with current understanding of genetic inheritance, such a hypothesis is plausible.

ENDOCRINE ABNORMALITIES

When analysing the considerable literature on endocrine abnormalities in endometriosis it is important to bear in mind some basic concepts. Firstly, the description of an endocrine abnormality does not prove that it is a cause of infertility *in vivo*. Secondly, in order to establish a causal link, such abnormalities should be shown to be consistently more common in endo-metriosis than in other infertile groups. Thirdly, the abnormalities should be shown to occur consistently from menstrual cycle to menstrual cycle, otherwise there is no evidence that they would significantly impair fertility over a long period of time. The three main areas in which endometriosis could affect endocrine function are in the hypothalamic–pituitary axis, in the developing follicle and in the corpus luteum.

Hypothalamic–pituitary axis

Cheeseman *et al.*[26] reported a bifid luteinizing hormone (LH) surge with daily urine monitoring in 26 out of 29 patients with endometriosis. In comparison with fertile controls there was an initial attenuated LH surge followed by a further surge 2–3 days later. This same abnormality was described in 2 out of 12 women with endometriosis monitored carefully throughout the cycle and compared with 6 fertile controls[27]. In a further 5 women there were elevated LH levels in the follicular phase; the remaining 7 showed no differences. It is not resolved in these papers whether these patients had other endocrine or ultrasound stigmata of polycystic ovary syndrome which would also explain the findings.

Raised plasma prolactin concentrations have been reported in women with endometriosis[28,29] and a controlled study showed the level after stimulation with thyrotropin-releasing hormone to be about twice that of women with unexplained infertility[30], although this did not reach statistical significance. An exaggerated and prolonged nocturnal peak of prolactin secretion has also been reported[31].

The follicle

The two main mechanisms by which endometriosis may affect follicular function are either by altering its growth or by changing the timing or quality of follicular rupture. Using a combination of temporal abnormalities of the menstrual cycle, abnormal endometrial biopsy, basal body temperature charts, ovarian morphology and negative progestogen withdrawal, anovulation was described in 17% of 350 cases[32] and 10.5% of 362 cases[33] of endometriosis. Women with endometriosis have been reported to have more and smaller follicles at the LH surge than normal controls[34]. However, there appear to be no reports of abnormal oestrogen secretion in women with endometriosis so caution must be exercised in concluding that endometriosis directly affects the function of the growing follicle. This is especially true because all the studies are on small numbers of patients — an inevitable consequence of the number of complex investigations required to adequately describe the menstrual cycle.

Much more work has been reported on abnormalities of follicular rupture, especially the luteinized unruptured follicle syndrome (LUF). In this latter syndrome, there is an apparently normal cycle both temporally and endocrino-logically, but following the LH surge there is no follicular rupture. The unruptured follicle does, however, behave like a normal corpus luteum, producing a picture of ovulatory infertility. The first reports made the diagnosis by observing the absence of an ovulation stigma on the corpus luteum at laparoscopy. Brosens et al.[35] reported absent stigma in 79% of 29 patients with endometriosis. Further evidence showed a higher incidence in moderate and severe disease compared with minimal endometriosis[36] and also a higher incidence (75%) than in fertile controls (21%)[37]. These observations combined with reported changes in the ovarian steroid concentrations in the peritoneal fluid led to the thesis that LUF was the cause of endometriosis[38,39]. However, criticisms of the specificity and reproducibility of the visual diagnosis were raised. Two controlled studies failed to find an association of LUF with endometriosis[40,41] and evidence was presented that the diagnosis could be frequently made in fertile women[42] and at laparoscopy in the luteal phase of conception cycles[43].

These uncertainties led investigators to use an ultrasound diagnosis of absent follicular rupture instead. A low incidence of LUF was described in apparently normal women[44] and, initially, a high incidence in those women with endometriosis[45]. However, more detailed studies combining ultrasonography with endocrine data have been unable to substantiate this finding[34,46,47]. In conclusion, there is little substantial evidence of an increased incidence of LUF in endometriosis and this negates the hypothesis that it causes the disease, although the hypothesis is appealing.

The corpus luteum

Grant first reported abnormalities of the luteal phase in 43 women out of 96 with endometriosis[48]. The diagnosis was made by abnormal basal body temperature charts or the presence of dysmature endometrium biopsied in the luteal phase. Recently there have been reports of a low mean mid-luteal phase progesterone concentration in 14 patients with endometriosis[29] and a slower rise in the luteal phase plasma progesterone concentration in 29 patients compared with 18 controls[26]. In the latter study the maximal luteal phase plasma progesterone was lower in the endometriosis group but this did not reach statistical significance. Most recently, Ayers et al.[49] showed that in 13 patients compared with 25 controls there was higher secretion of progesterone in the follicular phase. They suggested that this was due to a failure of luteolysis in endometriosis, which caused ovulatory asynchrony.

However, conflicting evidence has been produced that shows no abnormalities in the luteal phase in endometriosis. Radwanska and Dmowski[50] were unable to show any difference in mean luteal phase plasma progesterone concentration in 26 endometriotic patients compared with 28 controls. A larger study compared 68 patients with 75 controls and was unable to detect any difference in the rates of luteal phase defects, these being 9% and 5% respectively[51]. This lack of difference was also shown in 27 patients compared with 50 controls[52] and also in endometriotic patients on in vitro fertilization programmes when compared with those with tubal disease[53].

In conclusion, the weight of experimental evidence does not support reproductive endocrine abnormalities as the cause of infertility in endometriosis. With current knowledge it is difficult to explain how endometriosis may mediate these effects. It is most logical to assume that they occur secondarily to direct effects on the ovary, although the other possibility is that the disease secretes humoral signals that directly influence the hypothalamic–pituitary axis. There is some evidence that LH receptor expression is abnormal in the follicles and corpora lutea of women with endometriosis[54]. There is also evidence that peritoneal macrophages from women with endometriosis may modulate the secretion of progesterone from granulosa and luteal cells[55]. The importance of these observations remains to be proved. Overall the evidence in all aspects of reproductive endocrinology is conflicting and it is unknown whether any of these defects translates into decreased fertility in vivo.

ADVERSE FACTORS IN THE PERITONEAL FLUID

Many workers have investigated the peritoneal fluid and its contents as possible mediators of infertility in endometriosis. The subject is comprehensively reviewed by Bradley and Rock elsewhere in this volume and repetition serves no value. They describe changes in the volume of fluid and in the concentration of prostanoids and other peritoneal fluid proteins. They also describe changes in the activity of macrophages, growth factors, interleukins and lymphokines. However, they stress that overall much of the data is conflicting or that there are methodological difficulties in the studies. The inevitable conclusion is that there is little good evidence to show that the environment of the peritoneal fluid is causal in infertility.

It is interesting to speculate how this environment might affect fertility. Although sperm survival studies are interesting there is little evidence that fertilization is influenced by the peritoneal fluid. It occurs in the ampulla of the tube by sperm that will not have entered the peritoneal cavity. It is difficult to see how experimental sperm toxicity of peritoneal fluid is valid. The same criticism can be made of studies showing peritoneal fluid to be toxic to embryos. Perhaps the most appealing hypothesis is that the peritoneal fluid affects fimbrial function, which decreases the chance of successful oocyte retrieval. Suginami et al.[56] showed with an in vitro model in the golden hamster that fimbrial function disappeared more quickly in the presence of peritoneal fluid from women with endometriosis compared with controls. They postulated the presence of an 'oocyte capture inhibitor' to explain this. They later reported the finding of a membrane coating the fimbria when exposed to endometriotic peritoneal fluid[57]. Removal of this membrane by flushing appeared to restore fimbrial function. Although using an animal model, these observations provide an interesting possibility for a mechanism of infertility in endometriosis.

IMMUNE ABNORMALITIES

The role of immune abnormalities in the pathogenesis and maintenance of endometriosis is fully reviewed by Dmowski, Braun and Gebel elsewhere in this volume and, again, repetition serves no purpose. In summary, they report abnormalities in humoral and cell-mediated immunity in endometriosis and also in the immune function of macrophages in the peritoneal fluid. However, in view of the limitations of the available evidence, it cannot be extrapolated that any of these abnormalities are causal in infertility. It could be hypothesized that anti-endometrial antibodies impair implantation of the embryo. It is also possible that the immune abnormalities create an environment that is hostile to the fertilization of the oocyte and to the survival and development of an early pregnancy. Until more is known about the role of the immune system in normal reproduction and pregnancy, it will be difficult to prove that there is an immune mechanism in the infertility associated with endometriosis.

ABNORMAL OOCYTES

Fertilization rates in vitro allow a partially quantitative evaluation of oocyte function and normality. Wardle et al.[58] compared the fertilization rates per oocyte and per couple in patients with endometriosis with those in couples with unexplained infertility and tubal damage. They reported that the rate was significantly lower for both in the endometriotic patients ($p < 0.001$). They further reported improvement in the fertilization rate following treatment of the disease[59]. They concluded that there may be an unknown functional defect of the oocyte that could mediate the infertility. Since the publication of these reports there have been many studies of the effect of endometriosis on fertilization rates in IVF programmes (see later) and most fail to substantiate this finding. On balance, therefore, there is no definite evidence of an intrinsic abnormality in oocytes.

SPONTANEOUS ABORTIONS

An apparently higher risk of first-trimester miscarriage in women with endometriosis has been reported. Abortion rates of 46%[60] and 44.3%[61] have been described in retrospective studies of 65 and 263 patients with endometriosis. Petersohn[62] reported a 22% abortion rate that dropped to 8% following surgical therapy. In 65 patients a drop from 46% to 8% was reported following surgery[61]. There are methodological criticisms of these studies, especially as they tend to be retrospective and poorly controlled. More recent work has concluded that the high abortion rates can be explained by factors other than endometriosis[63]. This finding is confirmed by Regan *et al.*[64] who found, in a prospective study of 630 women, that the most important predictive factor for spontaneous abortion was the woman's past reproductive performance. As the previous reproductive performance will be an important confounding variable in patients with endometriosis, it is not possible to conclude that miscarriage is a mechanism for infertility.

IMPACT OF TREATMENT OF ENDOMETRIOSIS ON FUTURE FERTILITY

From the preceding section it can be seen that there are many postulated mechanisms by which endometriosis may cause infertility. However, there is virtually no evidence to show that any are causal *in vivo*. This is due to the major methodological difficulties of demonstrating this experimentally. In order to investigate the relationship further it is necessary to approach the problem from a different angle by reviewing the literature to see whether the treatment of endometriosis has been demonstrated to benefit future fertility. If this proves to be so, it is reasonable to conclude that the disease is causal in infertility.

There are many studies that appear to demonstrate a clear benefit to future fertility by treating endometriosis. These studies have major methodological problems in that they are either retrospective or uncontrolled. Often they quote pregnancy rates alone and make no attempt to relate these to the time required to conceive. Fertility can be defined as the chance of conception in a single menstrual cycle or the fecundability rate. In population terms this is best presented as a cumulative conception rate (CCR)[65]. Furthermore, interpretation of most of the pregnancy data is further complicated by the poor selection methods used for patients. In many studies the patients have other infertility factors and it is, therefore, impossible to calculate how important is the contribution of the endometriosis. For the sake of brevity, only those studies will be reviewed that are prospective, employ a control group who are not treated, have reasonable patient selection criteria and use the correct parameters for describing fertility.

The first prospective, randomized and controlled study appeared in 1982[66]. Sixty-five patients with minimal endometriosis were randomly allocated to either 6 months of danazol or 6 months of no treatment. There was no statistical difference in the pregnancy rates between the two groups. Eleven patients in the danazol group and 14 of those with no treatment had no other apparent infertility factors and the pregnancy rates were 36% in the treated and 57% in the non-treated groups. The same authors increased the size of the groups with no other infertility factors to 37 in the danazol group and 36 with no treatment and reported their findings in 1988[67]. The 12-month CCR was 37% in the danazol group and 57% in the non-treatment group. This difference was not statistically significant. Hull et al.[68] compared three groups of infertile patients who had no major explanation for their infertility except endometriosis. Thirty-six were allocated to medroxypro-gesterone acetate (MPA), 52 to danazol and 56 received no treatment. The CCR after 30 months was 71% in the MPA, 46% in the danazol and 55% in the control groups; none of these percentages was statistically significant. Badawy et al. were also unable to demonstrate any difference between danazol and expectant management in the effect on fertility[69].

There are only two studies that have used a placebo-controlled group. Thomas and Cooke[7] compared 20 patients treated with gestrinone for 6 months with 17 given placebo. The patients had been carefully selected so that they had no other explanation for their infertility except the presence of small amounts of asymptomatic endometriosis. The CCR at 12 months was 25% in the treatment and 30% in the placebo group. The absence or presence of residual endometriosis at the second laparoscopy did not affect future fertility and all the groups had a similar CCR to that of 23% in 26 women with unexplained infertility used as controls. Telimaa[70] reported results in three groups of patients; 18 prescribed danazol, 17 given MPA and 14 given placebo. Patient selection was not as rigorous as that by Thomas and Cooke, in that laparoscopic ablation of endometriosis was performed in some patients and there were 12 male partners with abnormal semen analysis. However, the 30-month CCR was 33% in the danazol, 42% in the MPA and 46% in the placebo group.

Controlled studies of the effect of surgical ablation of endometriotic deposits on future fertility are rare. A very recent study[71] compared the pregnancy rates after treatment of minimal endometriosis with danazol, laser ablation or a combination of both. There was no difference in the pregnancy rates whatever technique was used. The technique of laser laparoscopy, which is described by Sutton elsewhere in this book, is becoming more common. Although there are many obvious difficulties in controlling a laparoscopic study, including the ethical problem of sham operating, the data reported by Chong et al.[71] underline the need for such projects. This is especially important because there are other actions undertaken at laser laparoscopy, such as tubal insufflation and removal of the peritoneal fluid, which may benefit future fertility separately from ablation of the lesion.

At present it can only be concluded that no study that has been properly controlled has been able to show that the medical treatment of endometriosis improves future fertility. One[7] has also shown that successful treatment does not improve fertility compared with residual endometriosis or unexplained infertility. It is important to stress that all these studies are small and there is potential for a large false negative effect. It cannot, therefore, be said that treatment of endometriosis does not confer a small benefit to future fertility. Conversely, it is as likely to confer a small detriment and the fact that none of the studies has been able to demonstrate a positive benefit inevitably leads to the conclusion that no causal relationship between endometriosis and infertility has been proved.

One further exercise to investigate the relationship between infertility and endometriosis is to analyse the success rates of IVF, GIFT and donor insemination programmes and see whether the presence of the disease alters this. An initial report showing that endometriosis affects fertilization rates has already been discussed[58]. Since then there have been conflicting reports. Some authors report that there is a decreased success rate in patients with endometriosis compared with unexplained infertility[72] and others show the difference only in women with severe disease and explain that by the lower number of oocytes collected because of the mechanical difficulties[73]. These latter authors were unable to demonstrate any difference in the oestradiol or progesterone profiles in the follicular and luteal phases in patients with the disease compared to controls. Many other reports show no difference in success rates[74-77]. The balance of evidence favours the conclusion that the presence of endometriosis does not influence success on IVF/GIFT programmes unless there is mechanical damage. There are statistical limitations to all of these studies since the numbers of patients are small, so the same reservations as expressed before must apply. Jansen compared fertility between women with minimal endometriosis and those with no disease on a donor insemination programme[78] and there was a statistically better fecundability in the normal women. This is an important observation, although it must be noted that there is no detailed description of the indications for donor insemination. Conception rates after donor insemination are much higher in the partners of men with azoospermia than in those with oligozoospermia. As there were only seven patients in the minimal endometriosis group, there is a possibility that the semen characteristics of the men may have been different from those in the control group, thus biasing the results.

Clinicians are now faced with major dilemma because although they feel that there is a causal relationship between endometriosis and infertility it is not possible to demonstrate it *in vivo*. Furthermore, it has not been possible to demonstrate that any of the postulated mechanisms actually cause infertility *in vivo*. One argument could be that medical treatment does not completely obliterate endometriosis, that it continues to influence fertility, and that is why there is no effect of treatment. This is a possibility, although the comparability of pregnancy rates with women with unexplained infertility questions the validity of this. Whether this is true or not, there is still no evidence that medical treatment is of any benefit to future fertility and, therefore, there is little justification for prescribing it. This is especially true because the medication is potently contraceptive and has significant side-effects. However, it is known that these agents are effective in the treatment of endometriosis and before recommending that medication is not prescribed it is important to ensure that patients will not suffer from deterioration of the disease. To explore this problem further it is necessary to review our knowlege of the natural history of endometriosis and the effect of the drug therapy upon it.

THE IMPACT OF MEDICAL THERAPY UPON THE NATURAL HISTORY OF ENDOMETRIOSIS

The published literature describing the natural history of endometriosis is limited. This is because prior to the introduction of laparoscopy only symptomatic disease was treated and the symptoms could be used to define the progress of the disease and the effectiveness of therapy. Since laparoscopy, it has been possible to regularly visualize the effect of drugs on the disease. However, until the late 1980s no workers had verified that treatment had a beneficial effect compared to natural history of the disease. Telimaa et al.[79] reported a placebo-controlled trial of danazol and medroxyprogesterone acetate in which they showed that the disease deteriorated in 23% of those on placebo, which did not occur on either of the treatments. It only improved in 18% of those on placebo as compared with 60% of those on danazol and 63% of those on MPA. However, some of these patients also had laparoscopic electrocoagulation initially as treatment and therefore it is not a pure observation of the natural history of the phenomenon. Only one study has reported a placebo group that had no other treatment. Thomas and Cooke[80] performed a double-blind, randomized, placebo-controlled trial of gestrinone in asymptomatic endometriosis in infertile women. All patients had a pretreatment laparoscopy at which the disease was scored using the original American Fertility Society (AFS) score[81], and then a repeat laparoscopy in the final week of treatment. There was a significantly greater improvement in the treatment group compared with placebo. No patient on treatment deteriorated, whilst 8 out of the 17 on placebo did. In 3 this deterioration included the appearance of new periovarian and peritubal adhesions that may have mechanically impacted on fertility. The conclusion of this study was that the natural history of endometriosis was to deteriorate, that this deterioration was unpredictable, and therefore that there was good reason to treat on the finding of asymptomatic endometriosis even if it did not improve fertility.

However, there has been further evidence published that questions the validity of this recommendation. The frequency of the diagnosis of endometriosis appears to be increasing as our sensitivity to the visual diagnosis heightens. Dodge et al.[82] reported a high incidence of endometriosis in women presenting for reversal of sterilization who did not have the disease at the original procedure. This is a group that would previously have been expected to have a low incidence because of tubal occlusion and highlights the increased possibilities of diagnosis if the operator is alert and prepared to look carefully. Murphy et al.[83] described the microscopic finding of endometriosis in peritoneal mesothelium that had appeared normal when biopsied. Evidence was then presented that if great care was taken in selecting the site of biopsy then microscopic endometriosis did not appear[84]. These papers are not contradictory: one shows that random biopsies will demonstrate microscopic endometriosis while the other shows that you have to look very carefully not to find the disease. The final conclusion is still that the disease is common in the pelvic peritoneum and may be able to be found in all women if searched for rigorously.

A review article reported a frequency of 20% of the finding of pelvic endometriosis in patients with unexplained infertility who had a further laparoscopy 2 years after a normal laparoscopy[85]. This suggests that endometriosis may be constantly appearing and disappearing in the pelvis. Perhaps most important is the observation that the impact of medical therapy in endometriosis is only temporary. Evers[86] divided women who had equivalent amounts of endometriosis at the initial laparoscopy into two groups. The first group had the repeat laparoscopy in the final week of treatment and the second had the procedure delayed until the follicular phase of the second menstrual cycle after treatment was stopped. Resolution of the disease was significantly less in the second group, suggesting that the disease is not removed by medical therapy but is simply suppressed and reappears when oestrogen stimulation returns. All this new evidence makes it difficult to justify the medical therapy for asymptomatic endometriosis when the disease appears ubiquitous, is not removed by the treatment, and does not improve fertility.

CONCLUSIONS

The nature of the relationship between endometriosis and infertility remains unresolved. The balance of evidence is that, apart from mechanical damage, endometriosis does not cause infertility. The current knowledge of the natural history of the disease and the impact of drug therapy upon it does not allow us to recommend that the finding of endometriosis *per se* requires treatment. There is no proof that the medical or surgical treatment of endometriosis benefits future fertility unless it involves the lysis of peritubal or periovarian adhesions or the removal of ovarian endometriomas. The combination of these observations means that the use of therapy for asymptomatic disease in the infertile population cannot be justified, especially as it is contraceptive.

There seems little point in repeating drug trials of endometriosis in infertility. Research into the disease should now be focused towards an elucidation of its pathogenesis, its tissue of origin and the control of its growth. Only by such research will the significance of the visual finding of endometriosis be able to be placed in context.

REFERENCES

1. Strathy, J.H., Molgaard, C.A., Coulam, C.B. and Melton, L.J. (1982). Endometriosis and infertility: a laparoscopic study of endometriosis among fertile and infertile women. *Fertil. Steril.*, **38**, 667–672
2. Hasson, H.M. (1976). Incidence of endometriosis in diagnostic laparoscopy. *J. Reprod. Med.*, **16**, 135–135
3. Petersohn, E.P. and Behrman, S.J. (1970). Laparoscopy of the infertile patient. *Obstet. Gynecol.*, **36**, 363–367
4. Drake, T.S. and Grunert, G.M. (1980). The unsuspected pelvic factor in the infertility investigation. *Fertil. Steril*, **34**, 27–31
5. Goldenberg, R.L. and Magendantz, H.G. (1976). Laparoscopy and the infertility investigation. *Obstet. Gynecol.*, **47**, 410–414
6. Hull, M.G.R., Glazener, C.M.A., Kelly, N.J., Conway, D.I., Foster, P.A., Hinton, R.A., Coulson, C., Lambert, P.A., Watt, E. and Desai, K.M. (1985). Population study of causes,

treatment and outcome of infertility. *Br. Med. J.*, **291**, 1693–1697

7. Thomas, E.J. and Cooke, I.D. (1987). Successful treatment of asymptomatic endometriosis. Does it benefit infertile women? *Br. Med. J.*, **294**, 1117–1119

8. Schenken, R.S. and Asch, R.J. (1980). Surgical induction of endometriosis in the rabbit: Effects on fertility and concentrations of peritoneal fluid prostaglandins. *Fertil. Steril.*, **34**, 581–587

9. Schenken, R.S., Asch, R.J., Williams, R.F. and Hodgen, G.D. (1984). Etiology of infertility in monkeys with infertility: measurement of peritoneal fluid prostaglandins. *Am. J. Obstet. Gynecol.*, **150**, 349–353

10. Schenken, R.S., Asch, R.J., Williams, R.F. and Hodgen, G.D. (1984). Etiology of infertility in monkeys with endometriosis. Luteinized unruptured follicles, luteal phase defects, pelvic adjesions and spontaneous abortions. *Fertil. Steril*, **41**, 122–130.

11. Donnez, J., Wayemberg, M., Casanas-Roux, F., Karaman, Y., Willems, T. and Ferin, J. (1987). Effect on ovulation of surgically induced endometriosis in rabbits. *Gynecol. Obstet. Invest.*, **24**, 131–137

12. Kaplan, C.R., Eddy, C.A., Olive, D.L. and Schenken, R.S. (1989). Effect of ovarian endometriosis on ovulation in rabbits. *Am. J. Obstet. Gynecol.*, **160**, 40–44

13. Dmowski, W.P., Steele, R.W. and Baker, G.F. (1981). Deficient cellular immunity in endometriosis. *Am. J. Obstet. Gynecol.*, **141**, 377–383

14. Hahn, D.W., Carraher, R.P., Foldesy, R.G. and McGuire, J.L. (1986). Experimental evidence for failure to implant as a mechanism of infertility associated with endometriosis. *Am. J. Obstet. Gynecol.*, **155**, 1109–1113

15. Dunselman, G.A., Land, J.A., Bouckaert, P.X. and Evers, J.L. (1988). Effect of endometriosis on ovulation, ovum pickup, fertilization and tubal transport in the rabbit. *J. Reprod. Fertil.*, **82**, 193–197

16. Dunselman, G.A., Land, J.A., Dumoulin, J.C., Bouckaert, P.X. and Evers, J.L. (1988). Effect of endometriosis on early embryonic development in the rabbit. *Hum. Reprod.*, **3**, 459–461

17. Roddick, J.W., Conkey, G. and Jacobs, E.J. (1960). The hormonal response of endometrium in endometriotic implants and its relationship to symptomatology. *Am. J. Obstet. Gynecol.*, **79**, 1173–1177

18. Schweppe, K.W. and Wynn, R.M. (1981). Ultrastructural changes in endometriotic implants during the menstrual cycle. *Obstet. Gynecol.*, **58** 465–473

19. Vasquez, G., Cornillie, F. and Brosens, I.A. (1984). Peritoneal endometriosis. screening electron mircroscopy and histology of pelvic endometriotic lesions. *Fertil. Steril.*, **42**, 696–703

20. Janne, O., Kaupilla, A., Kokko, E., Lantto, T., Ronnberg, L. and Vikho, R. (1981). Estrogen and progesterone receptors in endometriosis tissue. Comparison with endometrial tissue. *Am. J. Obstet. Gynecol.*, **141**, 562–566

21. Gould, S.F., Shannon, J.M. and Cunha, G.R. (1983). Nuclear estrogen binding sites in human endometriosis. *Fertil Steril.*, **39**, 520–524

22. Haney, A.F., Handwerger, S. and Weinberg, J.B. (1984). Peritoneal fluid prolactin in infertile women with endometriosis: lack of secretory activity by endometrial implants. *Fertil. Steril.*, **42**, 935–938

23. McKenzie, W.F., Splitter, G.A. and Valerio, M.G. (1972). Endometriosis in primates. In *Medical Primatology*, Part 1, pp. 288–297. (Basel: Karger)

24. Simpson, J.L., Elias, S., Malinak, L.R. and Buttram, V.C. (1980). Hereditable aspects of endometriosis. 1. Genetic studies. *Am. J. Obstet. Gynecol.*, **137**, 327–331

25. Malinak, L.R., Buttram, V.C., Elias, S. and Buttram, V.C. (1980). Hereditable aspects of endometriosis. *Am. J. Obstet. Gynecol.*, **137**, 332–336

26. Cheeseman, K.L., Ben-Nun, I., Chatterton, R.T. and Cohen, M.R. (1982). The relationship of luteinizing hormone, pregnanediol-3-glucuronide and estriol-16-glucuronide in the urine of infertile women with endometriosis. *Fertil Steril.*, **38**, 542–548

27. Vaughan-Williams, C.A., Oak, M.K. and Elstein, M. (1987). Gonadotrophin reponses to oestrogen provocation in women with minimal endometriosis. *Clin. Reprod. Fertil.*, **5**, 119–126

28. Hirschowitz, J.S., Soler, N.G. and Worstman, J. (1978). The galactorrhea–endometriosis syndrome. *Lancet*, **1**, 896–898

29. Hargrove, J.T. and Abraham, G.E. (1980). Abnormal luteal function in endometriosis. *Fertil. Steril.*, **34**, 302

30. Muse, K., Wilson, E.A. and Jawad, M.J. (1982). Prolactin hyperstimulation in response to thyrotropin-releasing hormone in patients with endometriosis. *Fertil. Steril.*, **38**, 419–422

31. Radwanska, E., Henig, I. and Dmowski, W.P. (1987). Nocturnal prolactin levels in women with endometriosis. *J. Reprod. Med.*, **32**, 605–605

32. Soules, M.R., Malinak, L.R., Bury, R. and Poindexter, A. (1976). Endometriosis and anovulation: A coexisting problem in the infertile female. *Am. J. Obstet. Gynecol.*, **125**, 412–415

33. Dmowski, W.P., Chen, M.R. and Wilhelm, J.L. (1976). Endometriosis and ovulatory failure: Does it occur? Should ovulatory stimulating agents be used? In Greenblatt, R. (ed.) *Recent Advances in Endometriosis*, pp. 129–136. Excerpta Medica, International Congress Series, No. 368. (Amsterdam: Excerpta Medica)

34. Tummon, I.S., Maclin, V.M., Radwanska, E., Binor, Z. and Dmowski, W.P. (1987). Occult ovulatory dysfunction in women with minimal endometriosis or unexplained infertility. *Fertil. Steril.*, **50**, 716–720

35. Brosens, I.A., Koninckx, P.R. and Corvelyn, P.A. (1978). A study of plasma progesterone, oestradiol-17-beta, prolactin and LH levels, and of the luteal phase appearance of the ovaries in patients with endometriosis and infertility. *Br. J. Obstet. Gynaecol.*, **85**, 246–250

36. Donnez, J. and Thomas, K. (1982). Incidence of the luteinized unruptured follicle syndrome in fertile women and in women with endometriosis. *Eur. J. Obstet. Gynecol. Reprod. Biol.*, **14**, 187–190

37. Lesorgen, P.R., Wu, C.H., Green, W., Gocial, B. and Lerner, L.J. (1984). Peritoneal fluid and serum steroids in infertility patients. *Fertil. Steril.*, **42**, 237–242

38. Koninckx, P.R., Ide, P., Vanderbroucke, W. and Brosens, I.A. (1980). New aspects of the pathophysiology of endometriosis and associated infertility. *J. Reprod. Med.*, **24**, 247–260

39. Koninckx, P.R. and Brosens, I.A. (1982). The luteinized unruptured follicle syndrome. *Obstet. Gynaecol. Annu.*, **11**, 175–186

40. Dmowski, W.P., Rao, R. and Scommegna, A. (1980). The luteinized unruptured follicle syndrome and endometriosis. *Fertil. Steril.*, **33**, 30–34

41. Dhont, M., Serryn, R., Duvivier, P., Vanluchene, E., De Boevor, J. and Vanderkerkhove, D. (1984). Ovulation stigma and concentration of progesterone and estradiol in peritoneal fluid: relation with fertility and endometriosis. *Fertil. Steril.*, **41**, 872–877

42. Vanrell, J.A., Balasch, J., Fuster, J.S. and Fuster, R. (1982). Ovulation stigma in fertile women. *Fertil. Steril.*, **37**, 712–713

43. Portuondo, J.A., Pena, J., Otaola, C. and Echanojauregui, A.D. (1981). Absence of ovulation stigma in the conception cycle. *Int. J. Fertil.*, **28**, 52–54

44. Kerin, J.F., Kirby, C., Morris, D., McEvoy, M., Ward, B. and Cox, L.W. (1983). Incidence of the luteinized unruptured follicle syndrome in cycling women. *Fertil. Steril.*, **40**, 620–626

45. Liukonnen, S., Koskimies, A.I., Tenhunen, A. and Ylostalo, P. (1984). Diagnosis of luteinized unruptured follicle syndrome (LUF) by ultrasound. *Fertil. Steril.*, **41**, 26–30

46. Thomas, E.J., Lenton, E.A. and Cooke, I.D. (1986). Follicle growth patterns and endocrinological abnormalities in infertile women with minor degrees of endometriosis. *Br. J. Obstet. Gynaecol.*, **93**, 852–858

47. Holtz, G., Williamson, H.O., Mathur, R.S., Landgrebe, S.C. and Moore, E.E. (1985). Luteinized unruptured follicle syndrome in mild endometriosis. Assessment with biochemical parameters. *J. Reprod. Med.*, **30**, 643–645

48. Grant, A. (1966). Additional sterility factors in endometriosis. *Fertil. Steril.*, **17**, 514–519

49. Ayers, J.W., Birenbaum, D.L. and Menon, K.M. (1987). Luteal phase dysfunction in endometriosis: elevated progesterone levels in peripheral and ovarian veins during the follicular phase. *Fertil. Steril.*, **47**, 925–929

50. Radwanska, E. and Dmowski, W.P. (1981). Luteal function in infertile women with endometriosis. *Infertility*, **4**, 269–277

51. Pittaway, D.E., Maxson, W., Daniell, J., Herbert, C. and Wentz, A.C. (1983). Luteal phase defects in infertility patients with endometriosis. *Fertil. Steril.*, **39**, 712–713

52. Balasch, J. and Vanrell, J.A. (1985). Mild endometriosis and luteal function. *Int. J. Fertil.*, **30**, 4–6

53. Yovich, J.L., Matson, P.L., Richardson, P.A. and Hilliard, C. (1988). Hormonal profiles and embryo quality in women with severe endometriosis treated by in vitro fertilization and embryo transfer. *Fertil. Steril.*, **50**, 308–313

54. Ronnberg, L., Kauppila, A. and Ralaniemi, J. (1984). Luteinizing hormone receptor disorder in endometriosis. *Fertil. Steril.*, **42**, 64–68

55. Halme, J., Hammond, M.G., Syrop, C.H. and Talbert, L.M. (1985). Peritoneal macrophages modulate human granulosa-luteal cell progesterone production. *J. Clin. Endocrinol. Metab.*, **61**, 912–916

56. Suginami, H., Yano, K., Watanabe, K. and Matsuura, S. (1986). A factor inhibiting ovum capture by the oviductal fimbriae present in endometriosis peritoneal fluid. *Fertil. Steril.*, **46**, 1140–1146

57. Suginami, H. and Yano, K. (1988). An ovum capture inhibitor (OCI) in endometriosis peritoneal fluid: an OCI-related membrane responsible for fimbrial failure of ovum capture. *Fertil. Steril.*, **50**, 648–653

58. Wardle, P.G., McLaughlin, E.A., McDermott, A., Mitchell, J.D., Ray, B.D. and Hull, M.G.R. (1985). Endometriosis and ovulatory disorder: Reduced fertilization in vitro compared with tubal and unexplained infertility. *Lancet*, **2**, 236–239

59. Wardle, P.G., Foster, P.A., Mitchell, J.D., McLaughlin, E.A., Sykes, J.A.C., Corrigan, E., Hull, M.G.R., Ray, B.D. and McDermott, A. (1986). Endometriosis and IVF: Effect of prior therapy. *Lancet*, **1**, 276–277

60. Naples, J.D., Batt, R.E. and Sadigh, J. (1981). Spontaneous abortion rate in patients with endometriosis. *Obstet. Gynecol.*, **57**, 509–512

61. Olive, D.L., Franklin, R.R. and Gratkins, L.V. (1982). The association between endometriosis and spontaneous abortion. *J. Reprod. Med.*, **27**, 333–338

62. Petersohn, L. (1970). Fertility in patients with ovarian endometriosis before and after treatment. *Acta Obstet. Gynecol. Scand.*, **49**, 331–333

63. Pittaway, D.E., Vernon, C. and Fayez, J.A. (1988). Spontaneous abortion in women with endometriosis. *Fertil. Steril.*, **50**, 711–715

64. Regan, R., Braude, P.R. and Tembath, P.L. (1989). Influence of past reproductive performance on risk of spontaneous abortion. *Br. Med. J.*, **299**, 541–545

65. Cooke, I.D., Sulaiman, R.A., Lenton, E.A. and Parsons, R.J. (1981). Fertility and infertility statistics: Their importance and application. *Clin. Obstet. Gynaecol.*, **8**, 531–548

66. Seibel, M.M., Berger, M.J., Weinstein, F.G. and Taymor, M.D. (1982). The effectiveness of danazol on subsequent fertility in minimal endometriosis. *Fertil. Steril.*, **38**, 534–537

67. Bayer, S.R., Seibel, M.M., Saffan, D.S., Berger, M.J. and Taymor, M.L. (1988). Efficacy of danazol treatment for minimal endometriosis in infertile women. *J. Reprod. Med.*, **33**, 179–183

68. Hull, M.E., Moghissi, K.S., Magyar, D.F. and Hayes, M.F. (1987). Comparison of different treatment modalities of endometriosis in infertile women. *Fertil. Steril.*, **47**, 40–44

69. Badawy, S.Z., El Bakry, M.M., Samuel, F. and Dizer, M. (1988). Cumulative pregnancy rates in infertile women with endometriosis. *J. Reprod. Med.*, **33**, 757–760

70. Telimaa, S. (1988). Danazol and medroxyprogesterone acetate inefficacious in the treatment of infertility in endometriosis. *Fertil. Steril.*, **50**, 872–875

71. Chong, A.P., Keene, M.E. and Thornton, N.L. (1990). Comparison of three modes of treatment for infertility patients with minimal pelvic endometriosis. *Fertil. Steril.*, **53**, 407–410

72. Khan, I., Camus, M., Staessen, C., Wisanto, A., Devroey, P. and Van Steirteghem, A.C. (1988). Success rate in gamete intrafallopian transfer using low and high concentrations of washed spermatozoa. *Fertil. Steril.*, **50**, 922–927

73. Yovich, J.L., Matson, P.L., Richardson, P.A. and Hilliard, C. (1988). Hormonal profiles and embryo quality in women with severe endometriosis treated by in vitro fertilization and embryo transfer. *Fertil. Steril.*, **50**, 308–313

74. Yovich, J.L., Matson, P.L., Blackledge, D.G., Turner, S.R., Richardson, P.A., Yovich, J.M. and Edirisinghe, W.R. (1988). The treatment of normospermic infertility by gamete intrafallopian transfer (GIFT). *Br. J. Obstet. Gynaecol.*, **95**, 316–319

75. Wong, P.C., Ng, S.C., Hamilton, M.P., Anandakumar, C., Wong, Y.C. and Ratnam, S.S. (1988). Eighty consecutive cases of gamete intra-fallopian transfer. *Hum. Reprod.*, **3**, 231–233

76. Borerro, C., Ord, T., Balmaceda, J.P., Rojas, F.J. and Asch, R.H. (1988). The GIFT experience: an evaluation of the outcome of 115 cases. *Hum. Reprod.*, **3**, 227–230

77. Braeckmans, P., Devroey, P., Camus, M., Khan, I., Staessen, C., Smitz, J., Van Waesberthe, L., Wisanto, A. and Van Steirteghem, A.C. (1987). Gamete intra-Fallopian transfer: evaluation of 100 consecutive attempts. *Hum. Reprod.*, **2**, 201–205

78. Jansen, R.P.S. (1986). Minimal endometriosis and reduced fecundability: prospective evidence from an artificial insemination by donor program. *Fertil. Steril.*, **46**, 141–143

79. Telimaa, S., Puolakka, J., Ronnberg, L. and Kauppilla, A. (1987). Placebo-controlled comparison of danazol and high-dose medroxy progesterone acetate in the treatment of endometriosis. *Gynecol. Endocrinol.*, **1**, 13–23

80. Thomas, E.J. and Cooke, I.D. (1987). Impact of gestrinone on the course of asymptomatic endometriosis. *Br. Med. J.*, **294**, 272–274

81. American Fertility Society (1979). Classification of endometriosis. *Fertil. Steril.*, **32**, 633

82. Dodge, S.T., Pumphrey, R.S. and Miyazawa, K. (1986). Peritoneal endometriosis in women requesting reversal of sterilization. *Fertil. Steril.*, **45**, 774–777

83. Murphy, A.A., Green, W.R., Bobbie, D., de la Cruz, Z.C. and Rock, J.A. (1986). Unsuspected endometriosis documented by scanning electron microscopy in visually normal peritoneum. *Fertil. Steril.*, **46**, 522–524

84. Redwine, D.B. (1988). Is "microscopic" peritoneal endometriosis invisible? *Fertil. Steril.*, **50**, 665–666

85. Pepperell, R.J. and McBain, J.C. (1985). Unexplained infertility: a review. *Br. J. Obstet. Gynaecol.*, **92**, 569–580

86. Evers, J. (1987). The second look laparoscopy for the evaluation of the results of medical treatment of endometriosis should not be performed during ovarian suppression. *Fertil. Steril.*, **47**, 502–504

Section B
Clinical Aspects of Endometriosis

8
The classification of endometriosis: A comprehensive review

T. R. Groff

DESCRIPTIVE CLASSIFICATION OF ENDOMETRIOSIS

Most early medical classifications were descriptive, frequently devised by pathologists and physiologists who were interested in the aetiology and pathophysiology of specific disorders. The impact on clinical medicine caused Feinstein[1] to remark

> The organization of data and thought in modern clinical therapy is still based on a diagnostic classification of disease — the taxonomy of morbid anatomy — that was initiated almost 200 years ago. In preserving the diagnostic nomenclature of pathologic anatomy as the main contemporary system of identifying human ailments, clinicians perpetuate a mode of thinking that classifies morphologic form, but not clinical function; that classifies disease, but not people or illness; and that classifies clinical inferences, but not clinical observations.

Sampson first classified endometriosis when he described haemorrhagic cysts in the ovaries of 14 young women[2]. He catalogued haematomas of the ovary as follicular (including graafian follicle and atretic follicle), corpus luteal, stromal, and endometrial, and subsequently staged endometrial haematomas by their histological appearance[3]:

1. First, those consisting of glands, or tubules and dilated tubules, often lined by ciliated epithelium and without the characteristic stroma of normal endometrium, or with the stroma poorly developed. The structure resembles that of the mucosa of a primary adenomyoma of the tube, and strongly suggests that the implan-

131

tations might have been derived from the epithelium of the fallopian tube.

2. In the second group the adenomas consist of stroma and glands, similar to those of normal endometrium. The histological picture strongly suggests that these adenomas were derived from uterine epithelium escaping through the lumen of the fallopian tube, that is, from menstruation with back flow into the peritoneal cavity, or from portions of tubal mucosa which had reacted to menstruation.

3. In the third group the picture suggests a mixture of adenomas of tubal and uterine type, or represents transitional stages from one to the other.

Sampson reached beyond simple description by observing that haemorrhagic cysts in these patients were related to infertility and uterine fibroids, but not to distal tubal obstruction. Although he considered conservative surgery for superficial disease in women desiring to preserve fertility, he obtained maximum relief of pain from removal of uterus, tubes, ovaries and all adenomatous tissue.

Like Sampson, Wicks and Larson categorized endometriosis on the basis of the histological characteristics of resected lesions[4]. Their classification was based on Broder's grading of malignancy and is shown in Table 8.1. These authors recommended the grading of frozen section biopsy at the time of surgery, and they discouraged hysterectomy with bilateral oophorectomy, because most of their specimens demonstrated minimal histological activity. However, they did not correlate symptoms or clinical findings with the histological grade of their classification, but urged the gathering of such data.

Soon thereafter, Huffman reviewed the records of 300 private patients with endometriosis. He formulated a classification based on the presentation of gross disease and the similarity of endometriosis to metastatic disease[5]. He believed that endometriosis was a cause of sterility and he was the first to recommend treatment based on the stage of disease from a classification, as shown in Table 8.2. Huffman preserved fertility for patients in Stages I and

Table 8.1 Wicks and Larson's classification of endometriosis activity

Grade	Description
I	The wall of the cavity is lined by large bloated phagocytic cells containing blood pigment and cellular debris. The blood pigment and debris are most abundant on the inner side of the wall and these gradually blend out into the surrounding tissue.
II	The epithelium, or at least parts of it, remains and the individual epithelial cells appear atrophic. The stroma is partially or completely replaced by bloated phagocytic cells as described above.
III	Epithelium and stroma are both present. The epithelium may be a single flattened layer of cells or form atrophic glands. An endometrial type of stroma is easily recognized. Neither the epithelium nor the stroma appears to be materially influenced by the cyclic hormonal stimulation of the ovary.
IV	Lesions contain endometrium resembling that seen at some stage of the normal 28-day menstrual cycle as found in the uterus. Glands are always present and are supported by an abundant endometrial stroma.

Abstracted from Wicks, M.J. and Larson, C.P. (1949). Histologic criteria for evaluating endometriosis. *Northwest Med.*, **48**, 611–613

Table 8.2 Huffman's classification of endometriosis

Stage	Description
I	a. Limited to uterosacral ligaments and/or
	b. Limited to one ovary and/or
	c. Superficial peritoneal implants
II	a. Extensive involvement of one ovary, plus lesser involvement of second ovary and/or
	b. Superficial implants both ovaries and/or
	c. Superficial bowel implants and/or
	d. Infiltrating lesions of uterus or uterosacral ligaments
III	a. Extensive infiltrating both ovaries
	b. Bilateral ovarian endometriotic cysts
	c. Deeply invading rectovaginal lesions
	d. Infiltrating nonobstructing bowel implants
IV	a. Vesical invasion
	b. Intestinal invasion, obstructive
	c. Ureteral involvement

Modified from Huffman, J.W. (1951). External endometriosis. *Am. J. Obstet. Gynecol.*, **62**, 1243–1252. Reproduced with permission of the publisher, the C.V. Mosby Company.

II, and for selected patients in Stage III, with 47% becoming pregnant following conservative surgery. Despite Weitzman's impression that history and physical findings often formed the basis for the diagnosis of endometriosis, as culdoscopy and laparoscopy were not then in routine use[6], Huffman indicated that these patients were classified during inspection at laparotomy.

In 1954, Sturgis and Call published their study of pelvic pain based on the life cycle of endometriosis[7]. They divided endometriosis into three stages:

1. Early development by undetermined etiology,
2. active stage, and
3. the relatively symptom-free postmenopausal period of endometrial inactivity[7].

They believed that the deep fibrotic encapsulation of long-standing pelvic endometriosis was responsible for increasing pressure and chronic dysmenorrhoea. In addition, they considered the existence of microscopic nests of glands or stroma within the peritoneal scar in their recommendation for excision of both endometriotic implants and the resultant peritoneal scarring.

Norwood was concerned about an apparent increase in the occurrence of endometriosis in women under the age of 40 when he observed that 'no one has been able to develop standardized evaluation factors with which the assembled data can be weighed as to basic significance'[8]. He declared the need for standardized terminology for the description of endometriosis and urged the integration of clinical, anatomical, and histological data into a 'three-dimensional' classification. Norwood recorded the anatomical and pathological findings in a 'buck sheet', shown in Figure 8.1. His categorization specifically allowed for bilateral disease and endometriosis at extrapelvic sites. Although he suggested that his integrated data collection would permit a more definitive guide to treatment, he recommended individualized patient selection for conservative surgical therapy. His crude pregnancy rate was 94.4%.

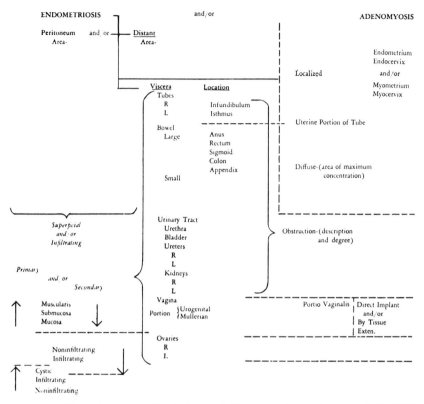

Figure 8.1 Three-dimensional 'buck sheet' of Norwood. (From Norwood, G.E. (1960). Sterility and fertility in women with pelvic endometriosis. *Clin. Obstet. Gynecol.*, **3**, 461. Reproduced with permission of the publisher, J.B. Lippincott Company)

Riva and co-workers announced their disappointment with their first attempt to categorize patients according to the severity of observed endometriosis[9]. Their measurements were ordinal; that is, they grouped the surgical findings from 156 patients according to the cumulative count of pelvic structures involved. They recommended that any future assessment of severity should consider 'the space occupied by lesions and the aggregate area of involvement as well as any associated disturbance of pelvic anatomy and physiology'.

Beecham later offered a simplified staging of endometriosis, shown in Table 8.3, based on the degree of involvement found at surgery in addition to findings on physical examination[10]. His intent was to simplify documentation of the initial assessment of endometriosis and of pelvic appearance after treatment. This was a purely descriptive classificiation. He offered no support for his staging, but he believed that effective observation of the long-term consequences of treatment demanded consistent description.

In 1971 Ranney described the treatment and outcome of 350 private patients with endometriosis[11]. He performed conservative surgery on 77;

134

Table 8.3 Beecham's suggested classification of endometriosis

Stage	Description
1	Scattered, small (1- to 2-mm) spots anywhere in the pelvis, diagnosed only at laparotomy
2	Uterosacral ligaments, broad ligaments, cervix, and ovaries are, collectively or individually, fixed, tender, nodular, and slightly enlarged.
3	The same as Stage 2, with ovaries at least twice normal size; uterosacral ligaments, rectum, and adnexa are confluent. The cul-de-sac is obliterated.
4	Massive involvement. Internal pelvic viscera cannot be clearly distinguished by palpation

Adapted from Beecham, C.T. (1966). Classification of endometriosis. *Obstet. Gynecol.*, **28**, 437, with permission of the author and the American College of Obstetricians and Gynecologists

removed the uterus but preserved ovarian function in 129; and removed uterus, adnexae and visible endometriotic implants in the remaining 144. He divided endometriosis into four categories within the last group:

1. Endometriosis of slight significance,
2. Endometriosis considered symptomatic,
3. Endometriosis in postmenopausal patients, and
4. Endometrioid carcinoma of the ovary.

Ranney did not report the effects of these surgical procedures, and did not present results for the first three groups.

PREDICTIVE CLASSIFICATIONS OF ENDOMETRIOSIS

In addition to clear and concise descriptions, the design of a classification for clinical use must be able to predict an effect, on the assumption that similar phases of a disorder will respond predictably to specific therapy. Ideally, such a classification would be based on findings at laparoscopy or laparotomy. It should permit a clear portrayal of the disease to simplify comparison between observers, unbiased selection of appropriate treatment, and indication of outcome with and without treatment and prediction of recurrence, and it must be simple to use[12].

Serious attempts to estimate outcome following selected treatment began in the early 1970s. In 1973, Acosta and co-workers presented laparoscopic data on 107 infertile patients undergoing conservative surgery for endometriosis, using a proposed classification shown in Table 8.4[13]. Although the assignment of visible peritoneal and ovarian abnormalities to stages was admittedly arbitrary, the pregnancy rate seemed to vary from 33% in severe disease to 75% for mild endometriosis.

The observations of endometrioid carcinoma of the ovary by Sampson and Ranney lent support to the taxonomy of Mitchell and Farber, who applied the staging for malignancy to endometriosis, as shown in Table 8.5[14]. They recommended surgical intervention in the presence of an ovarian mass (Stages III, IV and V) to rule out the possibility of malignancy. Conservative surgery, when performed for Stages I, II and III, resulted in a 32% pregnancy rate.

Dmowski and Cohen advised visual confirmation of endometriosis by

Table 8.4 Mitchell and Farber's classification of endometriosis

Stage	Description
I	One or more small superficial implants (less than 5 mm) on the pelvic peritoneum
II	Larger superficial implants involving uterosacral ligaments, rectovaginal septum, and/or ovaries
III	Endometriomas of the ovary greater than 5 cm in diameter with or without superficial involvement of broad ligament and adjacent organs
IV	Penetration of vagina, bowel, or urinary tract and distant metastases (lymph nodes, umbilicus, surgical wounds, and so forth)
V	Endometriomas giving rise to adenocarcinoma

Adapted from Mitchell, G.W. and Farber, M. (1974). Medical versus surgical management of endometriosis. In Reid, D.E. and Christian, C.D. (eds.) *Controversies in Obstetrics and Gynecology, II*, p. 631. (Philadelphia: W.B. Saunders)

Table 8.5 Acosta's proposed classification of pelvic endometriosis

Classification	Characteristics
Mild	1. Scattered, fresh lesions (i.e. implants not associated with scarring or retraction of the peritoneum) in the anterior or posterior cul-de-sac or pelvic peritoneum
	2. Rare surface implant on ovary, with no endometrioma, without surface scarring and retraction and without periovarian adhesions
	3. No peritubular adhesions
Moderate	1. Endometriosis involving one or both ovaries, with several surface lesions, with scarring and retraction, or small endometriomata
	2. Minimal periovarian adhesions associated with ovarian lesions described
	3. Minimal peritubular adhesions associated with ovarian lesions described
	4. Superficial implants in the anterior and/or posterior cul-de-sac with scarring and retraction. Some adhesions, but not sigmoid invasion
Severe	1. Endometriosis involving one or both ovaries with endometrioma greater than 2 × 2 cm (usually both)
	2. One or both ovaries bound down by adhesions associated with endometriosis, with or without tubal adhesions to ovaries
	3. One or both tubes bound down or obstructed by endometriosis; associated adhesions or lesions
	4. Obliteration of the cul-de-sac from adhesions or lesions associated with endometriosis
	5. Thickening of the uterosacral ligaments and cul-de-sac lesions from invasive endometriosis with obliteration of the cul-de-sac
	6. Significant bowel or urinary tract involvement

Reprinted from Acosta, A.A., Buttram, V.C., Besch, P.K., Malinak, L.R., Franklin, R.R. and Vanderheyden, J.D. (1973). A proposed classification of endometriosis. *Obstet. Gynecol.*, **42**, 21, with permission of the author and the American College of Obstetricians and Gynecologists.

endoscopic photography and by drawing observations on a preprinted outline of the pelvis[15]. Their findings were clustered in order to evaluate the results of treatment with the antigonadotropic steroid danazol (Danocrine®, Winthrop Pharmaceuticals, New York), as shown in Table 8.6. Three to eleven months of ovarian suppression seemed to result in symptomatic improvement and reduction in the distribution of disease observed at laparoscopy, but conception rates were not part of the report.

Ingersoll credited many of the previous authors with the concept of planning treatment based on the severity or the staging of disease[16]. He

Table 8.6 Dmowski's classification of endometriosis

Stage	Description
Mild	Small foci of endometriosis were recognized on one or more of the following structures: ovaries, uterosacral ligaments, vesicouterine peritoneal fold, or pelvic peritoneum elsewhere
Moderate	One ovary was enlarged by endometriosis
Severe	Both ovaries were enlarged by endometriomas

Abstracted from Dmowski, W.P. and Cohen, M.R. (1975). Treatment of endometriosis with an antigonadotropin, Danazol. *Obstet. Gynecol.*, **46**, 147, with permission of the author and the American College of Obstetricians and Gynecologists.

recommended that the American College of Obstetricians and Gynecologists and the American Fertility Society sponsor a classification that would permit direct comparison of various treatment plans for infertility and pain relief. He also proposed an expansion of Acosta's staging that is shown in Table 8.7. This system added Stage 0 for clinical suspicion and extended involvement to Stage IV, separating it from Acosta's severe stage.

Soon thereafter, Kistner and co-workers proposed equating the extent of endometriosis to treatment outcome by designing a classification based on the natural history of the disease, as shown in Table 8.8[17]. They believed that endometriosis extended from a peritoneal implantation stage to ovarian

Table 8.7 Ingersoll's classification of pelvic endometriosis

Classification	Characteristics
Stage 0	Pain, dyspareunia, suspicion of endometriosis
Stage I Mild	1. Scattered, fresh lesions (i.e. implants not associated with scarring or retraction of the peritoneum) in the anterior or posterior cul-de-sac or pelvic peritoneum 2. Rare surface implant on ovary, with no endometrioma, without surface scarring and retraction and without periovarian adhesions 3. No peritubular adhesions
Stage II Moderate	1. Endometriosis involving one or both ovaries, with several surface lesions, with scarring and retraction, or small endometriomata 2. Minimal periovarian adhesions associated with ovarian lesions described 3. Minimal peritubular adhesions associated with ovarian lesions described 4. Superficial implants in the anterior and/or posterior cul-de-sac with scarring and retraction. Some adhesions, but no sigmoid invasion
Stage III Severe	1. Endometriosis involving one or both ovaries with endometrioma larger than 2×2 cm (usually both) 2. One or both ovaries bound down by adhesions associated with endometriosis, with or without tubal adhesions to ovaries 3. One or both tubes bound down or obstructed by endometriosis; associated adhesions or lesions 4. Obliteration of the cul-de-sac by adhesions or lesions associated with endometriosis 5. Thickening of the uterosacral ligaments and cul-de-sac lesions from invasive endometriosis with obliteration of the cul-de-sac
Stage IV	Stage III plus extragenital involvement, bowel, bladder, ureter, etc

Modified from Ingersoll, F.M. (1977). Selection of medical or surgical treatment of endometriosis. *Clin. Obstet. Gynecol.*, **20**, 853, with permission of the publisher, J.B. Lippincott Company.

Table 8.8 Kistner's suggested classification of endometriosis

Stage	Description
I	Areas of endometriosis are present on the posterior pelvic peritoneum (cul-de-sac, uterosacral ligaments) or on the surface of the broad ligaments, but do not exceed 5 mm in diameter. Avascular adhesions may involve the tubes, but the fimbriae are free. The ovaries may show a few avascular adhesions, but there is no ovarian fixation. The surfaces of the bowel and the appendix are normal
IIA	Areas of endometriosis are present on the posterior pelvic peritoneum (cul-de-sac, uterosacral ligaments) and the broad ligaments, but do not exceed 5 mm in diameter. Avascular adhesions may involve the tubes, but the fimbria are free. Ovarian involvement by endometriosis has been subclassified as follows: IIA-1 Endometrial cyst or surface area 5 cm or less IIA-2 Endometrial cyst or surface area greater than 5 cm IIA-3 Ruptured endometrioma
IIB	The posterior leaf of the broad ligament is covered by adherent ovarian tissue. The tubes present adhesions not removable by endoscopic procedures. The fimbriae are free. The ovaries are fixed to the broad ligament and show areas of endometriosis greater than 5 mm in diameter. The cul-de-sac presents multiple implants, but there is no adherent bowel nor is the uterus in a fixed position. The bowel and the appendix are normal
III	The posterior leaf of the broad ligament may be covered by adherent tube or ovary. The tubal fimbriae are covered by adhesions. The ovaries are adherent to the broad ligament and tube and may or may not show surface endometriomas. The cul-de-sac shows multiple areas of endometriosis, but there is no evidence of adherent bowel or uterine fixation. The bowel and the appendix are normal
IV	Endometriosis involves the bladder serosa, and the uterus is fixed, third-degree retroversion. The cul-de-sac is covered by adherent bowel or is obliterated by the fixed uterus. The bowel is adherent to the cul-de-sac, uterosacral ligaments, or uterine corpus. The appendix may be involved by the endometriotic process

Modified from Kistner, R.W., Siegler, A.M. and Behrman, S.J. (1977). Suggested classification for endometriosis: relationship to infertility. *Fertil. Steril.*, **28**, 1008. Reproduced with permission of the publisher, the American Fertility Society.

involvement, then to tubo-ovarian involvement, and finally to anteroposterior pelvic spread. They did not provide for asymmetric involvement of the pelvis, and extrapelvic endometriosis was excluded from the proposal as being unrelated to infertility. They provided no data to support their position or results of treatment based upon this classification.

Buttram proposed a detailed and more precise taxonomy of endometriosis by revising the stages within Acosta's and Kistner's classifications[18]. He defined levels of increasing involvement within four anatomic stages, as shown in Table 8.9. He allowed for unilateral disease and, like Kistner, omitted extragenital endometriosis as being irrelevant to infertility. Buttram also provided a conversion table to relate this classification to that of Acosta. He did not offer data supporting this anatomic categorization until 1979. At that time, the results of 138 conservative pelvic procedures grouped according to this classification established pregnancy rates of 84%, 75%, and 56% for mild, moderate and severe disease, respectively[19]. He attributed the improvements in pregnancy rate to surgical technique.

Table 8.9 Buttram's expanded classification of endometriosis

Stage	Description

I (Peritoneal)
    A. No peritoneal involvement
    B. Scattered superficial, surface endometrial implants on the pelvic peritoneum (anterior or posterior cul-de-sac, uterosacral ligaments, or the broad ligaments) that do not exceed 5 mm in diameter. Neither tubal nor ovarian involvement
    C. Same as under B, but invasive endometriosis or plaques of endometrial implants > 5 mm in diameter. Fine, filmy adhesions may be present that may be lysed without great danger of resultant adhesions

II (Ovarian): 1, Right; 2, Left; 3, Bilateral
    A. No ovarian involvement
    B. Superficial surface endometrial implants of ovary < 5 mm in diameter that can be removed by scraping or fulguration without great danger of resultant adhesions. Fine, filmy adhesions may be present and can be lysed without great danger of resultant adhesions
    C. Invasive endometriosis (plaque or endometrioma) > 5 mm but < 2 cm and requiring surgical removal. Fine, filmy adhesions may be present and can be lysed without great danger of resultant adhesions
    D. Invasive endometriotic implants > 2 mm requiring surgical removal or a ruptured endometrioma of any size. Fine, filmy adhesions may be present and can be lysed without great danger of resultant adhesions
    E. B, C, or D with sufficient dense adhesions to fix ovary to adjacent tissue (usually posterior leaf of broad ligament)

III (Tubal): 1, Right; 2, Left; 3, Bilateral
    A. No tubal involvement
    B. Superficial surface endometrial implants on tube that do not exceed 5 mm in diameter and which can be removed by scraping or fulguration without great danger of resultant adhesions. Fine, filmy adhesions may be present and can be lysed without great danger of resultant adhesions
    C. Invasive endometriosis (plaque or endometrioma) requiring surgical removal. Fine, filmy adhesions may be present and can be lysed without great danger of resultant adhesions
    D. Tube involved with adhesions that distort tubal anatomy and/or limit tubal movement. Fimbriae are free and tube is patent. B or C may be present
    E. Fimbria are covered by adhesions or distal end of tube is occluded. B, C, or D may be present.

IV (Cul-de-Sac)
    A. Neither B nor C is present
    B. Invasive endometriosis of bladder or colon
    C. Posterior cul-de-sac obliterated and/or uterus fixed and retroverted. Bowel or adnexa may be adherent to cul-de-sac area. B is usually present

Modified from Buttram, V.C., Jr (1978). An expanded classification of endometriosis. *Fertil. Steril.*, **30**, 240. Reproduced with permission of the publisher, the American Fertility Society.

In 1979 Cohen proposed still another classification, shown in Table 8.10[20]. This, too, was based on the laparoscopic findings of severity and included categories for adenomyosis, distant organ involvement, and associated pelvic inflammatory disease. He recommended a variety of treatment plans, each determined by the stage of the disease, but he provided no data to support his classification or therapeutic plans.

Table 8.10 Cohen's classification of endometriosis

Stage		Description
Mild	I.	Superficial implants at one site
	II.	Superficial implants at two or more sites
Moderate	III.	Implants with puckering and fibrosis; mild ahesions
	IV.	Ovaries moderately adherent to endometrial implants
	V.	Multiple implants of ovaries, bladder peritoneum, ligaments with adhesions
Severe	VI.	Endometrial cyst, unilateral or bilateral, without tubal involvement
	VII.	Endometrial cyst, unilateral or bilateral, with tubal involvement
	VIII.	Adenomyomata
	IX.	Severe endometriosis plus pelvic inflammatory disease
	X.	Severe endometriosis and/or extragenital, bowel, urinary tract, distant organ involvement

Adapted from Cohen, M.R. (1978). Laparoscopy and the management of endometriosis. *J. Reprod. Med.*, **23**, 82, with permission of the author and the publisher.

Responding to the steady requests to sponsor one of a variety of classification proposals, the American Fertility Society convened a committee of authorities[21]. The 1979 report of their collaboration, presented in Figure 8.2, synthesizes portions of many earlier classifications with imagination and innovation. For example, distant disease was not scored, but asymmetric lesions were to be scored appropriately. An anatomical drawing was provided to depict the surgical findings, including extragenital implants. In addition, this was the first attempt to apply a weighted scale (ranging from 1 to 6 points) to the severity of endometriotic lesions involving the peritoneum, the ovary and the fallopian tube. Furthermore, the staging of the disease was arbitrarily determined by the cumulative count of these points.

Hasson pointed out a shortcoming of the American Fertility Society's 1979 classification: endometriosis causes pain as well as infertility, particularly when uterosacral ligament involvement is present[22]. He proposed a three-dimensional modification to increase the point scoring of uterosacral ligament involvement and nodular or cystic lesions of the peritoneum greater than 8 mm in depth, as shown in Figure 8.3.

Rock, Guzick, and co-workers presented the first comparative evaluation of the classification systems of Buttram, Kistner and the American Fertility Society[23]. They reported successful pregnancies in 54% of 214 patients undergoing conservative surgery for endometriosis. This evaluation failed to establish differences between the mild, moderate and severe categories of the American Fertility Society classification, and found that pregnancy rates were significantly reduced if large ovarian endometriomas were scored by this classification. When Guzick reviewed the point-scoring system of the American Fertility Society classification by dose–response monotonic estimation, he confirmed that the arbitrary point scores and the arbitrary divisions between stages failed to correlate the severity of endometriosis with the pregnancy rate after surgery[24]. He recommended the use of empirically-derived weights in place of the arbitrary category weights.

Brosens and colleagues pointed out that the American Fertility Society classification for endometriosis was not designed to assess the efficacy of medical treatment[25]. They believed that the number of visible implants, rather

AMERICAN FERTILITY SOCIETY CLASSIFICATION OF ENDOMETRIOSIS

Patient's name

Stage I   (Mild)   1–5
Stage II (Moderate)   6–15
Stage III (Severe)   16–30
Stage IV (Extensive) 31–54

Total

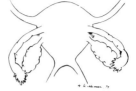

			<1 cm	1–3 cm	> 3 cm
PERITONEUM	ENDOMETRIOSIS				
			1	2	3
	ADHESIONS		filmy	dense w/ partial cul-de-sac obliteration	dense w/ complete cul-de-sac obliteration
			1	2	3
OVARY	ENDOMETRIOSIS		< 1 cm	1–3 cm	> 3 cm or ruptured endometrioma
		R	2	4	6
		L	2	4	6
	ADHESIONS		filmy	dense w/ partial ovarian enclosure	dense w/ complete ovarian enclosure
		R	2	4	6
		L	2	4	6
TUBE	ENDOMETRIOSIS		<1 cm	> 1 cm	tubal occlusion
		R	2	4	6
		L	2	4	6
	ADHESIONS		filmy	dense w/ tubal distortion	dense w/ tubal enclosure
		R	2	4	6
		L	2	4	6

Associated Pathology:

Figure 8.2 The American Fertility Society classification of endometriosis, 1979. (From the American Fertility Society (1979). Classification of endometriosis. *Fertil. Steril.*, **32**, 633. Reproduced with permission of the publisher, the American Fertility Society)

than their size, may be more relevant to the consequences of endometriosis. These authors also criticized the lack of data to support the scoring differential between superficial and deep peritoneal implants, and they urged the inclusion of physiopathological considerations in future revisions to the classification of endometriosis.

Buttram assessed the American Fertility Society's 1979 classification as 'helpful if for no other reason than to provide a standard classification for uniform use', but observed that inadequacies existed in the assessment of adhesive disease and disease of the cul-de-sac[26]. He introduced a revised classification intended to serve as a standard classification for gynaecologists, to permit aggregation of clinical data from various centres, to allow various treatment regimens to be compared, to assess infertile patients (also those not concerned with fertility), and to obtain more knowledge about endometriosis.

The American Fertility Society then submitted without comment their revised classification of endometriosis, shown in Figure 8.4[27]. Again, a

Name: _____

Age: _____ Parity: _____ Gravidity: _____

Method of observation:
Laparoscopy — Laparotomy

Stage I	(mild)	1-5
Stage II	(moderate)	6-15
Stage III	(severe)	16-30
Stage IV	(extensive)	31-54

ENDOMETRIOTIC LESIONS	SURFACE AREA OF PLAQUES			VOLUME OF NODULES OR CYSTS		Total Points
	< 1 cm	1-3 cm	> 3 cm	1-3 ml	> 3 ml.	
Peritoneum	1	2	3	2	4	
Uterosacral Ligaments — Rt.	1	2	3	2	4	
— Lt.	1	2	3	2	4	
Ovaries					(or ruptured endometrioma)	
— Rt.	1	2	3	4	6	
— Lt.	1	2	3	4	6	
Tubes					(or causing tubal occlusion)	
— Rt.	1	2	3	4	6	
— Lt.	1	2	3	4	6	
ADHESIONS:	FILMY		DENSE		EXTENSIVE	
Peritoneum		1	(w/partial cul de sac obliteration) 2		(w/complete cul de sac obliteration) 3	
Ovaries			(w/partial ovarian enclosure)		(w/complete ovarian enclosure)	
— Rt.		2	4		6	
— Lt.		2	4		6	
Tubes			(w/tubal distortion)		(w/tubal enclosure)	
— Rt.		2	4		6	
— Lt.		2	4		6	
TOTAL SCORE						

ASSOCIATED FINDINGS:

Figure 8.3 Hasson's recommended revision to the American Fertility Society classification of endometriosis. (From Hasson, H.M. (1981). Classification for endometriosis (Letter to the Editor). *Fertil. Steril.*, **35**, 368. Reproduced with permission of the publisher, the American Fertility Society)

weighted point system was used, arbitrarily divided into four stages based on the cumulative count of affected tubal, ovarian and peritoneal structures. Invasive endometriosis was given a greater point score than was superficial disease. Tubal adhesions were heaviliy weighted, whereas peritoneal adhesive disease and tubal endometriosis, albeit rare, were not scored. Endometriosis of the bowel, urinary tract, vagina, cervix, and skin lesions was not scored, to minimize awkwardness and detail. Clear and detailed examples of staging calculations were included.

Buttram, in 1985, presented a comparison of the classifications of Acosta, the American Fertility Society's original classification and the American Fertility Society's revised classification[28]. He found that none of these classification systems predicted resolution of endometriosis following danazol (Danacrine) treatment. Buttram pointed out that surgical removal of invasive endometriosis resulted in higher response rates than did suppressive therapy, but he was not able to correlate future pregnancy with gross evidence of the resolution of endometriosis, using these classifications. However, the American Fertility Society's revised classification did suggest a weak association between

Patient's Name _____ Date_____

Stage I (Minimal) · 1-5
Stage II (Mild) · 6-15
Stage III (Moderate) · 16-40
Stage IV (Severe) · >40
Total_____

Laparoscopy_____ Laparotomy_____ Photography_____
Recommended Treatment_____

Prognosis_____

PERITONEUM	ENDOMETRIOSIS	<1cm	1-3cm	>3cm
	Superficial	1	2	4
	Deep	2	4	6
OVARY	R Superficial	1	2	4
	Deep	4	16	20
	L Superficial	1	2	4
	Deep	4	16	20

	POSTERIOR CULDESAC OBLITERATION	Partial	Complete
		4	40

	ADHESIONS	<1/3 Enclosure	1/3-2/3 Enclosure	>2/3 Enclosure
OVARY	R Filmy	1	2	4
	Dense	4	8	16
	L Filmy	1	2	4
	Dense	4	8	16
TUBE	R Filmy	1	2	4
	Dense	4*	8*	16
	L Filmy	1	2	4
	Dense	4*	8*	16

*If the fimbriated end of the fallopian tube is completely enclosed, change the point assignment to 16

Additional Endometriosis _____ _____ | Associated Pathology _____ _____

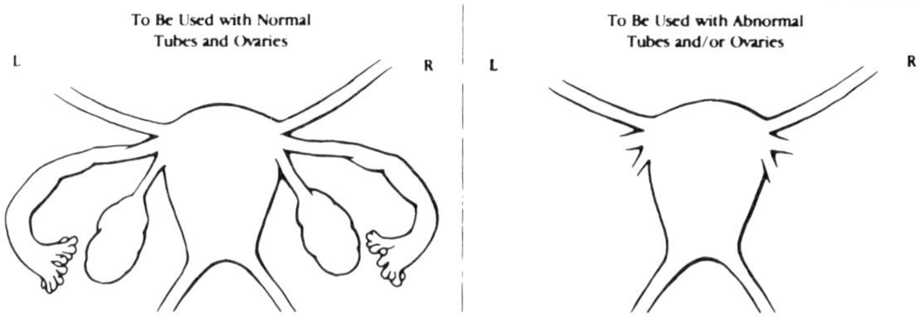

To Be Used with Normal Tubes and Ovaries

To Be Used with Abnormal Tubes and/or Ovaries

Figure 8.4 The American Fertility Society revised classification of endometriosis, 1985. (From the American Fertility Society (1985). Revised American Fertility Society classification of endometriosis: 1985. *Fertil. Steril.*, **43**, 351. Reproduced with permission of the publisher, the American Fertility Society)

the severity of endometriosis and the prognosis for successful pregnancy.

Modification of the American Fertility Society's revised classification of endometriosis is anticipated.

THE FUTURE CLASSIFICATION OF ENDOMETRIOSIS

The *de facto* goal of the classification and treatment of endometriosis to date seems to have narrowed to the rescue of fertility. This has been true since Beecham explored 49 of 58 women with endometriosis who presented with dysmenorrhoea, dyspareunia, lower abdominal pain, rectal pain and tenesmus, menorrhagia and metrorrhagia[29]. In reporting the results of conservative surgery, he cited a pregnancy rate of 37% rather than pain relief. As our understanding of the aetiology, pathophysiology and sequelae of treatment of endometriosis is limited, it seems apparent that the correlation of many fundamental conditions other than infertility must be considered during the evolution of an effective categorization of endometriosis. Malinak has observed that relief of *pelvic pain* after conservative surgery for endometriosis is consistent and immediate and the risk of recurrent disease is 12%[30]. He reported that pregnancy rates seemed to vary with coexisting infertility factors, in addition to the reported severity of endometriosis, but insufficient data existed to confirm the benefit of conservative surgery upon pelvic pain, on the basis of contemporary classification schemes. Metzger and co-workers reviewed the association between endometriosis and the risk of *spontaneous abortion*, reported to be as high as 63%[31]. Although they concluded that the actual spontaneous abortion rate in untreated endometriosis may be lower than suspected, no studies with well-defined controls have been conducted.

Location of endometriosis may influence the degree or prognosis of endometriosis, as the ovaries, the posterior broad ligament, the anterior and posterior cul-de-sacs, and the uterosacral ligaments seem to be particularly susceptible[32,33]. Wheeler and Malinak have presented a computerized anatomical model for the location of endometriotic implants and the results of conservative surgery[34]. This prototype provided a pelvic map of 17 zones into which the endometriosis findings are entered. Empirical projections of pregnancy and reoperation risk from clinical data can then be derived from frequency and lifetable analysis. This pelvic map can be shown in three dimensions by computer display with sufficient detail 'to distinguish recurrent endometriosis (i.e., re-growth of endometriosis at a previously treated site) versus persistent endometriosis (i.e., new growth of endometriosis previously treated)[35].

Furthermore, *extragenital and distant sites* of endometriosis should be considered in any attempt to categorize this disease. For example, endometriosis involving the cervix and some other extrapelvic structures is believed to decrease significantly the probability of pregnancy, even though not considered severe by the current system of classification[36].

However, endometriosis may be more widespread and varied in appearance than can be determined by direct visualization. Brosens *et al.*[37] and Vasquez *et al.*[38] have identified *unsuspected endometriosis* in normal-appearing peritoneum from 83% of patients with unexplained infertility. Murphy and co-workers suspect that conservative surgery for endometriosis is at best cytoreductive and that reoccurrence (or persistence) of disease may develop from unsuspected endometrial stroma and glands identified in grossly normal peritoneum[39]. Jansen has histologically identified the presence of endometriosis in non-pigmented peritoneal lesions, especially white, opacified peritoneum and red, flame-like lesions[40]. Knowledge of the role of ovarian steroids in the maintenance of endometriosis may be expanding. Although the involvement of oestrogen in the control of endometriosis has been well accepted, Dizerega and co-workers have shown that implantation may be independent of steroidal control and also that a new role for progesterone in the maintenance of endometriosis may exist, at least in the primate[41].

More recently, Muse reviewed the clinical manifestations of endometriosis, including infertility, pelvic pain and pelvic mass, in addition to the less common presentation of perimenstrual rectal pain, dysuria, haematuria, urinary obstruction, and spontaneous pneumothorax[42]. He observed that

> Future classification schemes may obviate these concerns [microscopic and unpigmented endometriosis] by incorporating, in addition to an anatomic assessment of disease distribution, a physiologic one. This may involve measuring prostaglandin production by the lesions, circulating CA-125 or antiendometriosis antibody levels, assessing ovulatory function, etc.

Barbieri and co-workers found significantly elevated serum concentrations of CA-125 in patients with endometriosis[43]. This cell surface antigen produced by coelomic epithelium surfaces seemed to vary with the severity of the disease. Badawy and co-workers have identified significant changes in peritoneal macrophages and lymphocytes with increases in acid phosphatase, prostaglandin $E_{2\alpha}$ and E_2, and complement components C_{3c} and C_4 in patients with endometriosis[44]. Vernon has identified a relationship between the morphological appearance of endometriotic implants and their capacity to synthesize prostaglandin $F_{2\alpha}$[45]. In a complex study of the peritoneal environment, Syrop and Halme found that peritoneal 6-keto-$PGF_{1\alpha}$, acid phosphatase, progestin-dependent endometrial protein and, possibly, peritoneal fluid volume, were elevated in infertile patients with endometriosis[46]. Recently, Fakih identified significant increases in peritoneal fluid volume and interleukin-1, a macrophage by-product known to induce prostaglandin synthesis and fibroblast proliferation, in infertile women with mild endometriosis[47].

The list of potential markers for peritoneal endometriosis is extensive.

THE BASIS OF A CLASSIFICATION FOR ENDOMETRIOSIS

Once such identifiers of endometriosis are defined and agreed upon, the spectrum of endometriosis must be divided into the aetiological, clinical, pathological, therapeutic, and functional parts, not unlike Norwood's 1960 proposal. Compounding the difficulty, some couples included in endometriosis studies may be sterile or subfertile through other factors. A recent study of 141 couples found that 40.4% presented with multiple infertility factors[48]. However, Verkoff observed a cumulative pregnancy rate, calculated by life-table analysis, of 55.1%, 62.2% and 58.3% for women with multiple factor, single factor and unexplained infertility, respectively, at 5 years from registration.

Additionally, Leridon pointed out that selection bias also affects the study of infertility patients[49]:

> First, couples are selected by the time they have been waiting for a conception without any success. A second selection is done by the physician, who has to decide which couples are good candidates for a specific treatment. The third selection, which is much more difficult to

control, is the self-selection determined by the couples themselves — when they decide to see a doctor, to change to another doctor, to accept or postpone treatment, etc.

Obviously, the development of a complete classification of endometriosis requires the gathering of these elements by carefully designed multicentred trials and precise statistical analysis. Although modern classifications have organized endometriosis by its anatomical distribution, Feinstein[50] insisted that 'a sick person cannot be classified properly unless the identification includes his distinguishing attributes in each of these different features' (laboratory data to describe the disease, personal data to describe the patient, and clinical data to describe the disease patient). He recommends grouping clinical disease into stages as follows[50]:

1. Collect pertinent clinical properties by surveying large numbers of patients,
2. Analyze results for frequency of appearance, sequence and timing,
3. Select aggregate properties to represent overlapping sets of the total clinical spectrum of the disease,
4. Divide sets or subsets or add new sets as needed, and
5. Select appropriate sets to compare with others determined in the laboratory or by clinical observations.

In this way, staging can divide heterogeneous mixtures into homogeneous groups. Cramer agreed that the first step in defining the severity of an infertility problem is obtaining a homogeneous group of patients for study, that is, classification by type and severity[51]. Many aspects must be evaluated, as the 'prognostic importance of each of these factors can only be determined by continuing clinical input, and it may require many years for a suitable classification scheme to evolve'[51].

Adamson and co-workers were able to identify areas of the pelvis most often involved with endometriosis[52]. They next applied *clustering techniques* to identify similar subgroups and determined which clusters were important in predicting outcome. However, they found that staging by the classification systems of Acosta and Kistner could not predict outcome. They recommended *life-table analysis* to correct for varying lengths of follow-up and losses to follow-up.

Alternatively, Gonella and colleagues proposed a 'staging' approach to measure disease severity that may apply to endometriosis[53]. They divided diseases into four categories of increasing severity borrowed from medical oncology[53]:

1. Conditions with no complications or with problems of minimal severity,
2. Problems limited to an organ or system and with a risk of complications significantly increased over stage 1,
3. Multiple site involvement, poor prognosis,
4. Death.

The proper application of statistics must establish the effectiveness of any classification scheme by its correlation with clinical success. Although frequently applied, crude pregnancy rates, or pregnancies per patient, may not be the most appropriate statistic to quantify success[54], Cramer proposed the use of life-table analysis to evaluate the treatment of infertility[51]. However, Guzick and Rock questioned his application of pure life-table analysis, because the outcome of infertility therapy is always less than 100% success[55]. By calculating the cure rate and the instantaneous probability of pregnancy among those patients *cured* of endometriosis, these authors developed a modified life-table model that more closely followed their clinical experience. Guzick later justified the application of the *likelihood-ratio test* to identify variation between cumulative pregnancy rates of dissimilar patient groups[56].

Olive and Lee believed this likelihood-ratio test was 'easily the most sophisticated attempt at modeling the success rates of a therapeutic fertility trial'. However, it requires large numbers of patients in each study group and assumes that the changes in pregnancy rate over time are exponential. Alternatively, these authors proposed use of the *Mantel–Byar analysis*, which eliminates the bias caused by delays between diagnosis and treatment and permits the transfer of individual patients between treatment programmes with near assumption-free analysis[57]. Olive and Lee's analysis suggests that severe disease by the Acosta classification was the only group to benefit from conservative surgery. However, a conservative operation was not considered beneficial for all other groups by the Acosta classification and other staging methods were not evaluated.

The use of these statistical models to correlate the many clinical and laboratory markers of patients with endometriosis with the treatment and outcome could provide the significance necessary to establish and validate a useful classification of endometriosis.

SUMMARY

The classification of endometriosis dates back to the original documentation of the disease. Precise description and development of a consistent vocabulary have been tedious, but necessary, first steps in the process. Weitzman and Buttram have recently provided an excellent review of many attempts to stage endometriosis[6]. Buttram found most recent proposals unsatisfactory and skilfully analysed their deficiencies[58]. Our inadequate understanding of endometriosis can be expanded by studying enormous quantities of pooled clinical findings via computerized data analysis and modern statistical tools. The effects of endometriosis (infertility, pelvic pain, menstrual abnormalities, spontaneous abortion); the visibility, histological type and activity, and location of the implants; the concomitant diagnoses; the chemical and cellular associations of the peritoneum and serum; the response to various pharmaceuticals or conservative surgery; and the risk of recurrence, must all be considered in the development of a complete classification of endometriosis. Eventually a classification (or classifications) of endometriosis can be empirically established, and an accurate prediction of the response of endometriosis to a specific treatment plan can then be realized.

REFERENCES

1. Feinstein, A.R. (1967). *Clinical Judgment*, pp. 72–73 (Huntington, NY: Robert E. Krieger)
2. Sampson, J.A. (1921). Perforating hemorrhagic (chocolate) cysts of ovary. *Arch. Surg.*, **3**, 245–323
3. Sampson, J.A. (1922). The life history of ovarian hematomas (hemorrhagic cysts) of endometrial (muellerian) type. *Am. J. Obstet. Gynecol.*, **4**, 451–512
4. Wicks, M.J. and Larson, C.P. (1949). Histologic criteria for evaluating endometriosis. *Northwest Med.*, **48**, 611–613
5. Huffman, J.W. (1951). External endometriosis. *Am. J. Obstet. Gynecol.*, **62**, 1243–1252
6. Weitzman, G.A. and Buttram, V.C., Jr (1989). Classification of endometriosis. *Obstet. Gynecol. Clin. North Am.*, **16**, 64–77
7. Sturgis, S.H. and Call, B.J. (1954). Endometriosis peritonei—relationship of pain to function activity. *Am. J. Obstet. Gynecol.*, **68**, 1421–1431
8. Norwood, G.E. (1960). Sterility and fertility in women with pelvic endometriosis. *Clin. Obstet. Gynecol.*, **3**, 456–471
9. Riva, H.L., Kawasaki, D.M. and Messinger, A.J. (1962). Further experience with norethynodrel in treatment of endometriosis. *Obstet. Gynecol.*, **19**, 111–117
10. Beecham, C.T. (1966). Classification of endometriosis. *Obstet. Gynecol.*, **28**, 437
11. Ranney, B. (1971). Endometriosis. III. Complete operations. *Am. J. Obstet. Gynecol.*, **109**, 1137–1144
12. Candiani, G.C. (1986). The classification of endometriosis: historic evolution, critical review and present state of the art. *Acta Eur. Fertil.*, **17**, 85–91
13. Acosta, A.A., Buttram, V.C., Besch, P.K., Malinak, L.R., Franklin, R.R. and Vanderheyden, J.D. (1973). A proposed classification of endometriosis. *Obstet. Gynecol.*, **42**, 19–25
14. Mitchell, G.W. and Farber, M. (1974). Medical versus surgical management of endometriosis. In Reid, D.E. and Christian, C.D. (eds.) *Controversy in Obstetrics and Gynecology, II*, pp. 631–636. (Philadelphia: W.B. Saunders)
15. Dmowski, W.P. and Cohen, M.R. (1975). Treatment of endometriosis with an antigonadotropin, Danazol. *Obstet. Gynecol.*, **46**, 147–154
16. Ingersoll, F.M. (1977). Selection of medical or surgical treatment of endometriosis. *Clin. Obstet. Gynecol.*, **20**, 849–864
17. Kistner, R.W., Siegler, A.M. and Behrman, S.J. (1977). Suggested classification for endometriosis: relationship to infertility. *Fertil. Steril.*, **28**, 1008–1010
18. Buttram, V.C. (1978). An expanded classification of endometriosis. *Fertil. Steril.*, **30**, 240–242
19. Buttram, V.C. (1979). Surgical treatment of endometriosis in the infertile female: a modified approach. *Fertil. Steril.*, **32**, 635–640
20. Cohen, M.R. (1979). Laparoscopy and the management of endometriosis. *J. Reprod. Med.*, **23**, 81–84
21. American Fertility Society (1979). Classification of endometriosis. *Fertil. Steril.*, **32**, 633–634
22. Hasson, H.M. (1981). Classification for endometriosis (Letter to the editor). *Fertil. Steril.*, **35**, 368–369
23. Rock, J.A., Guzick, D.S., Sengos, C., Schweditsch, M., Sapp, K.C. and Jones, H.W., Jr (1981). The conservative surgical treatment of endometriosis: evaluation of pregnancy success with respect to the extent of disease as categorized using contemporary classification systems. *Fertil. Steril.*, **35**, 131–137
24. Guzick, D.S., Bross, D.S. and Rock, J.A. (1982). Assessing the efficacy of the American Fertility Society's classification of endometriosis: application of a dose-response methodology. *Fertil. Steril.*, **38**, 171–176
25. Brosens, I.A., Cornille, F., Koninckx, P. and Vasquez, G. (1985). Evolution of the revised American Fertility Society classification of endometriosis. *Fertil. Steril.*, **44**, 714–716
26. Buttram, V.C. (1985). Evolution of the revised American Fertility Society classification of endometriosis. *Fertil. Steril.*, **43**, 347–350
27. American Fertility Society (1985). Revised American Fertility Society classification of endometriosis: 1985. *Fertil. Steril.*, **43**, 351–352
28. Buttram, V.C. (1987). Classification of endometriosis. *Contrib. Gynecol. Obstet.*, **16**, 73–83

29. Beecham, C.T. (1949). Surgical treatment of endometriosis. *Am. J. Obstet. Gynecol.*, **139**, 971–972
30. Malinak, L.R. (1980). Infertility and endometriosis: operative technique, clinical staging, and prognosis. *Clin. Obstet. Gynecol.*, **23**, 925–936
31. Metzger, D.A., Olive, D.L., Stohs, G.F. and Franklin, R.R. (1986). Association of endometriosis and spontaneous abortion: effect of control group selection. *Fertil. Steril.*, **45**, 18–22
32. Williams, T.J. and Pratt, J.H. (1977). Endometriosis in 1,000 consecutive celiotomies: incidence and management. *Am. J. Obstet. Gynecol.*, **129**, 245–250
33. Jenkins, S., Olive, D.L. and Haney, A.F. (1986). Endometriosis: pathogenic implications of anatomic distribution. *Obstet. Gynecol.*, **67**, 335–338
34. Wheeler, J.M. and Malinak, L.R. (1985). Application of computerized pelvic mapping to the conservative surgical treatment of endometriosis: analysis of anatomic areas in relations to prognosis for postoperative pregnancy. Presented at the *41st Annual Meeting of The American Fertility Society*, September 30, Chicago, Illinois
35. Wheeler, J.M. and Malinak, L.R. (1987). Computer graphic pelvic mapping, second look laparoscopy, and the distinction of recurrent versus persistent endometriosis. Presented at the *43rd Annual Meeting of The American Fertility Society*, September 28–30, Reno, Nevada
36. Wheeler, J.M. and Malinak, L.R. (1987). When "bad" endometriosis is not "severe": analysis of endometriosis of the bladder, ureter, cervix, vagina and vulva with implications current classification systems. Presented at the *43rd Annual Meeting of The American Fertility Society*, September 28–30, Reno, Nevada
37. Brosens, I., Vasquez, G. and Gordts, S. (1984). Scanning electron microscopy study of the pelvic peritoneum in unexplained infertility and endometriosis. *Fertil. Steril.*, **41** (suppl.), S21
38. Vasquez, G., Cornillie, F. and Brosens, I. (1984). Peritoneal endometriosis: scanning electron microscopy and histology of minimal pelvic endometriotic lesions. *Fertil. Steril.*, **42**, 696–703
39. Murphy, A.A., Green, W.R., Bobbie, D., dela Cruz, Z.C. and Rock, J.A. (1986). Unsuspected endometriosis documented by scanning electron microscopy in visually normal peritoneum. *Fertil. Steril.*, **46**, 522–524
40. Jansen, R.P.S. and Russell, P. (1986). Nonpigmented endometriosis: clinical, laparoscopic, and pathologic definition. *Am. J. Obstet. Gynecol.*, **155**, 1154–1159
41. Dizerega, G.S., Barber, D.L. and Hodgen, G.D. (1980). Endometriosis: role of ovarian steroids in initiation, maintenance and suppression. *Fertil. Steril.*, **33**, 649–653
42. Muse, K. (1988). Clinical manifestations and classification of endometriosis. *Clin. Obstet. Gynecol.*, **31**, 813–822
43. Barbieri, R.L., Niloff, J.M., Bast, R.C., Jr., Schaetzl, E., Kistner, R.W. and Knapp, R.C. (1986). Elevated serum concentrations of CA-125 in patients with advanced endometriosis. *Fertil. Steril.*, **45**, 630–634
44. Badawy, S.Z.A., Cuenca, V., Marshall, L., Munchback, R., Rinas, A.C. and Coble, D.A. (1984). Cellular components in peritoneal fluid in infertile patients with and without endometriosis. *Fertil. Steril.*, **42**, 704–708
45. Vernon, M.W., Beard, J.S., Graves, K. and Wilson, E.A. (1986). Classification of endometriotic implants by morphologic appearance and capacity to synthesize prostaglandin F. *Fertil. Steril.*, **46**, 801–806
46. Syrop, C.H. and Halme, J. (1987). Peritoneal fluid environment and infertility. *Fertil. Steril.*, **48**, 1–9
47. Fakih, H., Baggett, B., Holtz, G., Tsang, K., Lee, J.C. and Williamson, H.O. (1987). Interleukin-1: a possible role in the infertility associated with endometriosis. *Fertil. Steril.*, **47**, 213–217
48. Verkauf, B.S. (1983). The incidence and outcome of single-factor, multifactorial, and unexplained infertility. *Am. J. Obstet. Gynecol.*, **147**, 175–181
49. Leridon, J. and Spira, A. (1984). Problems in measuring the effectiveness of infertility therapy. *Fertil. Steril.*, **41**, 580–586
50. Feinstein, A.R. (1964). Scientific methodology in clinical medicine. II. Classification of human disease by clinical behavior. *Ann. Intern. Med.*, **61**, 757–781

51. Cramer, D.W., Walker, A.M. and Schiff, I. (1979). Statistical methods in evaluating the outcome of infertility therapy. *Fertil. Steril.*, **32**, 80–86
52. Adamson, G.D., Drison, L. and Lamb, E.J. (1982). Endometriosis: studies of a method for the design of a surgical staging system. *Fertil. Steril.*, **38**, 659–666
53. Gonnella, J.S., Hornbrook, M.C. and Louis, D.Z. (1984). Staging of disease. *J. Am. Med. Assoc.*, **251**, 637–644
54. Olive, D.L. (1986). Analysis of clinical fertility trials: a methodologic review. *Fertil. Steril.*, **45**, 157–171
55. Guzick, D.S. and Rock, J.A. (1981). Estimation of a model of cumulative pregnancy following infertility therapy. *Am. J. Obstet. Gynecol.*, **140**, 573–578
56. Guzick, D.S., Bross, D.S. and Rock, J.A. (1982). A parametric method for comparing cumulative pregnancy curves following infertility therapy. *Fertil. Steril.*, **37**, 503–507
57. Olive, D.L. and Lee, K.L. (1986). Analysis of sequential treatment protocols for endometriosis-associated infertility. *Fertil. Steril.*, **154**, 613–619
58. Buttram, V.C., Reiter, R.C. and Ward, S. (1985). Treatment of endometriosis with danazol: report of a 6-year prospective study. *Fertil. Steril.*, **43**, 353–360

9
Extrapelvic endometriosis

S. M. Markham

INTRODUCTION

Although endometriosis was initially described in the mid nineteenth century[1], little interest in this pathological process was apparent until the early twentieth century when Sampson presented his classic theory on menstrual reflux as the aetiology of peritoneal endometriosis[2]. Since that time, endometriosis has proved to be both one of the most fascinating, yet most frustrating, pathological conditions of the female reproductive tract. Clinicians and researchers alike have shared in an intense interest in the aetiology and the most effective management of women with endometriosis of the true pelvis or of extrapelvic sites.

Sampson originally divided endometriosis into two main groups: (a) direct (internal) and (b) indirect (external)[2]. The first group included what is now referred to as adenomyosis while the second group included all other endometriosis that was 'not continuous with normally situated mullerian mucosa'[2]. More recently, because of the variety of locations in which endometriosis has been found, it has been useful to divide Sampson's indirect (external) endometriosis into two separate groups: (a) pelvic endometriosis and (b) extrapelvic endometriosis. Pelvic endometriosis is defined as endometriotic lesions involving the uterus, fallopian tubes, ovaries and the surrounding peritoneum in the anterior and posterior cul-de-sac and on the pelvic side walls. Extrapelvic endometriosis is defined as endometriotic-like lesions elsewhere in the body[3]. Extrapelvic endometriosis has been identified in virtually every organ system and tissue in the human female body (Figures 9.1 and 9.2). The exception may be the spleen, which seems to express an unusual resistance to endometriotic involvement.

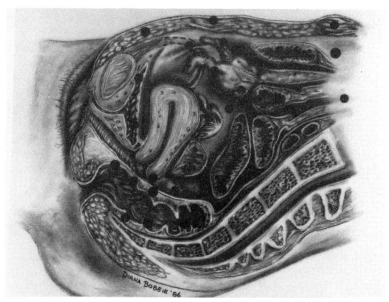

Figure 9.1 Sites of reported endometriosis in the abdominal cavity not including the uterus, fallopian tubes, ovaries or surrounding peritoneum. From Rock, J.A. and Markham, S.M. (1987). Extrapelvic endometriosis. In Wilson, E.A. (ed.) *Endometriosis*, p. 185. New York: Alan R. Liss, with permission

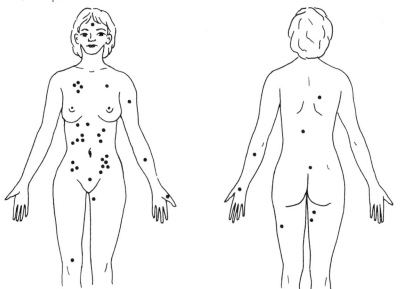

Figure 9.2 Sites of reported extrapelvic endometriosis. From Markham, S.M., Carpenter, S.E. and Rock, J.A. (1989). Extrapelvic endometriosis *Obstet. Gynecol. Clin. North Am.*, **16**(I), 192, with permission

This chapter will concentrate on a review of extrapelvic endometriosis as presented in the medical literature along with personal observations. The intention is to focus on the location and symptoms of extrapelvic disease and to review diagnostic techniques and management modalities that have proved to be most effective. A similar review of endometriosis limited to the pelvis will be found in earlier chapters of this book.

INCIDENCE

The reported incidence of extrapelvic endometriosis (Table 9.1) would suggest a substantially smaller occurrence than that of pelvic disease (Table 9.2). The incidence of endometriosis, both pelvic and extrapelvic, might not be accurately diagnosed if only gross examination and histological sections of suspected tissue were utilized in making a diagnosis. Using scanning electron microscopy (SEM), submicroscopic endometriosis can be detected in otherwise normal-appearing peritoneum[4]. This impression has been refuted in a study using only light microscopy (LM)[5]. Occult endometriosis does, however,

Table 9.1 Incidence of extrapelvic endometriosis

Author	Site	Incidence %
Barbieri and Kistner (1986)[86]	Small intestine	0.1–0.2 (women with endometriosis)
Williams (1985)[89]	Omentum	0.6
	Small intestine	0.2
	Appendix	1.4
	Rectovaginal septum	1.6
	Rectovaginal septum with rectosigmoid involvement	3.9
	Rectovaginal septum with vaginal involvement	1.8
	Sigmoid	0.8
	Cervix	2.5
	Inguinal area	0.8
	Umbilical area	0.8
	Incisional, ventral	0.8
	Incisional, vulvar	0.2
Gitelis et al. (1985)[90]	Lung and pleura	51.0 (extra-abdominal endometriosis)
Yates-Bell et al. (1972)[91]	Urinary tract	1.0 (women with endometriosis)
Ball and Platt (1962)[92]	Urinary tract	0.5 (women with endometriosis)
Macafee and Greer (1960)[93]	Intestine	12.0 (7177 cases of endometriosis reviewed)
Lane (1960)[94]	Appendix	< 1.0 endometriosis cases)
Scott and TeLinde (1950)[95]	Appendix	1.4 (cases of endometriosis)

From Markham, S.M., Carpenter, S.E. and Rock, J.A. (1989). Extrapelvic endometriosis. *Obstet. Gynecol. Clin. North Am.*, **16**(1), 193, with permission

Table 9.2   Incidence of pelvic endometriosis

Author	Incidence
Cramer (1987)[85]	5.6–7.9% of women hospitalized with genital disorders other than pregnancy
Barbieri and Kistner (1986)[86]	5–15% of women between 25 and 35 years of age undergoing laparotomy
Ranney (1980)[87]	4–17% of menstruating women
Meyers et al. (1979)[32]	8–15% of women
Williams and Pratt (1977)[84]	38% of women
Meigs (1941)[88]	36% of 400 consecutive patients at laparotomy

From Markham, S.M., Carpenter, S.E. and Rock, J.A. (1989). Extrapelvic endometriosis. *Obstet. Gynecol. Clin. North Am.*, **16**(1), 193, with permission

provide an interesting explanation for the observed high recurrence rate in treated disease.

AETIOLOGIES OF EXTRAPELVIC ENDOMETRIOSIS

The aetiology of endometriosis has generally been attributed to theories of (1) endometrial particle transport (transport theory), or (2) coelomic metaplasia (metaplasia, Meyer theory)[6]. The transport theory has been further subdivided into (a) retrograde regurgitation of endometrial fragments (Sampson theory)[2], (b) vascular transport of endometrial fragments[3], and (c) lymphatic transport of endometriotic fragments (Halban theory)[3]. The higher incidence of endometriosis in the abdominal and pelvic cavity would favour retrograde menstruation with passage of viable endometriotic tissue into the pelvis and abdomen and subsequent attachment to, and growth on, the recipient tissue. Indeed, animal studies involving transection of the uterus through the cervix, with retention of the uterus giving rise to menstruation into the abdominal cavity, have resulted in gross endometriosis in 70% of the animals[8]. Additionally, it has been a common observation that women with obstructed outflow tracts share a higher incidence of endometriosis presumed to be secondary to retrograde menstruation.

Considering the vastly different locations of reported extrapelvic endometriosis, it would appear that no single theory can adequately explain the origin of all observed disease either inside or outside of the pelvis. Furthermore, data now exist to support the theory that, no matter what the cause, the immune system of the body is significantly involved in the pathophysiologic development and progression of endometriosis[7]. The presence of autoantibodies to endometrial antigens observed in serum, in peritoneal fluid and on endometriotic implants of patients with active endometriosis[9] strongly suggests a 'multifactorial' theory in considering the aetiology and management of extrapelvic disease.

LOCATIONS OF EXTRAPELVIC ENDOMETRIOSIS

For anatomical reasons it is beneficial to group endometriosis outside of the pelvis into four separate groups: (1) intestinal tract endometriosis, (2) urinary tract endometriosis, (3) pulmonary and thoracic endometriosis and (4) endometriosis of other sites. Such a subdivision simplifies an understanding of reported cases of extrapelvic disease and is helpful in considering the diagnosis and management of cases under review.

A recently introduced new classification and staging system of extrapelvic endometriosis (Table 9.3)[3], dividing lesions into areas of involvement, size, volume of involvement and physiological impact of surrounding tissues and organs, may in the future allow for a more accurate reporting and assessment of management modalities.

Intestinal tract endometriosis

Endometriosis of the intestinal tract, including endometriosis of the bowel within the pelvis as well as of the rectovaginal and rectocervical areas, reflects the most common site of endometriosis outside of the female reproductive organs[6]. In one of the more extensive reviews of locations of endometriosis, Masson reported on 2686 cases of endometriosis operated upon at the Mayo Clinic between 1923 and 1945[10]. Of this group, 360 patients were identified as having involvement of the sigmoid, rectum, and rectosigmoid (13.4%), 67 of the rectovaginal septum (2.5%), 37 of the abdominal wall (1.4%), 35 of the small bowel (1.3%) and 15 of the appendix (0.6%) (Table 9.4). Utilizing the

Table 9.3 Classification and stages of extrapelvic endometriosis

Classification of extrapelvic endometriosis	
Class I:	Endometriosis involving the intestinal tract
Class U:	Endometriosis involving the urinary tract
Class L:	Endometriosis involving the lung and thoracic cage
Class O:	Endometriosis involving other sites outside the abdominal cavity
Staging of extrapelvic endometriosis	
Stage I	*No organ defect*
1.	Extrinsic: surface of organ (serosa, pleura)
	(a) < 1 cm lesion
	(b) 1–4 cm lesion
	(c) > 4 cm lesion
2.	Intrinsic: mucosal, muscle, parenchyma
	(a) < 1 cm lesion
	(b) 1–4 cm lesion
	(c) > 4 cm lesion
Stage II	*Organ defect*[a]
1.	Extrinsic: surface of organ (serosa, pleura)
	(a) < 1 cm lesion
	(b) 1–4 cm lesion
	(c) > 4 cm lesion
2.	Intrinsic: mucosal, muscle, parenchyma
	(a) < 1 cm lesion
	(b) 1 to 4 cm lesion
	(c) > 4 cm lesion

From Markham, S.M., Carpenter, S.E. and Rock, J.A. (1989). Extrapelvic endometriosis. *Obstet. Gynecol. Clin. North Am.*, **16**(1), 193, with permission
[a]Organ defect would depend on the organ of involvement and would include but not be limited to obstruction and partial obstruction of the urinary tract and the intestinal tract and haemothorax, haemoptysis, and pneumothorax resulting from pulmonary involvement

Table 9.4 Endometriosis of the intestinal tract

Author	Site	Number of cases	Percentage of total cases	Comment
Masson (1945)[10]	Sigmoid, rectum and rectosigmoid	360	13.4	Of 2686 cases found to have endometriosis
	Rectovaginal septum	67	2.5	
	Cervix	45	1.7	
	Vaginal wall	44	1.6	
	Abdominal wall	37	1.4	
	Small intestine	35	1.3	
	Caecum	18	0.7	
	Appendix	15	0.6	
	Umbilicus	11	0.4	
	Femoral hernia	2	> 0.1	
	Vesicovaginal septum	1	> 0.1	
Williams and Pratt (1977)[84]	Rectosigmoid	172	35.5	Of 485 patients found to have endometriosis in 1000 consecutive coeliotomies
	Appendix	19	3.9	
	Ileum	9	1.9	
Weed and Ray (1987)[11]	Colonic lesions	121	4.0	Of 3037 laparotomies found to have endometriosis
	Appendiceal lesions	22	0.7	
	Ileocaecal lesions	20	0.7	

Adapted with revision from Markham, S.M., Carpenter, S.E. and Rock, J.A. (1989). Extrapelvic endometriosis. *Obstet. Gynecol. Clin. North Am.*, **16**(1), 193, with permission current definition of extrapelvic endometriosis, 706 of Masson's 2686 cases had extrapelvic endometriosis (26.3%) and, of this number, over half were of sigmoid, rectum, and rectosigmoid involvement. An equally impressive series published by Weed and Ray in 1987 reported on 3037 cases of endometriosis operated upon at the Ochsner Foundation Hospital between 1955 and 1985[11]. Their data revealed that 163 of the 3037 cases were found to have involvement of the colon (4.0%), 22 of the appendix (0.7%) and 20 of the ileocaecum (0.7%). Though these data indicate some variation in reported incidence rates, sufficient data exist to document the fact that intestinal tract endometriosis is the most common location for extrapelvic endometriosis. Considering the transport theory, intestinal tract involvement, because of the close proximity to the fallopian tubes, would be expected to represent a high probability area of extrapelvic disease.

Presenting complaints of patients with intestinal tract endometriosis include (1) abdominal pain, (2) distension, (3) bowel function defects, and (4) rectal bleeding (Table 9.5). Intestinal obstruction is a frequent finding in more advanced disease and seems to favour the sigmoid, rectosigmoid and ileocaecal areas. With obstruction there is generally an extension of endometriotic growth through the bowel wall from the serosa to the mucosa. Non-obstructive lesions are usually limited to the serosa surface but may extend into the muscularis. A few cases have been reported in which massive ascites have also been present[12].

Management of intestinal endometriosis should be based on an accurate assessment of the location of the disease, the extent of involvement and the degree of physiological malfunction. Intestinal obstruction serves as an appropriate dividing point between institution of essential surgical intervention and the option of utilizing medical suppressive therapy or surgery. When obstructive lesions are not present, medical suppressive therapy is rec-ommended (Table 9.6). Although continuous (acyclic) birth control pills or progestins for a 6-month course have been utilized with good success, testosterone derivatives such as danazol have received much attention and have enjoyed a high success rate and are one of the more common forms of medical management at the present time[14]. More recent studies suggest that gonadotropin-releasing hormone (GnRH) analogues also provide good results in the suppression of endometriosis[13,14], but with the added advantage of none of the androgenic side-effects seen with testosterone derivatives. GnRH agonists, therefore, are proving to be an effective and desirable management option in spite of the parenteral routes of administration. It must be kept in mind, however, that recurrence of endometriosis is a possibility following any form of medical suppressive therapy.

Intestinal obstruction due to endometriosis requires immediate surgical intervention to relieve the obstruction. Additionally, lesions not responding to medical management or those of a more advanced level require a surgical approach. It is recommended that conservative surgery utilizing resection of individual endometriotic lesions be accomplished rather than more extensive approaches where possible. In cases of more advanced disease, segmental bowel resection or possibly an anterior resection may be required. Because of the possibility of the need for more extensive surgery, an aggressive bowel

Table 9.5 Case reports — intestinal tract endometriosis

Author	Age (years)	Abdominal/intestinal symptoms	Gynaecological symptoms	Operative procedure/ medical therapy	Diagnosis
Markham (1989, unpublished)	29	Constipation and rectal bleeding	Pelvic pressure and pelvic pain (some increase with menses)	(Danazol for 8 months followed by luprolide acetate for 20 months.) Laparoscopy followed by laparotomy with anterior resection and end-to-end anastomosis	Endometriosis of proximal rectum (Class I, Stage II2b) (see Table 9.3)
Ledley et al. (1988)[20]	38	Crampy abdominal pain, bloody diarrhoea and fever	(Hx vaginal hysterectomy for dysmenorrhoea)	Sigmoidoscopy, exploratory laparotomy with sigmoid resection and end-to-end reanastomosis, left partial S&O[a]	Endometrioma of the sigmoid colon with perforation and abscess formation
Thiel (1986)[21]	41	Abdominal and back pain, vomiting	None	Drainage of right ovarian cyst, partial right hemicolectomy	Endometriosis of the appendix and caecum
Naraynsingh et al. (1985)[22]	24	Abdominal distension and discomfort	Dysmenorrhoea	Laparotomy with biopsy of omentum (Depo-Provera)	Omental endometriosis with ascites
Halme et al. (1985)[12]	23	Abdominal distension and pain	None	Laparotomy with peritoneal biopsy (danazol)	Peritoneal endometriosis with ascites
Mann et al. (1984)[23]	41	None	Abnormal uterine bleeding, dysmenorrhoea, dyspareunia	Hysterectomy, left salpingo-oophorectomy and appendectomy	Left ovarian endometrioma, intussusception of appendix with endometriosis
	58	Abdominal distension, pelvic mass	None	Previous TAH[b] and Bil S&O[a], laparotomy with resection of nodules, rectosigmoid and appendix	Recurrent endometrioid carcinoma, appendix with intussusception and endometriosis

Table 9.5 Continued

Author	Age (years)	Abdominal/intestinal symptoms	Gynaecological symptoms	Operative procedure/ medical therapy	Diagnosis
Floberg et al. (1984)[24]	34	Abdominal pain	Early postpartum acute abdominal pain	Laparotomy with resection of left ovarian abscess, segment of sigmoid and fistulous tract	Left ovarian abscess with fistula to colon, rupture of colon, endometriosis of the colon
Caccese et al. (1984)[25]	37	Recurrent rectal bleeding, loose stools	None	Flexible sigmoidoscopy (management unknown)	Endometriosis of the colon
Langsam et al. (1984)[26]	32	Abdominal pain, nausea and vomiting	Symptoms worse with menses	Laparotomy with excision of left ovarian cystectomy and appendectomy	Left ovarian endometrioma, intussusception and endometriosis of the appendix
Hardy et al. (1983)[27]	40	Mid-abdominal pain, distension, diarrhoea and vomiting	None	Laparotomy with resection of terminal ileum and caecum	Endometriosis of the terminal ileum
Forsgren et al. (1983)[28]	43	Obstruction and diarrhoea	Unknown	Anterior resection	Endometriosis of the colon and rectum
	40	Obstruction and abdominal pain	Unknown	Laparotomy and colpotomy	Endometriosis of the colon and rectum
	51	Obstruction	Unknown	Laparotomy with dissection of segment of sigmoid	Endometriosis of the colon and rectum
	45	Obstruction, diarrhoea and abdominal pain	Unknown	Anterior resection (failed hormone therapy)	Endometriosis of the colon and rectum
	40	Obstruction, rectal bleeding and abdominal pain	Symptoms worse with menses	No operation (management unknown)	Endometriosis of the colon and rectum
	40	Obstruction and abdominal pain	Symptoms worse with menses	Laparotomy with dissection of rectal obstruction	Endometriosis of the colon and rectum

159

Table 9.5 Continued

Author	Age (years)	Abdominal/intestinal symptoms	Gynaecological symptoms	Operative procedure/medical therapy	Diagnosis
Teunen et al. (1982)[29]	47	Diarrhoea and constipation	None	Oophorectomy	Endometriosis of anterior rectal wall
	29	None	Infertility	Resection of endometriosis	Endometriosis of the rectosigmoid colon
	47	Increased urinary frequency	None	Resection of endometriosis	Endometriosis of the rectosigmoid colon
	60	Right lower quadrant pain	None	No operation (diet management only)	Endometriosis of the rectosigmoid colon
	33	None	Dysmenorrhoea, menometrorrhagia	No operation (progestins)	Endometriosis of the sigmoid colon
	47	Constipation	Dysmenorrhoea	No operation (diet management only)	Endometriosis of the sigmoid colon
	38	None	Dysmenorrhoea, menometrorrhagia	Resection of endometriosis	Endometriosis of the sigmoid colon
	48	Constipation, left lower quadrant pain (renal insufficiency)	Menometrorrhagia	Presacral neurectomy, urine deviation and haemodialysis (progestins)	Endometriosis of the sigmoid colon
	37	Left lower quadrant pain, constipation, diarrhoea and rectal bleeding	Symptoms worse with menses, secondary infertility	Resection of endometriosis (progestins, danazol and diet)	Endometriosis of the sigmoid colon
	40	Left lower quadrant pain, constipation, diarrhoea and rectal bleeding	None	Resection of endometriosis (progestins and diet management)	Endometriosis of the sigmoid colon
	41	Constipation, rectal bleeding	None	(progestins)	Endometriosis of the sigmoid colon
	41	Constipation, diarrhoea	Symptoms worse with menses, dysmenorrhoea	(progestins)	Endometriosis of the sigmoid colon
	38	Left lower quadrant pain, rectal bleeding	Infertility, dysmenorrhoea, symptoms worse with menses	Resection of endometriosis	Endometriosis of the sigmoid colon
	33	None	Infertility	Appendectomy	Endometriosis of the appendix, serosa of ileum

Table 9.5 Continued

Author	Age (years)	Abdominal/intestinal symptoms	Gynaecological symptoms	Operative procedure/ medical therapy	Diagnosis
	28	None	Infertility, dysmenorrhoea	Ileocaecal resection	Endometriosis of the appendix, ileocaecum and ascending colon
	39	Diarrhoea, rectal bleeding	Infertility, symptoms worse with menses	Resection of endometriosis (progestins)	Endometriosis of the ileum
	33	None	Infertility	Resection of endometriosis (progestins)	Endometriosis of the ileum
	45	Right lower quadrant pain, cyclic small bowel obstruction	Symptoms worse with menses	Ileocaecal resection	Endometriosis of ileocaecal angle
Honore (1980)[30]	48	Abdominal pain, postoperative small bowel obstruction	None	Excision of Meckel's diverticulum	Endometriosis of Meckel's diverticulum
Farinon et al. (1980)[31]	42	None	Multiple uterine fibromas	Hysterectomy with left salpingo-oophorectomy (progestins)	Endometriosis of the rectum
	41	None	Uterine fibroids left ovarian cyst	Hysterectomy with left salpingo-oophorectomy (progestins)	Endometriosis of the rectosigmoid
	36	Pelvic pain	Left ovarian cyst	Myomectomy with left oophorectomy (progestins)	Endometriosis of the sigmoid colon
Meyers et al. (1979)[32]	44	Intermittent pain, constipation and rectal bleeding	Vaginal bleeding	Previous TAH[b] and unilateral oophorectomy, resection of endometriosis and oophorectomy	Endometriosis of the sigmoid colon
	31	Abdominal pain, constipation, diarrhoea, rectal bleeding	Dyspareunia, symptoms worse with menses	TAH[b] with Bil S&O[a] (progestins)	Endometriosis of the colon Stage IV pelvic endometriosis

Table 9.5 Continued

Author	Age (years)	Abdominal/intestinal symptoms	Gynaecological symptoms	Operative procedure/ medical therapy	Diagnosis
	36	Episodic abdominal pain, diarrhoea and rectal bleeding	Menometrorrhagia and dyspareunia, some symptoms worse with menses	TAH with Bil S&O[a] hemicolectomy (hormone suppression)	Endometriosis of the transverse and descending colon
	29	Episodes of bloody diarrhoea, abdominal pain, rectal bleeding	Dysmenorrhoea and dyspareunia	Anterior resection with TAH[b] and Bil S&O[a] (hormone suppression)	Endometriosis of the descending and sigmoid colon
	47	Episodic abdominal pain, constipation and pressure	(Previous history of hysterectomy and right oophorectomy for pelvic endometriosis)	Sigmoid colectomy and left oophorectomy	Endometriosis of the sigmoid colon
	33	Episodic mucoid, bloody stools and abdominal pain	Menometrorrhagia (in past)	Sigmoid colectomy, TAH[b] with bilateral salpingo-oophorectomy	Endometriosis of the sigmoid colon
	40	Abdominal pain and rectal bleeding	(Previous history of hysterectomy and left salpingo-oophorectomy for pelvic endometriosis)	Resection of endometriosis with right salpingo-oophorectomy	Endometriosis of the sigmoid colon

Adapted with revision from Rock, J.A. and Markham, S.M. (1987). Extrapelvic endometriosis. In Wilson, E.A. (ed.) *Endometriosis*, p. 185. (New York: Alan R. Liss) with permission
[a]S&O = salpingo-oophorectomy (Bil = bilateral); [b]TAH = Total abdominal hysterectomy

Table 9.6 Medical management of extrapelvic endometriosis[a]

1. *Continuous (acyclic) combined oestrogen–progestin*
   (a) Ethinyl oestradiol 0.035–0.050 mg p.o., with norethindrone 0.4–1.0 mg p.o.
       continuously (Ovcon 35, Norinyl 1 + 35, Modicon, Ovcon 50)
   (b) Ethinyl oestradiol 0.030–0.050 mg p.o., with norgestrel 0.3–0.5 mg p.o.
       continuously (Lo/Ovral, Ovral)
   (c) Ethinyl oestradiol 0.050 mg p.o., with norethindrone acetate 1.0 mg p.o.
       continuously (Norlestrin 1/50)
2. *Continuous progestins*
   (a) Medroxyprogesterone acetate 40–60 mg p.o. daily (Provera); 200 mg i.m. every 2
       weeks (Depo-Provera)
   (b) Norethindrone acetate 30 mg p.o. daily (Norlutate)
   (c) Megestrol acetate 20–40 mg p.o. daily (Megase)
3. *Continuous testosterones*
   (a) 17-Ethinyl testosterone derivatives (danazol), 400–800 mg p.o. daily (Danocrine)[19]
   (b) 19-Nortestosterone derivatives 2.5–5.0 mg p.o. 2 or 3 times/week (gestrinone)[19]
   (c) Methyltestosterone 5–10 mg s.l. daily[18]
4. *Gonadotropin-releasing hormone (GnRH) analogues*
   (a) Buserelin 300 μg i.n. 3 times/day[16]
   (b) Luprolide 0.5 mg s.c. daily (Lupron); 7.5 mg i.m. monthly (Lupron Depot)
   (c) Nafarelin 200–400 μg i.n. 2 times/day[17]

Adapted with revision from Markham, S.M., Carpenter, S.E. and Rock, J.A. (1989). Extrapelvic endometriosis. *Obstet. Gynecol. Clin. North Am.*, **16**(1), 193, with permission
[a]p.o. = per os; i.m. = intramuscularly; s.l. = sublingually; i.n. = intranasally; s.c. = subcutaneously

preparation should be accomplished before any surgical resection of the intestinal tract for endometriosis is undertaken. The primary goal of any surgical approach should be complete resection of all endometriotic lesions. When both the intestinal tract and the reproductive organs are involved, conservation of the reproductive organs is acceptable if the involvement is minimal and can be completely excised or destroyed by electrocoagulation or vaporization at the time of bowel surgery. When more definitive surgery is needed, because of extensive endometriosis, it is unwise to leave a single ovary even though it is free of involvement. Past data would suggest that such an action is frequently followed by additional surgery for removal of the remaining ovary at a later date[3].

In cases of conservative management, a combined approach utilizing medical suppression following surgery appears to be more effective than either approach alone[15]. When more extensive involvement of the reproductive organs is found, or when the patient has no desire for additional childbearing, a total abdominal hysterectomy and bilateral salpingo-oophorectomy with appropriate bowel surgery is the treatment of choice.

Urinary tract endometriosis

Urinary tract endometriosis, including lesions of the pelvic ureter and the urinary bladder, is less common than intestinal tract disease but is significantly more common that extrapelvic endometriosis of other sites (Table 9.1). Although unilateral involvement of the ureter and kidney is the most common form of the disease, bilateral involvement of the urinary tract has been reported[34,35]. Endometriosis of the urinary tract may occur at any location, with the highest incidence in the bladder followed by the lower ureter, the upper ureter and the kidney[36,37].

Endometriosis of the urinary tract is best considered by dividing its occurrence into intrinsic and extrinsic types[3]. Intrinsic disease commonly presents with haematuria no matter where the area of involvement. Presenting symptoms of vesical endometriosis frequently include dysuria, urgency and frequency, while ureteral and kidney endometriosis more commonly present with haematuria and abdominal and flank pain (Table 9.7). Intrinsic ureteral endometriosis leads to a relatively high incidence of partial or complete obstruction of the ureter[35]. By far the most significant complication of obstruction is the loss of a kidney, which may occur in as many as 25% of patients with ureteral obstruction[37,38]. Extrinsic disease is less threatening but is often masked by symptoms of other pelvic involvement, including menometrorrhagia, dysmenorrhoea and dyspareunia. Isolated endometriosis of the kidney is infrequent[39]. Endometriosis of both the lower and upper urinary tract is only slightly more common. Diagnosis of endometriosis of the kidney is difficult and frequently confused with carcinoma.

The management of urinary tract endometriosis depends on the presence or absence of ureteral obstruction. When obstruction is present, a surgical approach with segmental resection and implantation, diversion or an end-to-end re-anastomosis is required. In cases of non-obstruction or partial obstruction, either a surgical or a medical management plan can be utilized. Past experience would suggest the use of medical management as a first approach with resort to surgical intervention only for non-responsive disease or cases where surgery is required for other pelvic involvement. Medical literature has little data directed exclusively to the medical management of urinary tract endometriosis or to extrapelvic endometriosis of any site. There is no reason to believe, however, that pelvic disease responds differently from extrapelvic endometriosis and, therefore, medical management with progestins, testosterone derivatives or gonadotropin-releasing hormone analogues (Table 9.6) would be expected to be effective. Success in the treatment of ureteral endometriosis has been reported using danazol, 400–600 mg/day[40] or with Depo-Provera, 400 mg twice per week[33]. GnRH analogues represent a more effective method of disrupting ovarian steroidogenesis, without the side-effects of progestins and testosterone derivatives and, therefore, the use of GnRH agonists can be expected to be as effective in suppressing extrapelvic endometriosis of the urinary tract as with pelvic disease[41].

Management of renal endometriosis would depend on the presenting symptoms and would include surgery, since carcinoma cannot be excluded effectively by any current means.

Pulmonary and thoracic endometriosis

Endometriosis of the lungs and thorax represent an uncommon site of extrapelvic endometriosis. The diagnosis is difficult because symptoms of thoracic endometriosis are similar to those of other more common pulmonary

Table 9.7 Case reports — urinary tract endometriosis

Author	Age (years)	Urinary tract symptoms	Gynaecological symptoms	Operative procedure/medical therapy	Diagnosis
Koszczuk et al. (1989)[36]	28	Intermittent cystitis, haematuria and low abdominal pain	None	Cystourethroscopy. Laparotomy with excision of bladder endometrioma (Danazol postop)	Endometriosis of the bladder wall
	45	Intermittent haemorrhagic cystitis and low abdominal pain	Dyspareunia (Hx of pelvic endometriosis treated by TAH[a])	Cystourethroscopy and biopsy. Bilateral salpingo-oophorectomy (Progestins)	Endometriosis of the bladder involving the trigone
	46	Gross haematuria, intermittent retention	None (Hx of previous TAH[a] and bilateral S&O[b] for unrelated problem)	IVP[c] = left ureteral obstruction. Laparotomy with left nephroureterectomy	Left ureteral endometriosis with obstruction
	27	Urgency and frequency, lower lumbar pain extending to right anterior thigh	Pelvic pain, dysmenorrhoea, dyspareunia (Hx Stage 3 pelvic endometriosis recently diagnosed)	Cystourethroscopy. Laparotomy with excision of endometriosis, lysis of adhesions and right salpingo-oophorectomy (Danazol pre- and postoperatively)	Endometriosis of the bladder wall and trigone
	43	Haematuria, dysuria and urgency	None (Hx of extensive pelvic endometriosis recently made)	Laparotomy with TAH and bilateral S&O[a] and left ureteral exploration with excision of endometriosis	Endometriosis of the left ureter, extensive pelvic endometriosis
Buka (1988)[42]	32	None	Dysmenorrhoea (Hx of previous caesarean section)	Cystoscopy and biopsy. Laparotomy with TAH[a] and excision of bladder endometriosis	Endometriosis of the bladder (post caesarean section)
Kiely et al. (1988)[43]	70	Right loin pain (status post percutaneous removal of right renal and upper ureteric calculi)	Post-menopausal	Exploration with a right nephroureterectomy and lysis of adhesions	Endometriosis of the right ureter

165

Table 9.7 Continued

Author	Age (years)	Urinary tract symptoms	Gynaecological symptoms	Operative procedure/ medical therapy	Diagnosis
Lucero et al. (1988)[44]	31	Cyclic right flank pain	Symptoms worse before menses	Laparoscopy, laparotomy with TAH[a] and bilateral S&O[b], left ureterolysis and right ureteroneocystostomy (post op cyclic oestrogen)	Endometriosis of the right ureter (intrinsic and extrinsic)
	42	Left costovertebral tenderness	Symptoms worse with menses	Laparotomy with TAH[a] and bilateral S&O[b], left ureteroneocysostomy	Endometriosis of the left ureter with partial obstruction
	27	Right flank pain, right hydronephrosis	Hx of right adnexal cyst	Laparotomy with right ovarian cystectomy and right salpingectomy, excision of bladder endometriosis (postop cyclic oestrogen)	Endometriosis of the bladder with pelvic endometriosis
Foster et al. (1987)[45]	27	Cyclic suprapubic pain exacerbated by voiding	Severe dysmenorrhoea (Hx of previous TAH[a] with biopsy of right ovary)	Laparotomy with partial cystectomy (acyclic oestrogen/progestin postop)	Endometriosis of the bladder
Al Saleh (1987)[46]	29	Intermittent left lower abdominal and flank pain	Dysmenorrhoea and infertility	Laparotomy with excision of ovarian endometriomas, exploration of left ureter, ureterotomy with reimplantation into the bladder	Endometriosis of the left ureter (with duplex), moderate pelvic endometriosis
Mourin-Jouret et al. (1987)[34]	41	End-stage renal failure (consideration of renal transplant)	Menometrorrhagia	Transplantation of cadaver kidney in left lower quadrant — native ureter dilated. Ipsilateral ureteronephrectomy	Endometriosis of the left ureter with obstruction
Thomsen et al. (1987)[47]	41	Haematuria and left hydronephrosis	None	Laparotomy with resection of endometriosis and left ureteroureterostomy	Endometriosis of the left ureter (intrinsic)

166

Table 9.7 Continued

Author	Age (years)	Urinary tract symptoms	Gynaecological symptoms	Operative procedure/ medical therapy	Diagnosis
Plous et al. (1985)[48]	74	Gross haematuria, dysuria and frequency	None	Exploration with ureterotomy and reimplantation of the right ureter	Endometriosis of the right ureter
Porena et al. (1985)[49]	54	Persistent microhaematuria, left flank pain	Hx of oestrogen replacement therapy in past	Exploration with left nephroureterectomy and lymph node excision	Endometriosis of the left ureter with obstruction and atrophy of the left kidney
Vermesh et al. (1985)[50]	39	Intermittent gross haematuria, dysuria, frequency and urgency	Hx of previous vaginal hysterectomy for prolapse	Resection of bladder tumours transurethrally (danazol postop)	Endometriosis of the bladder wall
Matsuura et al. (1985)[40]	21	Increasing body weight	Dysmenorrhoea and cyclic abdominal pain	Laparotomy with left salpingo-oophorectomy, biopsy of abdominal and pelvic lesions (Danazol postop)	Endometriosis of the left ureter, pelvic endometriosis
Gantt et al. (1981)[33]	26	None	Low abdominal pain, worse during menses	Laparotomy with resection left ovarian endometriomas (Depo-Provera postop)	Endometriosis of the left ureter, pelvic endometriosis
Bazaz-Malik et al. (1980)[39]	40	Right loin pain, right hydronephrosis	None	Exploration with left nephrectomy	Endometriomas of the right kidney
Moore et al. (1979)[35]	43	Backache, left hydronephrosis	Dysmenorrhoea	Laparotomy with TAH[a] and bilateral S&O[b], resection of distal third of left ureter and left ureteroneocystotomy	Endometriosis of the left ureter, pelvic endometriosis
	30	Obstruction distal to left ureter	Dysmenorrhoea, infertility	Laparotomy with TAH[a] and left salpingo-oophorectomy, ureteral lysis	Pelvic endometriosis

Table 9.7 Continued

Author	Age (years)	Urinary tract symptoms	Gynaecological symptoms	Operative procedure/ medical therapy	Diagnosis
	32	Premenstrual dysuria, hydronephrosis and hydroureter	Dysmenorrhoea and low abdominal pain	Laparotomy with TAH[a] and bilateral S&O[b] and bilateral ureteral lysis (progestins postop)	Endometriosis of ureters, bilateral. Pelvic endometriosis with intestinal tract involvement
	25	Right flank pain, haematuria and right hydronephrosis	Dysmenorrhoea	Laparotomy with TAH and bilateral S&O, right ureteroneocystotomy	Endometriosis of the right ureter, pelvic endometriosis
	33	Left hydronephrosis	Dyspareunia, pelvic mass	Exploration with resection of left kidney and left ureter, resection of pelvic endometriosis	Endometriosis of the left ureter, pelvic endometriosis
	26	Dysuria with menses	Dysmenorrhoea with left lower quadrant pain	Laparotomy with open resection of the bladder, right ureteral lysis and segmental resection of the transverse colon	Endometriosis of the bladder, pelvic endometriosis with involvement of the intestinal tract
	44	Right hydronephrosis	Right lower quadrant pain (Hx of right salpingo-oophorectomy, resection of pelvic endometriosis and segmental small bowel resection)	Laparotomy with proximal right ureterostomy, ureteral lysis, resection of bladder wall endometriosis	Endometriosis of the bladder and right ureter, extensive pelvic endometriosis
	21	Impaired drainage of right ureter	Dysmenorrhoea	Laparotomy with right ureterolysis, resection of endometrioma of uterosacral ligaments	Pelvic endometriosis with endometriosis of the right uterosacral ligament

Adapted with revision from Rock, J.A. and Markham, S.M. (1987). Extrapelvic endometriosis. In Wilson, E.A. (ed.) *Endometriosis*, p. 185. (New York: Alan R. Liss), with permission

[a]TAH = Total abdominal hysterectomy; [b]S&O = salpingo-oophorectomy; [c]IVP = intravenous pyelogram

pathologies. Presenting symptoms and signs usually include chest pain, pneumothorax, haemothorax, or haemoptysis, usually concomitant with menses[6] (Table 9.8). An additional presenting sign of asymptomatic pulmonary nodule(s) has also been noted in some cases[51]. Previous reviews have conveniently divided this disease into four distinct categories: (a) catamenial pneumothorax, (b) catamenial haemothorax, (c) catamenial haemoptysis, and (d) asymptomatic pulmonary nodules[3,51]. A review of recently reported cases indicates, however, that not all cases have catamenial symptoms. More important is the fact that in those cases with catamenial symptoms a histological diagnosis cannot always be made. In these patients a diagnosis was made by exclusion, noting the cyclicity of symptoms and the regression of symptoms with removal of the ovaries or with medical suppression of the menstrual cycle. A review of 84 cases of thoracic endometriosis found that 22% of patients with catamenial pneumothorax had documented pelvic endometriosis[51]. All of those with catamenial haemothorax and none of the patients with catamenial haemoptysis were found to have concurrent pelvic endometriosis. Cases reported in Table 9.8 showed a 71% incidence of pelvic endometriosis occurring with pulmonary disease and, when pelvic endometriosis was present, it was usually of a more advanced stage. Karpal's review further showed that the right chest was more likely involved in cases of catamenial pneumothorax and exclusively involved in the cases of catamenial haemothorax. Of the patients with asymptomatic pulmonary nodules, three of five involved only the right lung and one of five involved both lungs. None of the nodules were noted to vary with the menstrual cycle. Clearly, the right lung and chest cage are more frequently involved with extrapelvic endometriosis than the left. Such a finding would tempt the conclusion that pulmonary endometriosis has, as its origin, the transport of endometriotic fragments through a rent or perforation in the right diaphragm, a defect which is less frequently found on the left. Rents or fenestrations of the diaphragm have been reported in the past and are located more commonly in the right diaphragm[52]. Additionally, a theory has been proposed of a continuous current of peritoneal fluid circulating clockwise in the abdomen from the pelvis to the right upper quadrant[3]. Such theories can not be entirely proved as the sole cause of pulmonary endometriosis; nor can the idea of diaphragmatic implantation followed by infiltration and subsequent perforation. Other possibilities of pulmonary spread could be by passage of endometriotic fragments through lymphatics to the lung[53].

Management of pulmonary endometriosis, based on a review of past medical literature, would favour surgical intervention with thoracotomy, excision of endometriotic lesions and/or pleurodesis[6]. More recent data, however, have suggested an increasing role for primary medical therapy utilizing ovarian suppressing drugs such as danazol, particularly in cases of catamenial haemoptysis[52,54]. Medical therapy in conjunction with surgery has been commonly utilized in more extensive disease and in the presence of pelvic endometriosis. Hysterectomy with bilateral salpingo-oophorectomy has been considered necessary in progressive or recurrent disease[6].

As with other forms of extrapelvic endometriosis, a treatment plan for pulmonary disease should take into consideration the location and extent of

Table 9.8 Case reports — pulmonary and thoracic cage endometriosis

Author	Age (years)	Pulmonary symptoms	Gynaecological symptoms	Operative procedures/ medical therapy	Diagnosis
Balasingham et al. (1986)[55]	30	Breathlessness and chest pain, pneumothorax	Symptoms associated with menses	Thoracostomy, thoracotomy with pleural ablation (preop acyclic oestrogen/progestin)	Catamenial pneumothorax
Wilkins et al. (1985)[56]	32	Dyspnoea, cough, pleural effusion (bloody)	Symptoms not associated with menses (Hx of PID)	Pleural biopsy, right chest tube thoracostomy, laparotomy (with presumed TAH[a] and bil S&O[b])	Pleural endometriosis with recurrent haematothorax, pelvic endometriosis severe
Suginami et al. (1985)[57]	25	Haemoptysis with severe cough	Symptoms associated with menses, menorrhagia (Hx elective abortion)	Laparoscopy, bronchoscopy and biopsy of lung (danazol). Thoracotomy with resection of upper lobe of right lung	Endometriosis of the right lung, pelvic endometriosis
Karpel et al. (1985)[51]	25	Right-sided pleuritic chest pain, dyspnoea (Hx spontaneous pneumothorax)	Symptoms associated with menses	Chemical pleurodesis, thoracotomy with closure of diaphragmatic perforations and abrasive pleurodesis	Catamenial pneumothorax
	42	Dyspnoea, right shoulder pain, right pneumothorax, right pleural effusion	Symptoms associated with menses	Thoracostomy (danazol), pleurodesis, thoracotomy, excision of haemorrhagic cyst, pleural decortication TAH with bil S&O[b]	Catamenial haemothorax, pelvic endometriosis
	31	Haemoptysis, pleuritic chest pain	Symptoms associated with menses (Hx of 2 normal pregnancies)	Bronchoscopy with washings	Catamenial haemoptysis
Rosenberg and Riddick (1981)[54]	37	Recurrent haemoptysis	Symptoms associated with menses	Bronchoscopy with biopsy (danazol)	Catamenial haemoptysis, pelvic endometriosis

Table 9.8 Continued

Author	Age (years)	Pulmonary symptoms	Gynaecological symptoms	Operative procedures/ medical therapy	Diagnosis
Foster et al. (1981)[52]	30	Right-sided chest pain, spontaneous pneumothorax (right)	Symptoms associated with menses, infertility	Pleuroscopy (danazol), thoracotomy, apical pleurectomy, excision of endometrial nodules (pleura)	Catamenial pneumothorax, pelvic endometriosis, mild to moderate
	24	Dyspnoea, opacification of the right lung field	Low abdominal pain, pelvic mass. Symptoms associated with menses	Thoracentesis, laparotomy (danazol), thoracotomy with pleurectomy, excision of implants of the diaphragm, closure of diaphragmatic defects	Pleural endometriosis, pelvic endometriosis
	36	Recurrent haemoptysis, chest pain	Symptoms associated with menses	Bronchoscopy with washings (danazol)	Catamenial haemoptysis
Charles (1981)[58]	42	Dyspnoea, pain in left chest, pleural effusion	Symptoms not associated with menses, dysmenorrhoea, dyspareunia, umbilical mass	Pleural aspirations laparotomy with TAH[a] and bil S&O[b], resection of umbilical mass (postop oral progestin)	Pelvic endometriosis, severe, with pleural effusion
Hibbard et al. (1981)[59]	48	Intermittent right upper chest pain, chronic bronchitis, bronchiectasis and right empyema	Symptoms associated with menses	(Depo-Provera) D&C (Premarin) laparotomy with TAH[a] and bil S&O[b] (cyclic oestrogens)	Catamenial chest pain, pelvic endometriosis severe
	28	Recurring haemorrhagic pleural effusion	(Presumed cyclic symptoms associated with menses)	Thoracocentesis, open lung biopsy, pleural needle biopsies, bronchoscopy, pulmonary arteriography, laparotomy with appendectomy, laparotomy with subtotal hysterectomy and attempted bil S&O[b] (postop Depo-Provera)	Catamenial haemothorax, pelvic endometriosis, severe

Adapted with revision from Rock, J.A. and Markham, S.M. (1987). Extrapelvic endometriosis. In Wilson, E.A. (ed.) Endometriosis, p. 185. (New York: Alan R. Liss), with permission
[a]TAH = Total abdominal hysterectomy; [b]S&O = salpingo-oophorectomy (bil = bilateral)

the disease, the patient's age and the desire for future childbearing. Acute complications such as pneumothorax or haemothorax would require prompt surgical intervention. Once the patient has been stabilized, then diagnostic procedures such as thoracentesis, bronchoscopy and biopsy may be appropriately followed with conservative medical management. If satisfactory response is not achieved or the disease recurs or progresses, surgical intervention with thoracotomy, excision of lesions, lysis of adhesions, and/or pleurodesis with either chemical or abrasive means is the treatment of choice. Thoracotomy should be accomplished in cases of pulmonary nodules, symptomatic or asymptomatic, for purposes of diagnosis and for surgical management.

In cases of progressive or recurrent disease treated by a total abdominal hysterectomy and bilateral salpingo-oophorectomy, low-dose oestrogen replacement therapy has been effective in managing oestrogen-deprivation symptoms without significant stimulation of recurrent disease[6]. It should be noted that radiation therapy as a means of castration in cases of pulmonary or pleural endometriosis offers no advantage over hormone suppressive therapy or surgery[6]. Increasing experience with GnRH analogues may soon prove that these agents will be a treatment of choice over hormone suppression as primary therapy or in conjunction with surgical intervention with more advanced disease[41].

Endometriosis of other sites

Extrapelvic endometriosis of sites other than the intestinal tract, the urinary tract and the lungs represents only a small number of cases. Patients reported in this group share several common factors: (a) the disease is frequently misdiagnosed for a prolonged period of time; (b) the symptoms are generally cyclic in nature and related to the menstrual period; and (c) surgical excision has been the management of choice. Virtually all tissues and organ systems in the female body have been reported to have had endometriotic involvement (Table 9.9), with the exception of the spleen. A review of surgical pathology specimens at The Johns Hopkins Hospital between 1938 and 1988 failed to identify a single case of splenic endometriosis. Cases of splenosis mimicking endometriosis have, however, been reported[60]. The spleen seems to enjoy a uniquely privileged status which in the future may be important in the understanding of the aetiology, growth and progression of both pelvic and extrapelvic disease.

Most extrapelvic endometriosis outside the abdominal and chest cavities presents as a palpable mass, generally causing pain, and usually more symptomatic at the time of the menses. Abdominal and episiotomy scars, along with the umbilical and inguinal areas, are the most frequent sites of involvement; however, any mass progressing in size and fluctuating with the menstrual cycle should be suspect of extrapelvic endometriosis.

Because of the small number of cases available for review and because of the vastly different tissue structures involved, management must be based on individual factors, including size of lesion, location of involvement, symptoms and the desire for future reproduction. Case reports of extrapelvic endomet-

172

Table 9.9 Case reports — endometriosis of other sites

Author	Age (years)	Non-gynaecological symptoms	Gynaecological symptoms	Operative procedure/ medical therapy	Diagnosis
Thibodeau et al. (1987)[61]	20	Generalized seizures, right occipital headache	Symptoms not associated with menses	Right parieto-occipital craniotomy, excision of cystic lesion of posteroinferior parietal lobe (postop danazol)	Cerebral endometriosis
Hibbard et al. (1984)[64]	40	Right foot drop, pain in right hip radiating into right leg	None (Hx of previous TAH and right salpingo-oophorectomy for pelvic endometriosis)	Computerized tomographic scan, exploration of right sciatic nerve	Endometriosis of the right sciatic nerve
Salazar-Grueso et al. (1986)[65]	24	Episodic back and right leg pain, right foot drop and constant right buttock pain	None (Hx of previous TAH[a] and right salpingo-oophorectomy for pelvic endometriosis). Symptoms not associated with menses prior to TAH	Computerized tomographic scan, surgical exploration with neurolysis, lysis of adhesions, resection of endometriosis and piriformis muscle (postop progestin) (later underwent a left S&O[b])	Endometriosis of the right sciatic nerve
Michowitz et al. (1983)[66]	43	Periumbilical pain, periumbilical mass	Symptoms worse with menses	Excision of periumbilical mass	Endometriosis of the umbilicus
Blumenthal et al. (1981)[67]	46	Umbilical lump and pain	Symptoms worse with menses (no evidence of pelvic endometriosis)	Excision of umbilical mass	Endometriosis of the umbilicus
Sataloff et al. (1989)[68]	37	Bulge in right groin, non-reducible	Mass increased in size with menses (No hx of pelvic endometriosis)	Exploration of inguinal region with excision of mass and right round ligament	Endometriosis of the right groin
	33	Lump in superior aspect of caesarean section scar	(Hx of two caesarean sections)	Excision of abdominal wall mass	Endometriosis of incisional scar
Brzezinski and Durst (1983)[69]	41	Right inguinal mass and tenderness	Mass increased in size with menses	Excision of right inguinal hernia and mass	Endometriosis of the right inguinal canal

Table 9.9 Continued

Author	Age (years)	Non-gynaecological symptoms	Gynaecological symptoms	Operative procedure/ medical therapy	Diagnosis
Wolf and Kopecky (1989)[70]	30	Pain and swelling in caesarean section scar	Symptoms worse with menses (Hx of two previous caesarean sections)	Computerized tomographic scan, resection of anterior abdominal wall mass	Endometriosis of the anterior abdominal wall
Kennedy et al. (1988)[71]	27	Anterior abdominal wall mass and pain	Hx of dysmenorrhoea and dyspareunia, hx of TAH[a] for termination of pregnancy	(Preop nafarelin acetate). Excision of anterior abdominal wall mass	Endometrioma of the anterior abdominal wall
Rovito and Gittleman (1986)[72]	29	Pain in caesarean section scar, tenderness in scar, mass in same area	Pain related to menstrual cycles	Exploration of scar with excision of mass	Endometrioma of caesarean section scar
	35	Pain in old caesarean section scar, mass in same area	No relation to menses (Hx of two previous caesarean sections)	Exploration with excision of anterior rectus sheath mass	Endometriosis of caesarean section scar
Finkel et al. (1986)[62]	21	Episodic sharp, epigastric pain, nausea and vomiting, right subcostal mass	Symptoms not related to menses	Exploration with drainage and partial excision of an intrahepatic cyst (postop danazol)	Endometrioma of the liver
Goswami et al. (1986)[73]	40	Recurrent episodes of left flank pain	None	Exploration with left radical nephrectomy, distal pancreatectomy and splenectomy	Endometriosis of the pancreas

174

Table 9.9 Continued

Author	Age (years)	Non-gynaecological symptoms	Gynaecological symptoms	Operative procedure/ medical therapy	Diagnosis
Marchevsky et al. (1984)[74]	36	Mild epigastric pain (Hx previous acute pancreatitis)	None	Exploratory laparotomy with distal pancreatectomy and splenectomy	Endometrioma of the pancreas
Gupta (1985)[75]	42	Pain and bleeding from left thumb	Symptoms occurred during menses and began at menarche	Excision of mass from tip of left thumb	Endometriosis of the thumb
Patel et al. (1982)[63]	32	Painful swelling of lateral aspect of right knee	Swelling increased during menses	Exploration of knee with biopsy (postop danazol)	Endometriosis of the knee
Giagnarra et al. (1987)[76]	25	Pain in left thigh (Hx of previous excision of cavernous haemangioma from right knee)	Pain increased before menses	Exploration of thigh with excision of mass	Endometriosis of the biceps femoris
Pellegrini et al. (1981)[77]	36	Intermittent pain in right groin, tenderness, mass over pubic tubercle	Symptoms more prominent before menses	Excision of pubic mass	Endometrioma of pubis
	30	Intermittent pain in right groin and hip, tender mass over right pubic tubercle	Symptoms worse before menses	Excision of pubic mass	Endometrioma of pubis

Adapted with revision from Rock, J.A. and Markham, S.M. (1987). Extrapelvic endometriosis. In Wilson, E.A. (ed.) *Endometriosis*, p. 185. (New York: Alan R. Liss), with permission
[a]TAH = Total abdominal hysterectomy; [b]S&O = salpingo-oophorectomy

riosis would suggest surgical excision as the most effective means of therapy. Postoperative hormonal suppression may be of added benefit when the endometriosis is not completely excised or when it is in a critical area or in a contained space[61-63]. In difficult cases or when future childbearing is no longer an issue, oophorectomy with or without hysterectomy may be the treatment of choice[3].

DISCUSSION

Of the disease processes involving the human body, endometriosis generates a degree of fascination unique in medicine. This interest occurs because of the lack of complete knowledge as to the origin of the disease, the poor understanding of its progression and the vastly different areas of occurrence. Classical theories of aetiology of endometriosis must now be tempered with the possibility of a multifactorial phenomenon with a possible immunological basis as a primary contributor to occurrence and progression. Involvement of tissues outside the abdominal cavity generally cannot be explained by Sampson's classic retrograde menstruation theory. Involvement of such distal areas as the brain and extremities would also not be fully explained purely by lymphatic or haematogenous spread without other tissues being equally involved.

An immunological relationship to the origin and progression of endometriosis is a most attractive theory considering the known increase in immunoglobulin levels and the high frequency of autoantibodies found in patients with endometriosis[78]. Additionally, danazol, which effectively suppresses endometriosis, is known to inhibit autoantibody production[79]. The possibility exists, therefore, that endometriosis is an autoimmune disease not dissimilar to systemic lupus erythematosus, with which there has been a frequent association[80].

No matter what the true aetiology of endometriosis, the common denominator appears to be the presence of oestrogen. The fact that endometriosis occurs almost without exception during the reproductive years in patients with functional ovaries supports this view. Additionally, patients with ovarian dysgenesis, such as Turner's syndrome, have not been reported to have had endometriosis except when they have received oestrogen replacement therapy[81,82]. Data have also suggested that patients with endometriosis do not develop recurrent disease following hysterectomy and oophorectomy unless residual ovarian function is present or they have received oestrogen replacement therapy[83].

Pelvic and extrapelvic endometriosis are different only in (a) their occurrence rate and (b) their anatomical location. The frequency of occurrence appears to decrease as the distance from the uterus and fallopian tubes increases[84]. There are no data to support an impression that endometriosis of the pelvis and of extrapelvic sites differ in origin, progression, or response to medical or surgical management. The incidence of pelvic endometriosis is felt to be between 10% and 15% of women in the reproductive age group[3], while the incidence of extrapelvic disease represents less than 12% of reported cases of endometriosis[6]. In spite of a considerably smaller occurrence of extrapelvic endometriosis, such a disease process is significant to the gynaecologist and surgeon because of the potential for major organ involvement with complications such as intestinal or urinary tract obstruction or pulmonary emergencies such as pneumothorax or haemothorax.

Endometriosis of the intestinal tract represents the highest incidence of extrapelvic disease with the most frequent area of involvement being the sigmoid colon and rectum, followed by the iliocaecal area and appendix. Less common is involvement of the transverse colon and the small bowel. Management of intestinal tract endometriosis without obstruction is best accomplished utilizing medical suppressive therapy (Table 9.6). This would include hormone suppression with progestins such as medroxyprogesterone (Provera, Depo-Provera) and megestrol acetate (Megase) or suppression with testosterones such as 17-ethinyltestosterone derivatives (danazol) and 19-nortestosterone derivatives (gestrinone). Recently, impressive results have been achieved with GnRH agonists such as luprolide, buserelin and nafarelin; however, government (US FDA) approval for utilization of GnRH agonists in the management of endometriosis is still under consideration. It should be noted that endometriomas or adhesive disease do not respond to medical management with either GnRH agonists or with hormone suppression. Intestinal tract endometriosis with obstruction or involvement not responding to medical management requires surgical intervention that should include excision of all lesions and possible segmental bowel resection. Total abdominal hysterectomy with bilateral salpingo-oophorectomy is also indicated in advanced disease or in progressive disease. There is no merit in leaving a single uninvolved ovary. In reported cases utilizing a unilateral oophorectomy, removal of the remaining ovary at a later date becomes necessary in a majority of cases (Table 9.5). Though recurrence of endometriosis has been reported following hysterectomy and oophorectomy when oestrogen replacement has been implemented, it is felt that the benefits of oestrogen replacement with physiological doses of conjugated oestrogen (Premarin 0.625 mg/day) far outweigh the risk of recurrent disease, particularly in the symptomatic patient.

Extrapelvic endometriosis of the urinary tract is less common than intestinal tract disease but is no less important. Ureteral obstruction represents the most serious complication and not infrequently results in loss of a kidney. The highest frequency of urinary tract involvement occurs in the bladder followed by the lower ureter, the upper ureter and the kidney. Cases without obstruction are best managed by medical suppression similarly to intestinal tract disease. In cases of obstruction, or cases not responding to medical management, surgical intervention is necessary and should include excision of all endometriotic lesions and possible ureteral resection with anastomosis or reimplantation. Hysterectomy and oophorectomy should be included in cases of more advanced disease with obstruction and in patients not interested in future childbearing.

Endometriosis of the lung and thorax represent the most common site of extrapelvic endometriosis outside the abdominal cavity. Involvement of this area is conveniently divided into four categories: (a) catamenial pneumothorax,

(b) catamenial haemothorax, (c) catamenial haemoptysis, and (d) asymptomatic pulmonary nodules. Though therapy in the past has been primarily surgical, it now appears that once life-threatening events such as pneumothorax and haemothorax have been stabilized, medical suppressive therapy is appropriate, leaving operative intervention for advanced disease or for patients with failed medical management. Operative intervention should include thoracotomy, excision of endometriotic lesions, lysis of chest cage adhesions and/or pleurodesis. Hysterectomy with oophorectomy should be included only in progressive disease or when pelvic indications would suggest the need for removal of the reproductive organs.

Extrapelvic endometriosis of other sites is so infrequent that management decisions should be individually based on location of the disease, extent of involvement and the existence of organ/tissue malfunction. Unlike the other types of extrapelvic endometriosis, disease outside the abdominal and thoracic cavities generally is best treated by surgical excision. The need for postoperative medical suppression should also be considered when involvement of major organs has occurred or when incomplete resection is suspected.

Accurate diagnosis and management of extrapelvic endometriosis, as with any other disease process, rests to some degree on knowledge of other cases of the same disease and their management and follow-up. In pelvic endometriosis, a standardized staging system introduced by the American Fertility Society in 1985 has been of benefit in the evaluation of cases presented for review. No similar staging system was present for extrapelvic disease until 1989, when a new classification and staging system was introduced[3] (Table 9.3). This system divides extrapelvic endometriosis into four classes dependent on location: Class I, endometriosis of the intestinal tract; Class U, endometriosis of the urinary tract; Class L, endometriosis of the lung and thoracic cage; and Class O, endometriosis involving other sites. Involvement is further divided into Stage I (no organ defect) and Stage II (organ defect). Finally, the classification divides the disease into intrinsic and extrinsic involvement and into the size of the involvement (< 1 cm; $1-4$ cm; and > 4 cm).

The tables presented in this chapter represent a review of the more significant cases of extrapelvic endometriosis reported in the last decade (1979–1989). Had a classification and staging system been available and utilized in these case reports, perhaps a more meaningful assessment of therapies would have been possible.

The current hormonal and surgical management of extrapelvic endometriosis may in the future be replaced with GnRH analogues because of their superior ability to disrupt ovarian steroidogenesis and to suppress oestrogen production. Additionally, use of immunological therapy modalities such as autoantibody inhibitors may well augment the benefits of GnRH regimens. These new approaches will be limited to mild and moderate disease, however, since more extensive disease with obstruction or endometriomas and adhesions will continue to require a surgical approach.

Finally, the issue of risks and benefits of post-oophorectomy oestrogen replacement therapy, or concurrent low-dose oestrogen replacement with GnRH therapy, in the management of extrapelvic endometriosis needs further evaluation. It has been an observation that oestrogen replacement using conjugated oestrogens does not stimulate recurrent endometriosis in the same manner as endogenous oestrogen from ovaries left in place. It is therefore felt that the practice of oestrogen replacement under these circumstances is safe; however, it should be kept in mind that recurrence has been reported and close surveillance is necessary. The possibility of using concurrent low-dose oestrogen during GnRH analogue suppression is presently being evaluated and it is possible that such a combination will allow a longer therapeutic course with improved results.

REFERENCES

1. Saleh, N. and Daw, E. (1980). Endometriosis in non-gynecological sites. *Practitioner*, **224**, 1189
2. Sampson, J.A. (1940). The development of the implantation theory for the origin of peritoneal endometriosis. *Am. J. Obstet. Gynecol.*, **40**, 549
3. Markham, S.M., Carpenter, S.E. and Rock, J.A. (1989). Extrapelvic endometriosis. *Obstet. Gynecol. Clin. North Am.*, **16**(1), 193
4. Murphy, A.A., Green, W.R., Bobbie, D., dela Cruz, Z.C. and Rock, J.A. (1986). Unsuspected endometriosis documented by scanning electron microscopy in visually normal peritoneum. *Fertil. Steril.*, **46**(3), 522
5. Redwine, D.B. (1988). Is 'microscopic' peritoneal endometriosis invisible? *Fertil. Steril.*, **50**(4), 665
6. Rock, J.A. and Markham, S.M. (1987). Extrapelvic endometriosis. In Wilson, E.A. (ed.) *Endometriosis*, p. 185. (New York: Alan R. Liss)
7. Dmowski, W.P. (1987). Immunological aspects of endometriosis. *Cont. Gynecol. Obstet.*, **16**, 48
8. TeLinde, R.W. and Scott, R.B. (1950). Experimental endometriosis. *Obstet. Gynecol.*, **60**, 1147
9. Mathur, S., Garza, E.E., Chihal, H.J., Rust, P.F., Homm, R.S. and Williamson, H.O. (1988). Endometrial antigens involved in the autoimmunity of endometriosis. *Fertil. Steril.*, **50**(6), 860
10. Masson, J.C. (1945). Present conception of endometriosis and its treatment. *Trans. West. Surg. Assoc.*, **53**, 35
11. Weed, J.C. and Ray, J.E. (1987). Endometriosis of the bowel. *Obstet. Gynecol.*, **69**(5), 727
12. Halme, J., Chafe, W. and Currie, J.L. (1985). Endometriosis with massive ascites. *Obstet. Gynecol.*, **65**(4), 591
13. Schriock, E., Monroe, S.E., Henzl, M. and Jaffe, R.B. (1985). Treatment of endometriosis with a potent agonist of gonadotropin-releasing hormone (nafarelin). *Fertil. Steril.*, **44**(5), 583
14. Yee, B. (1986). A preliminary report on the comparative use of Buserelin (hoe 766) and Danazol in the treatment of endometriosis: The University of Southern California. *Prog. Clin. Biol. Res.*, **222**, 175
15. Wheeler, J.M. and Malinak, L.R. (1989). The surgical management of endometriosis. *Obstet. Gynecol. Clin. North Am.*, **16**(1), 147
16. Jelley, R.Y. and Magill, P.J. (1986). The effects of LHRH agonist therapy in the treatment of endometriosis. *Prog. Clin. Biol. Res.*, **225**, 227
17. Henzl, M.R., Corson, S.L., Moghissi, K.S., Buttram, U.C., Berquist, C. and Jacobson, J. (1988). Administration of nasal Nafarelin as compared with oral Danazol for endometriosis. *N. Engl. J. Med.*, **318**, 485
18. Hammond, M.G., Hammond, C.B. and Parker, R.T. (1978). Conservative treatment of endometriosis externa: The effects of methyltestosterone therapy. *Fertil. Steril.*, **29**, 651
19. Barbieri, R.L. and Hornstein, M.D. (1987). Medical therapy for endometriosis. In Wilson, E.A. (ed.) *Endometriosis*, p. 111. (New York: Alan R. Liss)
20. Ledley, G.S., Shenk, I.M. and Heit, H.A. (1988). Sigmoid colon perforation due to

endometriosis not associated with pregnancy. *Am. J. Gastroenterol.*, **83**(12), 1424

21. Thiel, C.W. (1986). Endometriosis of the appendix and cecum. *Minn. Med.*, **69**, 20
22. Naraynsingh, V., Raju, G.C. and Wong, J. (1985). Massive ascites due to omental endometriosis. *Postgrad. Med. J.*, **61**, 539
23. Mann, W.J., Fromowitz, F., Saychek, T., Madariaga, J.R. and Chalas, E. (1984). Endometriosis associated with appendiceal intussusception. *J. Reprod. Med.*, **29**(8), 625
24. Floberg, J., Backdahl, M., Silfersward, C. and Thomassen, P.A. (1984). Postpartum perforation of the colon due to endometriosis. *Acta Obstet. Gynecol. Scand.*, **63**, 183
25. Caccese, W.J., McKinley, M.J., Bronzo, R.L. (1984). Endoscopic confirmation of colonic endometriosis. *Gastrointest. Endosc.*, **30**(3), 191
26. Langsam, L.B., Raj, P.K. and Galag, C.F. (1984). Intussusception of the appendix. *Dis. Colon Rectum*, **27**(6), 387
27. Hardy, R.F. and Kaude, J.V. (1983). Invasive endometriosis of the terminal ileum: A case of small bowel obstruction of obscure origin. *South. Med. J.*, **76**(2), 253
28. Forsgren, H., Lindhagen, J., Melander, S. and Wagermark, J. (1983). Colorectal endometriosis. *Acta Chir. Scand.*, **149**, 431
29. Teunen, A., Ooms, E.C.M. and Tytgat, G.N.T. (1982). Endometriosis of the small and large bowel. *Neth. J. Med.*, **25**, 142
30. Honore, L.H. (1980). Endometriosis of Meckel's diverticulum associated with intestinal obstruction — a case report. *Am. J. Proctol.*, **31**(2), 11
31. Farinon, A.M. and Vadora, E. (1980). Endometriosis of the colon and rectum: An indication for preoperative colonoscopy. *Endoscopy*, **12**, 136
32. Meyers, W.C., Kelvin, F.M. and Jones, R.S. (1979). Diagnosis and surgical treatment of colonic endometriosis. *Arch. Surg.*, **114**, 169
33. Gantt, P.A., Hunt, J.B. and McDonough, P.G. (1981). Progestin reversal or ureteral endometriosis. *Obstet. Gynecol.*, **57**, 665
34. Mourin-Jouret, A., Squifflet, J.P., Cosyns, J.P., Pirson, Y. and Alexandre, G.P.J. (1987). Bilateral ureteral endometriosis with end-stage renal failure. *Urology*, **29**(3), 302
35. Moore, J.G., Hibbard, L.T., Growdon, W.A. and Schifrin, B.S. (1979). Urinary tract endometriosis: Enigmas in diagnosis and management. *Am. J. Obstet. Gynecol.*, **134**(2), 162
36. Koszczuk, J.C., Fogliette, M., Perez, J.F., Dono, F.V. and Thomas, R.J. (1989). Urinary tract endometriosis. *J. Am. Osteopath. Assoc.*, **89**(1), 83
37. Kerr, S.W. (1966). Endometriosis involving the urinary tract. *Clin. Obstet. Gynecol.*, **9**, 331
38. Stanley, K.E., Utz, D.C. and Dockerty, M.D. (1965). Clinically significant endometriosis of the urinary tract. *Surg. Gynecol. Obstet.*, **120**, 491
39. Bazaz-Malik, G., Saraf, V. and Rana, B.S. (1980). Endometrioma of the kidney: Case report. *J. Urol.*, **123**, 422
40. Matsuura, K., Kawasaki, N., Oka, M., II, H. and Maeyama, M. (1985). Treatment with Danazol of ureteral obstruction caused by endometriosis. *Acta Obstet. Gynecol. Scand.*, **64**, 339
41. Erickson, L.D. and Ory, S.J. (1989). GnRH analogues in the treatment of endometriosis. *Obstet. Gynecol. Clin. North Am.*, **16**(1), 123
42. Buka, N.J. (1988). Vesical endometriosis after cesarean section. *Am. J. Obstet. Gynecol.*, **158**(5), 1117
43. Kiely, E.A., Grainger, R., Kay, E.W. and Butler, M.R. (1988). Post-menopausal ureteric endometriosis. *Br. J. Urol.*, **62**, 91
44. Lucero, S.P., Wise, H.A., Kirsh, G., Devoe, K., Hess, M.L., Kandawalla, N. and Crago, J.R. (1988). Ureteric obstruction secondary to endometriosis: Report of three cases with a review of the literature. *Br. J. Urol.*, **61**, 201
45. Foster, R.S., Rink, R.C. and Mulcahy, J.J. (1987). Vesical endometriosis: Medical or surgical treatment. *Urology*, **29**(1), 64
46. Al Saleh, B.M.S. (1987). Endometriosis: an unusual cause of obstruction in duplex ureters. *Br. J. Urol.*, **60**, 467
47. Thomsen, H. and Schroder, H.M. (1987). Simultaneous external and internal endometriosis of the ureter. *Scand. J. Urol. Nephrol.*, **21**, 241
48. Plous, R.H., Sunshine, R., Goldman, H. and Schwartz, I.S. (1985). Ureteral endometriosis in post-menopausal women. *Urology*, **26**(4), 408

49. Porena, M., Mearini, E., Vespasiani, G., Micali, F. and Virgili, G. (1985). Ureteral endometriosis: an endoscopic diagnosis. *Urology*, **26**(6), 566
50. Vermesh, M., Zbella, E.A., Menchaca, A., Confino, E. and Lipshitz, S. (1985). Vesical endometriosis following bladder injury. *Am. J. Obstet. Gynecol.*, **153**(8), 894
51. Karpel, J.P., Appel, D. and Merav, A. (1985). Pulmonary endometriosis. *Lung*, **163**, 151
52. Foster, D.C., Stern, J.L., Buscema, J., Rock, J.A. and Woodruff, J.D. (1981). Pleural and parenchymal pulmonary endometriosis. *Obstet. Gynecol.*, **58**, 552
53. Doshi, N. and Fujikura, T. (1978). Squamous cell passage from the peritoneal cavity to lymph glands and pulmonary lymphatics in a malformed infant: A mechanism for endometriosis and pulmonary metastasis. *Am. J. Obstet. Gynecol.*, **131**, 221
54. Rosenberg, S.M. and Riddick, D.H. (1981). Successful treatment of catamenial hemoptysis with Danazol. *Obstet. Gynecol.*, **57**(1), 130
55. Balasingham, S., Arulkumaran, S., Nadarajah, K. and Jayaratnam, F.J. (1986). Catamenial pneumothorax. *Aust. N.Z. Obstet. Gynecol.*, **26**, 88
56. Wilkins, S.B., Bell-Thomson, J. and Tyras, D.H. (1985). Hemothorax associated with endometriosis. *J. Thoracic Cardiovasc. Surg.*, **89**(4), 636
57. Suginami, H., Hamada, K. and Yano, K. (1985). A case of endometriosis of the lung treated with Danazol. *Obstet. Gynecol.*, **66**(3), 68S
58. Charles, S.X. (1981). Pelvic and umbilical endometriosis presenting with hemorrhagic pleural effusion: A case report. *Int. Surg.*, **66**, 277
59. Hibbard, L.T., Schumann, W.R. and Goldstein, G.E. (1981). Thoracic endometriosis: A review and report of two cases. *Am. J. Obstet. Gynecol.*, **140**(2), 227
60. Watson, W.J., Sundwall, D.A. and Benson, W.L. (1982). Splenosis mimicking endometriosis. *Obstet. Gynecol.*, **59**, 51S
61. Thibodeau, L.L., Prioleau, G.R., Manuelidis, E.E., Merino, M.J. and Heafner, M.D. (1987). Cerebral endometriosis. *J. Neurosurg.*, **66**, 609
62. Finkel, L., Marchevsky, A. and Cohen, B. (1986). Endometrial cyst of the liver. *Am. J. Gastroenterol.*, **81**(7), 576
63. Patel, V.C., Samuels, H., Abeles, E. and Hirjibehedin, P.F. (1982). Endometriosis at the knee. *Clin. Orthop. Related Res.*, **171**, 140
64. Hibbard, J. and Schreiver, J.R. (1984). Footdrop due to sciatic nerve endometriosis. *Am. J. Obstet. Gynecol.*, **149**(7), 800
65. Salazar-Grueso, E. and Roos, R. (1986). Sciatic endometriosis: A treatable sensorimotor mononeuropathy. *Neurology*, **36**, 1360
66. Michowitz, M., Baratz, M. and Stavorovsky, M. (1983). Endometriosis of the umbilicus. *Dermatologica*, **167**, 326
67. Blumental, N.J. (1981). Umbilical endometriosis. *S. Afr. Med. J.*, **59**, 198
68. Sataloff, D.M., LaVorgna, K.A. and McFarland, M.M. (1989). Extrapelvic endometriosis presenting as a hernia: Clinical reports and review of the literature. *Surgery*, **105**(1), 109
69. Brzezinski, A. and Durst, A.L. (1983). Endometriosis presenting as an inguinal hernia. *Am. J. Obstet. Gynecol.*, **146**(8), 982
70. Wolf, G.C. and Kopecky, K.K. (1989). MR Imaging of endometriosis arising in cesarean section scar. *J. Comput. Assist. Tomogr.*, **13**(1), 150
71. Kennedy, S.H., Brodribb, J., Godfrey, A.M. and Barlow, D.H. (1988). Pre-operative treatment of an abdominal wall endometrioma with nafarelin acetate. Case report. *Br. J. Obstet. Gynaecol.*, **95**, 521
72. Rovito, P. and Gittleman, M. (1986). Two cases of endometrioma in cesarean scars. *Surgery*, **100**, 118
73. Goswami, A.K., Sharma, S.K., Tandon, S.P., Malik, N., Mathur, R.P., Malik, A.K. and Bapna, B.C. (1986). Pancreatic endometriosis presenting as a hypovascular renal mass. *J. Urol.*, **135**, 112
74. Marchevsky, A.M., Zimmerman, M.J., Aufses, A.H. and Weiss, H. (1984). Endometrial cyst of pancreas. *Gastroenterology*, **86**, 1589
75. Gupta, S.D. (1985). Endometriosis in the thumb. *J. Indian Med. Assoc.*, **83**, 122
76. Giagnarra, C., Gallo, G., Newman, R. and Dorfman, H. (1987). Endometriosis in the biceps femoris. *J. Bone Joint Surg.*, **69A**(2), 290
77. Pellegrini, V.D., Pasternak, H.S. and Macaulay, W.P. (1981). Endometrioma of the pubis: A differential in the diagnosis of hip pain. *J. Bone Joint Surg.*, **63A**(8), 1333

78. Dmowski, W.P., Gebel, H.M. and Rawlins, R.G. (1981). Immunologic aspects of endometriosis. *Obstet. Gynecol. Clin. North Am.*, **16**(1), 93
79. El-Roiety, A., Dmowski, W.P., Gleicher, N., Binor, Z., Radwanska, E. and Tummon, I. (1988). Effect of danazol and GnRH agonists (GnRH-a) on the immune system in endometriosis (abstract 448). Presented at the *35th Annual Meeting of the Society for Gynecologic Investigation*, March 17–20, Baltimore
80. Grimes, D.A., Lebolt, S.A., Grimes, K.R. and Winco, P.A. (1985). Systemic lupus erythematosus and reproductive function: A case control study. *Am. J. Obstet. Gynecol.*, **153**, 179
81. Binns, B.A.O. and Banerjee, R. (1983). Endometriosis with Turner's syndrome treated with cyclical oestrogen/progestogen. Case report. *Br. J. Obstet. Gynaecol.*, **90**, 581
82. Peress, M.R., Sosnowski, J.R., Mathur, R.S. and Williamson, H.O. (1982). Pelvic endometriosis and Turner's syndrome. *Am. J. Obstet. Gynecol.*, **144**(4), 474
83. Dmowski, W.P., Radwanski, E. and Rana, N. (1988). Recurrent endometriosis following hysterectomy and oophorectomy: the role of residual ovarian fragments. *Int. J. Gynecol. Obstet.*, **26**, 93
84. Williams, T.J. and Pratt, J.H. (1977). Endometriosis in 1,000 consecutive celiotomies: Incidence and management. *Am. J. Obstet. Gynecol.*, **129**, 245
85. Cramer, D.W. (1987). Epidemiology of endometriosis. In Wilson, E.D. (ed.) *Endometriosis*, p. 5. (New York: Alan R. Liss)
86. Barbieri, R. and Kistner, R.W. (1986). Endometriosis. In Kistner, R.W. (ed.) *Gynecology: Principles and Practice*, 4th edn., p. 393. (Chicago: Year Book Medical Publishers)
87. Ranney, B. (1980). Endometriosis: Pathogenesis, symptoms and findings. *Clin. Obstet. Gynecol.*, **23**, 965
88. Meigs, J.V. (1941). Endometriosis: Its significance. *Ann. Surg.*, **114**, 866
89. Williams, T.J. (1985). Endometriosis. In Mattingly, R.F. and Thompson, J.D. (eds.) *TeLinde's Operative Gynecology*, 6th edn., p. 257. (Philadelphia: J.B. Lippincott)
90. Gitelis, S., Petasnick, J.P., Turner, D.A., Ghiselli, R.W. and Miller, A.W. (1985). Endometriosis simulating a soft tissue tumor of the thigh: CT and MR evaluation. *J. Comput. Assist. Tomogr.*, **9**, 573
91. Yates-Bell, A.J., Molland, E.A. and Pryor, J.P. (1972). Endometriosis of the ureter. *Br. J. Urol.*, **44**, 58
92. Ball, T.L. and Platt, M.A. (1962). Urologic complications of endometriosis. *Am. J. Obstet. Gynecol.*, **84**, 1516
93. Macafee, C.H. and Greer, H.L. (1960). Intestinal endometriosis. A report of 29 cases and a survey of the literature. *J. Obstet. Gynaecol. Br. Emp.*, **67**, 538
94. Lane, R.E. (1960). Endometriosis of the vermiform appendix. *J. Obstet. Gynecol.*, **79**, 372
95. Scott, R.B. and TeLinde, R.W. (1950). External endometriosis: The scourge of the private patient. *Ann. Surg.*, **131**, 697

10
Macro- and microsurgical treatment of endometriosis

J. M. Wheeler

INTRODUCTION

The surgical treatment of endometriosis is in rapid evolution, some would say revolution, owing to advances in microsurgical instrumentation, endoscopic methods, and operative adjuncts including adhesion inhibitors. Standards of treatment are difficult to define, perhaps better referred to as accepted treatment options. This chapter, summarizing one surgeon's approach to endometriosis surgery, can at best be a snapshot in time of accepted operative methods; in fact, the degree of being accepted varies, as there continues ample controversy regarding optimum treatment of this confusing disease. Hopefully, in 5 to 10 years, some of the principles described in this chapter will seem overly simplistic, much as we now view the previous standard of hysterectomy and castration for all endometriosis patients. The history of endometriosis treatment may provide useful perspective, however, in the 'modern approach' to surgical treatment. In the following section, a brief overview of historical trends will suggest where surgical treatment is heading, as well as give proper credit to the work of surgeons who pioneered new options in endometriosis therapy.

HISTORICAL PERSPECTIVE

Respected medical journals today bind together a large number of peer-reviewed, heavily edited, overly brief, forcibly under-referenced condensations of what the authors would really like to communicate to their readers. Authors and editors alike, myself included[1], call for improved methodology and statistical analyses of clinical research in endometriosis therapy. We seem to have lost the eloquence and penchant for detail found in the surgical journals of the pre-Medline era. Witness the length and detail of Sampson's collected series — illustrated, personal and comprehensive communications of case histories and treatments. It is in these early works that we have the best documentation of the natural history of endometriosis.

Early on, endometriosis was identified as a histologically benign disease that nevertheless had the biological potential to invade adjacent tissues and distort normal anatomy[2]. Surgical treatment was designed to remove all tissues involved with endometriosis en bloc, along with the causative uterus and ovaries. In the first 40 years of endometriosis surgery, treatment was deemed 'conservative' if any ovarian tissue was preserved, regardless of the patient's age or reproductive goals. Today, ovaries are more likely to be preserved in the reproductive-aged woman for potential use at *in vitro* fertilization (IVF).

'Conservative' surgery as we know it today began in the 1960s, a classic example is Rogers' and Jacobs' article published in 1968[3]. Probably not coincidentally, contraceptive advances in the 1960s finally gave women control over their own reproduction. During the same period, women no longer accepted the universal recommendation for hysterectomy as cure, a theme that has extended itself to the entire issue of hysterectomy for benign disease. Surgical procedures were developed to remove endometriosis and adhesions, yet preserve some chance of having children.

In the 1970s, conservative surgery for endometriosis at laparotomy (CSEL) became popular and widespread. The increased availability of IVF has encouraged even more aggressive preservation of ovarian tissue at time of CSEL. Whereas the appropriateness of CSEL for severe cases of ovarian endometriomata is not questioned, the indications for CSEL were extended to women with only a few spots of endometriosis as well. Now, with the realization that mild endometriosis may simply be a variant of normal anatomy rather than representing true 'disease'[4,5], treatment with laparotomy is rarely warranted.

In reviewing the endometriosis literature, one can detect a cyclicity in the popular treatments of endometriosis[6]. Over the last 30 years, it has seemed that either surgical or medical therapy has been held in more regard than the other. The late 1980s and early 1990s mark the first time when significant advances were made concomitantly in both medical and surgical treatments. Well-designed prospective randomized trials have demonstrated the efficacy and safety of GnRHa's when compared to danazol in the medical treatment of endometriosis[7,8]; however, implants do seem to return to their full activity with withdrawal of the drug. Newer yet on the horizon are GnRH antagonists, which will lack the paradoxical ovarian stimulation phase of the agonists and thus have the advantage of faster achievement of hypo-oestrogenism[9]. Agonists and antagonists in depot form will offer convenience and improved compliance in treating patients. Treatment protocols of GnRHa plus add-back steroids (e.g. oestrogen, progestins, danazol) are being evaluated that may allow longer use of the GnRHa's with less concern about bone loss.

Concomitant with these advances in medical treatment, the development of endoscopic instrumentation has proliferated. In trained hands, almost all cases of endometriosis can be treated laparoscopically. Although patients recuperate faster, it has yet to be proved that endoscopic treatment has improved efficacy in treating endometriosis than laparotomy. This topic will be explored in more detail below.

In the 1980s, laparoscopic treatment of endometriosis became more widespread, with some predicting the death of the laparotomy for conditions causing infertility[10]. Laparoscopic treatment will be discussed subsequently in this chapter and by Sutton in Chapter 11.

Finally, in addition to rapid development of medical therapy and endoscopic instrumentation, the 1980s also saw improvement in perioperative adjuncts to limit adhesion inhibition, including Interceed TC-7[11], tissue plasma activators[12], and others[13]. Most adhesion inhibition work has been done in animal models. More studies are needed to completely define the role of these adhesion inhibitors in endometriosis surgery, particularly laparoscopic surgery.

Further advances in treatment are likely in the 1990s. Most cases of endometriosis will be treated laparoscopically, although probably not necessarily with lasers in preference to cautery, scissors or thermal coagulation. More cases will be treated with combined medical–surgical protocols; preoperative treatment will help with the most severe cases, and postoperative treatment may improve pregnancy rates and lessen recurrence rates in moderate and severe cases[14,15]. Depot forms of GnRH agonists will dominate in the 1990s, with either shorter periods of use (3–4 months) or longer use associated with hormonal add-backs to minimize toxicity. Hopefully, we will have better understanding of the causes of and cures of endometriosis through the work described in Chapters 1–7 in this book. While we await further advances in understanding the pathophysiology and treatment of endometriosis, the remainder of this chapter describes the current status of surgical therapy.

DIAGNOSIS AND SURGICAL STAGING

In usual clinical practice, endometriosis is diagnosed visually at the time of laparoscopy performed for the evaluation of pelvic pain or infertility. Unfortunately, visual diagnosis is neither the most specific nor the most sensitive method of diagnosis, it is simply the method most often used. The most specific definition requires histological demonstration of ectopic endometrial glands and stroma. The demonstration of endometrial glands by electron microscopy[16] probably adds an extra degree of sensitivity to microscopic diagnosis, but the clinical significance of these peritoneal lesions is uncertain. Further complicating the problem of visual against microscopic diagnosis is the accepted range of visual appearances of endometriosis — from clear vesicles to petechial lesions to the classic blue-black implants[17]. Endometriosis continues to be best diagnosed surgically, preferably with biopsy confirmation of the surgeon's suspicion of disease. Other tissue may visually appear to be endometriosis, yet lack histological confirmation, including small venules, previous sutures, and areas of adhesions and fibrosis unassociated with endometriosis. The discrepancy between visual and histological criteria for endometriosis may be resolved by steroid receptor research as described by Bergqvist in Chapter 3.

Serum markers for endometriosis diagnosis such as CA-125 lack the sensitivity to be particularly good screening tools. CA-125 levels also lack specificity, as many adnexal processes cause elevated levels of that antigen. Currently, if the CA-125 level is elevated prior to surgery and then falls with surgical treatment, it may prove useful in early diagnosis of recurrent endometriosis. The roles of serum markers are likely to expand with the active work under way into the immunological aspects of host response to endometriosis. The most useful serum marker may prove to be an endometriosis-specific protein or messenger that is detected with the amplification techniques of the polymerase chain reaction. Non-invasive diagnosis and follow-up of patients with endometriosis will be a notable advance in the care of women.

Accurate description of the extent of endometriosis found at operative diagnosis is an important responsibility of the surgeon. Not only should the number, size and location of lesions be identified, but some assessment of the lesions' biological activity as well. For example, are the tissues inflamed, fibrotic, or relatively normal? Are the implants invasive and nodular, or do they appear as very superficial bumps upon the native tissue? Associated adhesions may range from clinically insignificant filmy contacts to dense, obliterative tissue lacking any dissection plane. Although several classifications for endometriosis have been proposed (see Chapter 8), none has been demonstrated to be superior as a prognostic tool for pregnancy or recurrence. Until data are obtained demonstrating the value of arbitrary numbers assigned to endometriosis extent, the most useful aspect of current classification systems is the use of a carefully detailed diagram of the surgical findings[18]. A simple computer-based method of recording surgical details has been described[5], and is being used prospectively to determine which anatomical aspects of endometriosis impart change in prognosis for either pregnancy or recurrence.

CHOOSING A TREATMENT STRATEGY

Endometriosis treatment is individualized, depending upon the presenting symptoms and reproductive goals of the patient herself. An algorithm summarizing most current options in endometriosis treatment has been described previously[6], and is modified in Table 10.1. Treatment options within the algorithm are ranked, with similarly efficacious options receiving the same rank within each clinical cell. For women with stage I or II disease and somatic complaints, surgical treatment at time of diagnosis offers the greatest likelihood of prompt relief; most reproductive surgeons today would treat these women laparoscopically. Surgery is the treatment of choice in women with stage III or IV disease, whether the presenting symptoms are pain or infertility.

Our bias in favour of primary surgical therapy is apparent, and is similar to the bias of most other reproductive surgeons. Many surgeons have adapted a treatment approach to endometriosis that resembles the approach to malignant epithelial tumours of the ovary. After all, endometriosis behaves like ovarian carcinoma in terms of its peritoneal spread, ovarian distortion, and potential for unbridled growth. Like ovarian cancer, the diagnosis of endometriosis requires surgery, despite advances in tomographic and magnetic resonance imaging and new serum markers. Once the diagnosis of either disease is made, preferably histologically, surgical treatment is directed towards removal of as much gross disease as possible. In severe endometriosis cases, complete removal may include bowel resection and ureteral dissection, just like ovarian cancer cases. In the presence of known or strongly suspected residual endometriosis, postoperative adjunctive medical therapy is elected. A primary surgical approach seems to be more efficacious than medical treatment for most advanced cases of endometriosis; however, this opinion has not been tested by a properly performed prospective randomized clinical trial. Despite advances in GnRH agonists and antagonists, it is unlikely that medical treatment will have anything but transient results on invasive, nodular implants or ovarian endometriomata.

The treatment algorithm also includes a role for assisted reproductive technologies such as *in vitro* fertilization (IVF) and gamete intrafallopian transfer (GIFT). Success rates with IVF or GIFT for women with endometriosis seem to follow disease severity to some degree. Women with mild endometriosis, with no other aetiology of their infertility, behave much like those couples classified as having unexplained infertility, whereas those women with severe disease behave much like women with tuboperitoneal factor due to previous pelvic infection. Except in the unusual circumstances of advanced age or concomitant significant male factor, IVF continues to be the end-stage treatment for most women with endometriosis.

Contraindications to surgery for endometriosis are the same as for gynaecological surgery in general, i.e. when severe co-morbidity and excessive anaesthesia risks outweigh potential benefits of surgery. In clinical practice, the most commonly encountered contraindication to endometriosis surgery is incomplete evaluation of the male or of ovulation in the infertile couple. Because the optimum time to conceive after surgery is the first 12–18 months, the infertile couple should be completely evaluated, with surgery for endometriosis delayed until these other factors are evaluated and treated, if necessary.

Despite the admitted surgical bias within this chapter, there are many women for whom either medical therapy or expectant management are appropriate and sometimes preferred. Particularly, women with mild endometriosis who present with infertility may be managed expectantly, with equal success expected as compared to medical or surgical therapy. Medical aspects of endometriosis treatment are covered in detail elsewhere in the book.

LAPAROSCOPY VERSUS LAPAROTOMY FOR SURGICAL TREATMENT

Laparoscopy continues to be the mainstay of endometriosis diagnosis and staging, and is becoming increasingly important in the treatment of many cases as well. Many surgeons have noticed a decrease in the relative proportion of particularly severe endometriosis cases, which may reflect improved sensitivity by gynaecologists in the early diagnosis and treatment of endometriosis. Whatever the cause of this spectral shift towards milder disease, there has been a concomitant improvement in endoscopic instrumentation and training. Some surgeons perform most endometriosis surgery laparoscopically, yet the choice of laparoscopy against laparotomy is probably less important than these surgical objectives:

- Complete resection of macroscopic endometriosis and adhesions.
- Minimum tissue handling; most grasping is done on tissues actually removed.
- Restoration of normal tubo-ovarian anatomic relations.
- Complete haemostasis, but minimal suturing.
- Massive irrigation to remove deposited fibrin.
- Appropriate use of adhesion inhibitors, particularly newly approved barriers, e.g Interceed, TC-7.

If these principles are maintained, laparoscopic treatment is likely to be as successful as treatment at laparotomy. In the situation of particularly severe disease (e.g. invasive colonic or bladder implants), or inaccessibility of the patient to a trained reproductive laparoscopist, laparotomy will continue to be appropriate treatment. Although the advantages of a laparoscopic approach include shorter hospitalization and overall recovery time, and potentially less adhesions, there is no properly performed trial demonstrating superiority of operative laparoscopy over laparotomy, or vice versa. A perfect prospective, randomized trial is unlikely, as the issue of performance bias would be nearly impossible to resolve; most surgeons have already judged what type of cases are most amenable to laparoscopic treatment as opposed to laparotomy.

Laparoscopic methods

Whereas diagnostic laparoscopy is typically a one- or two-puncture technique, operative laparoscopy for endometriosis typically involves two to four puncture sites. For mild to moderate disease, two punctures are typical; for cul-de-sac obliteration, ovarian endometriomata, and appendix involvement, three punctures are used — laser laparoscope at the umbilicus, and secondary 5- or 10-mm ports at the lateral edge of each abdominis rectus muscle.

Several methods of endometriosis destruction or removal are amenable to laparoscopic use. Again, the specific tool chosen is less important than the surgeon and his or her overall technique. Dissection with scissors is as likely to remove a peritoneal plaque of endometriosis as is a laser; many surgeons prefer the laser owing to the potential of improved haemostasis and, theoretically, 'sterilizing' the edges of the dissection of any residual endo metriosis. The careful use of uni- or bi-polar cautery would confer this same advantage to the surgeon using scissors. In fact, with the recent development of improved electrocautery instruments for use at laparoscopy, there may be less laparoscopic use of lasers by the year 2000 than might be predicted today. Although laser laparoscopy is covered in detail in Chapter 11, it is appropriate to state here the main advantage in the use of any laser laparoscopically is its potential for multiple functions, including scalpel/scissors and coagulator. Again, the choice of the laser as a tool is less important than the training and experience of the surgeon holding the tool in the properly selected patient.

Pelviscopy, as taught by Semm[19], requires the use of a vast array of graspers, scissors, an irrigator/aspirator, and endocoagulator. The pelviscopy instruments are unique in design and utility for advanced operative laparo-scopic procedures of adnexectomy or appendectomy, but for most cases of endometriosis the only instruments used are an atraumatic grasper, a toothed grasper, hooked scissors, irrigator/aspirator and a coagulation device. Many surgeons prefer the bipolar forceps owing to its faster action than the endocoagulator. Thus, for most endometriosis cases, only a few of the pelviscopy instruments are usually needed. Unfortunately, one rarely knows how severe the case is likely to be prior to diagnostic laparoscopy; thus, we do request the full complement of pelviscopic instruments when endometriosis or adhesions are suspected.

Another advantage of the pelviscopy instrumentation is the ability to suture laparoscopically. Just as fewer sutures are placed at laparotomy for endometriosis, it is unusual for sutures to be placed at laparoscopic treatment of endometriosis, except for endoloop placement at adnexectomy. The ability to endosuture with 4-0 polydiaxanone does come in handy for the occasional bleeding bed after removal of an endometriosis implant.

Figures 10.1(a), (b) and (c) summarize the laparoscopic approach to endometriosis treatment. A thorough search is made throughout the abdomen and pelvis for endometriosis and accompanying adhesions; for illustration purposes, the case presented has superficial endometriosis overlying the left ureter in multiple foci, bilateral uterosacral invasive nodules, and a 1-cm endometrioma of the right ovary. As seen in Figure 10.1 (b), the margins of dissection are outlined with the laser beam (typically a carbon dioxide laser at 15 watts, superpulse mode, spot size 0.2 mm), before the natural topography is disturbed by dissection. Once the lesion is outlined, the edge of the peritoneum can be grasped and undercut with scissors or laser; sometimes, dissection with water pressure from the irrigator/aspirator will aid the dissection of the peritoneum.

Whatever method is selected, the goals include removal of peritoneum and endometriosis *in toto* to the level of the preperitoneal fat, with 2–3 mm of clear margin around each lesion. The location of the ureters must be recognized, just as at laparotomy, and, depending upon the experience of the surgeon, does not specifically contraindicate a laparoscopic dissection. Each uterosacral nodule is excised; the one on the right required deeper dissection than did the left. The ovarian lesion is managed by simply vaporizing the endometrioma through to the level of subcortical ovary; dissection is difficult with these small endometriomata, so they are better vaporized. The easiest endometriomata to open, irrigate, and peel from the ovary are 3–5 cm in size. After vaporization or dissection of all visible endometriosis, the beds of dissection are amply irrigated and assessed for haemostasis. Typically, 2–6 litres of lactated Ringer's solution are used per endoscopic case; the last litre includes 5000 units of heparin. In the patient at risk of adhesion formation, such as the patient in Figure 10.1(c), where the right ovarian lesion is immediately juxtaposed to the uterosacral injury, Interceed is applied to cover the wound with a 2–3 mm margin. The first few applications of Interceed laparoscopically are difficult; the easiest way seems to be to roll the material like a cigar over the atraumatic grasper or the 3 mm needle holder of Semm. Then, the material is introduced via the 10-mm second puncture, and unrolled over the lesion while being held in place by the blunt probe through a 5-mm third puncture. Although not desirable, the only known effect of the edges being folded back on themselves is slower absorption — taking perhaps 6 weeks rather than the usual 28 days[20]. The material is wetted with the heparin-containing buffer, and covered by the bowel under visualization to make sure it does not slip away; it is not sutured in place at laparoscopy or laparotomy. Because the efficacy of Interceed at laparoscopic surgery is unknown, it may be advisable to apply it only to those cases strongly suspected of being at risk of serious adhesion formation. For example, the woman in Figure 10.1 is more likely to benefit from the membrane over the right uterosacral and ovarian lesions than over the left uterosacral defect.

CONSERVATIVE SURGERY FOR ENDOMETRIOSIS AT LAPAROTOMY (CSEL)

As suggested in Table 10.1, the indications for CSEL include:

- Persistence of somatic symptoms or infertility in women after a suitable trial of expectant, medical or laparoscopic treatment.
- Severity of endometriosis or adhesions exceeding the training or available instrumentation of a laparoscopic surgeon.
- Presence of pathology more amenable to treatment at laparotomy, e.g. invasive bowel nodule requiring resection.

Following diagnosis and staging at laparoscopy, most patients prefer CSEL under the same general anaesthesia, although for special circumstances, the laparotomy may be delayed for up to several months without an obvious decrement in success[21]. Some surgeons will delay CSEL in the worst of cases to allow pre-laparotomy medical suppression for 3 months. A No. 8 paediatric Foley catheter is placed within the endometrial cavity to effect chromotubation; this is typically performed even in the pelvic pain patient who desires preservation of childbearing potential. Low transverse incisions are usually elected; midline incisions are used in the very obese or those with pre-existing midline incisions.

As outlined above, a minimal-touch technique is used once the abdomen is opened. The wound edges are draped with moistened sponges, and care is taken that the self-retaining retractor is not overly compressing the abdominal wall or the iliopsoas muscles. Magnification with 2.5 × or 4 × loupes is useful; the microscope with laser attached is elected by some surgeons. Near-constant irrigation is performed with warmed lactated Ringer's

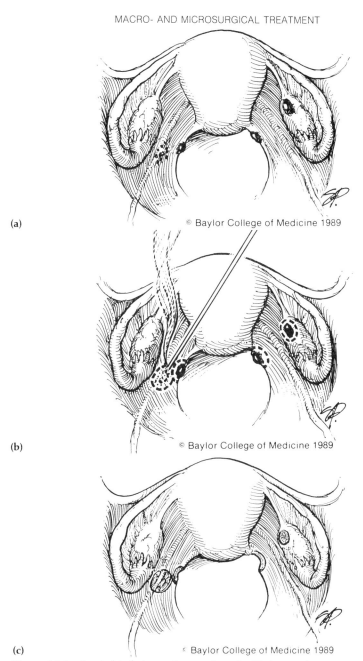

(a)

© Baylor College of Medicine 1989

(b)

© Baylor College of Medicine 1989

(c)

© Baylor College of Medicine 1989

Figure 10.1 Surgical technique using a carbon dioxide laser at laparoscopy or laparotomy. (a) All lesions are identified, as are important anatomic structures such as the ureters. (b) Lesions are outlined with the laser, with 2–3 mm circumferential margins of uninvolved tissue. (c) Lesions are removed *in toto* to the thickness of normal underlying tissue. Haemostasis is assured, and sutures are minimized. Consideration is given to use of Interceed for each defect in the peritoneum or ovarian cortex (Reproduced by kind permission of Mosby Yearbook Inc.)

Table 10.1 Treatment options in endometriosis patients[a]

AFS stage	Desires preservation of childbearing potential		Childbearing completed
	Presenting complaint		Pelvic pain
	Infertility	Pelvic pain	
I and II	1. Expectant	1. Laparoscopic	1. Laparoscopic
	2. Laparoscopic	2. Medical	2. Medical
	2. Medical	2. CSEL ± PSN	3. TAH ± BSO
	3. CSEL ± PSN		3. CSEL + PSN
	4. IVF/ET		
III	1. Laparoscopic	1. Laparoscopic	1. Laparoscopic
	1. CSEL ± PSN	1. CSEL + PSN	2. Medical
	2. Medical	2. Medical	3. TAH ± BSO
	3. IVF/ET		3. CSEL + PSN
IV	1. CSEL + medical	1. CSEL, PSN, medical	1. TAH ± BSO
	2. CSEL ± PSN	2. Medical	2. CSEL, PSN, medical
	3. Laparoscopic + medical	3. Laparoscopic + medical	2. Laparoscopic + medical
	4. IVF/ET		

[a]Treatment options are ranked per cell; same ranks suggest similar efficacy. Abbreviations: Medical = 3–6 months of treatment with danazol or GnRH agonist; CSEL = conservative surgery for endometriosis at laparotomy; PSN = presacral neurectomy; TAH = total abdominal hysterectomy; BSO = bilateral salpingo-oophorectomy; IVF/ET = *in vitro* fertilization/embryo transfer, or other assisted reproductive technology. '±' denotes an adjunctive treatment option that may be elected on an individualized basis.

solution, each litre of which is supplemented with 5000 units of heparin. Gentle traction, with fingers or Teflon-coated retractors, is preferred to grasping instruments. The CSEL is an orchestrated procedure between surgeon and support team; the first component performed is typically presacral neurectomy.

Presacral neurectomy, in most published series, seems to relieve or decrease pelvic pain in the majority of patients[22]. The posterior peritoneum is opened in the mid-sagittal plane for 3–4 cm. Lateral margins of dissection are the right ureter and the left inferior mesenteric vessels in the sigmoid mesocolon. A 1-cm length of hypogastric plexus is removed, thus avoiding encroachment upon either the aortic/vena caval bifurcations or the hollow of the sacrum with its massive venous plexuses. Sometimes, the median sacral artery and vein may require ligation prior to neurectomy. Haemostasis is assured prior to closure of the posterior peritoneum.

Next, an organized approach is taken to dissection of all visible endometriosis and adhesions. Preference is given to excision of adhesions rather than incision; similarly, endometriosis is excised preferentially to superficial carbonization with the laser. The uterosacral ligaments are excised only to the point of involvement with disease; uterosacral ligament plication is rarely indicated today with the development of adhesion barriers.

Invasive bowel lesions are individualized. Serosal lesions may be excised from unprepped bowel; muscularis and mucosal lesions are more safely treated by excision, sometimes requiring segmental resection, in bowel prepared with antibiotic and mechanical cleansing. Thus, diagnostic laparoscopy must carefully assess the rectosigmoid when deciding to perform immediate versus delayed CSEL.

Complications from CSEL are unusual, but include infection, excessive blood loss, and visceral injury. Presacral neurectomy has a small risk of injury to the great vessels, ureters, and sacral venous plexus. Complications would be expected to be more common in severe, invasive disease of the ureters or colon, necessitating careful dissection.

CSEL for pelvic pain is typically at least 80% successful in eliminating or reducing pain. In infertile women, CSEL is associated with pregnancy rates of 50% in severe cases, 65% in moderate, and 75% in mild cases; very similar numbers are seen with laparoscopic surgery, suggesting that it is the technique, rather than the method of access, that dictates likelihood of pregnancy postoperatively. Recurrence after CSEL may occur in 15% of patients within 3 years and 35% within 5 years.

PERIOPERATIVE MEDICAL THERAPY

There are a few small series supporting the use of perioperative danazol or GnRHa following primary surgical therapy (refs. 14, 15; for review see ref. 23). This support comes from largely retrospective case series, but does seem to suggest the value of medical therapy as an adjunct to surgery in more severe cases. Preoperative therapy has less of a record in the literature than postoperative therapy; preop medication for 3 months is helpful in the most severe of cases treated by CSEL[23]. More frequently, at CSEL or laparoscopic therapy, severe cases are treated with 3 months of postoperative therapy. Several companies have expressed interest in funding definitive study of perioperative medical therapy. Clearly, one arm of a large trial would include operative laparoscopy followed by postoperative medical therapy, perhaps in comparison to CSEL alone.

SECOND-LOOK LAPAROSCOPY

Again, the data supporting second-look laparoscopy (SLL) in endometriosis treatment are derived from clinical case series with the potential for significant bias. Currently, SLL is recommended to patients with severe endometriosis, especially if extensive dissection is required in the ovaries of posterior cul de sac. SLL is performed 4–12 weeks after CSEL; if postoperative medical suppression is used, SLL is delayed for 2–4 weeks after completing medical treatment[24].

COMPLETE OPERATIONS

As seen in Table 10.1, hysterectomy may be indicated in the woman with significant somatic symptoms who has completed her childbearing. Fortunately, with improvements in surgical and medical therapies, including IVF, it is currently quite unusual to be forced to perform hysterectomy in a woman with severe disease prior to some attempt at conception.

The treatment algorithm in Table 10.1, for the sake of simplicity, lists hysterectomy as 'TAH'. Vaginal hysterectomy is desirable for less hospitalization and shorter recovery time. Many patients are amenable to a combined operative laparoscopic/vaginal hysterectomy approach. Laparoscopic-aided vaginal hysterectomy offers the same completeness of inspection as does abdominal hysterectomy, takes about the same amount of time, and offers the patient faster recovery time. Although many surgeons are now performing laparoscopy/vaginal hysterectomy for endometriosis or adhesions, data are still forthcoming to demonstrate hard evidence of improvement over the current standard of total abdominal hysterectomy.

Total abdominal hysterectomy (TAH) is typically performed via a low transverse incision; the Maylard modification of the low transverse incision is preferable to the Pfannenstiel or even a vertical incision to gain access to the pelvic sidewalls. Similar methods as at CSEL are recommended: careful inspection for disease, using magnification, complete removal of disease, careful tissue handling. As suggested in Figure 10.2, an *en bloc* approach to involved areas is useful in maintaining anatomical perspective while ensuring the removal of diseased tissue. In Figure 10.2, the left ovary is removed because of a large endometrioma, along with invasive nodules of the anterior cul de sac and posterior uterine serosa; the right ovary is preserved because it is visually and palpably normal in this young patient. Preservation of the

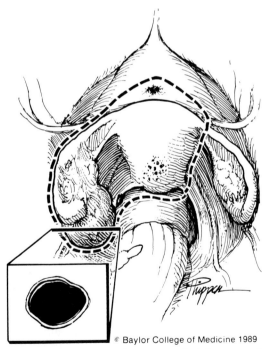

© Baylor College of Medicine 1989

Figure 10.2 *En bloc* removal of severe endometriosis. The left ovary with endometrioma is removed with uterus and invasive anterior cul-de-sac lesion as a 'field' of dissection (Reproduced by kind permission of Mosby Yearbook Inc.)

ovaries is always discussed with patients, regardless of their age; in the woman with endometriosis of sufficient severity to indicate TAH, many surgeons suggest complete removal of the adnexa. Others suggest that the perfectly normal adnexum may be conserved in the young woman (the age threshold varies between surgeons from 35 to 40 years), as illustrated in Figure 10.3. The utero-ovarian ligament is triplicated with the remaining segment of round ligament, thus pexing the adnexum on the lateral abdominal wall, with care taken not to kink the infundibulopelvic ligament. Thus, the ovary is high above the vaginal cuff, less likely to be bumped during intercourse.

Similarly to CSEL, all areas involved with endometriosis are treated. Invasive nodules of the bowel are treated as completely as the degree of preoperative bowel preparation permits; transmural lesions are preferably treated by segmental resection and anastomosis.

Hormone replacement in the castrated woman with endometriosis offers the same advantages of less coronary artery disease and osteoporosis complications as in women without endometriosis. If known residual disease remains, post-hysterectomy danazol may be prescribed for 3–6 months, with known effects to inhibit bone loss. GnRHa's are contraindicated, as their mechanism is to induce hypo-oestrogenism indirectly via the pituitary and

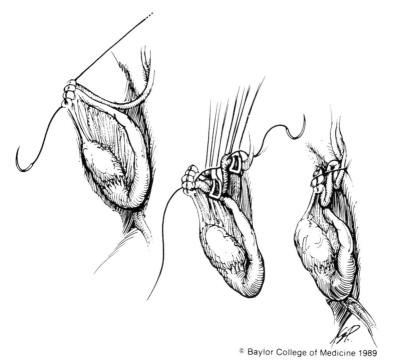

© Baylor College of Medicine 1989

Figure 10.3 Suspension of the normal, preserved ovary high on the abdominal wall away from the vaginal cuff (Reproduced by kind permission of Mosby Yearbook Inc.)

ovaries, now removed. If there is no suspicion of residual disease, physiological hormone replacement usually imparts much greater health benefits compared to the risk of stimulating endometriosis. The topic of hormonal replacement in these patients is discussed in much greater detail in Chapter 15.

SUMMARY

For the first time in the 100 years of endometriosis treatment, significant advances have recently been made in both medical and surgical treatments of this disease. The GnRH agonists and antagonists are likely to replace danazol as primary medical therapy for endometriosis; yet their usefulness as perioperative adjuncts will first have to be demonstrated to be similar to that of danazol. Also, the GnRHA's are likely to be used for short-term therapy only, unless steroid add-back strategies can be demonstrated to impede bone loss associated with agonist use. We might see a resurgence in the use of progestins, either alone or with GnRHa's, as medical therapy for endometriosis; as inexpensive agents, progestins never did get properly evaluated in comparative trials when danazol first appeared in the 1970s. Despite these advances in medical treatment theory and practice, endometriosis continues to be largely a surgical disease. Advances in operative laparoscopic techniques, coupled with a decline in the proportion of cases that are severe, are prominent trends in surgical treatment. However, laparoscopic treatment has not been unequivocally demonstrated to have similar or better efficacy in relieving pain, producing pregnancy, or reducing recurrence risk. Finally, the roles of second-look laparoscopy and perioperative medical therapy must be evaluated by improved prospective studies in the future. Until then, clinicians must individualize treatment, in consultation with the patient herself, using the many options available today.

ACKNOWLEDGEMENTS

The figures contained within this chapter resulted from the excellent work of Spencer Phippen of Baylor's Department of Medical Illustration. The editorial assistance of Lisa Wheeler is noted and appreciated.

REFERENCES

1. Wheeler, J.M. (1990). The emperor (or, rather, his statistician) has new clothes. *Fertil. Steril.*, **53**, 220–223
2. Sampson, J.A. (1940). Development of the implantation theory of origin of peritoneal endometriosis. *Am. J. Obstet. Gynecol.*, **40**, 549–561
3. Rogers, S.F. and Jacobs, W.M. (1968). Infertility and endometriosis: conservative surgical approach. *Fertil. Steril.*, **19**, 529–536
4. Malinak, L.R. and Wheeler, J.M. (1988). Does mild endometriosis cause infertility? *Semin. Reprod. Endo.*, **6**, 239–248
5. Wheeler, J.M. (1990). The epidemiology of endometriosis-associated infertility. *J. Reprod. Med.*, **34**, 41–46
6. Wheeler, J.M. and Malinak, L.R. (1989). The surgical management of endometriosis. *Obstet.*

Gynecol. Clin. North. Am., **16**, 147–156

7. Henzl, M.R., Corson, L.L., Moghissi, K.S., Buttram, V.C., Berquist, C. and Jacobson, J. (1988). Administration of nasal nafarelin as compared with oral danazol for endometriosis. *N. Engl. J. Med.*, **318**, 485–489
8. Wheeler, J.M., Malinak, L.R., Miller, J., Knittle, J. and the Depot Lupron study group, (1990). A randomized, placebo controlled comparison of depot leuprolide acetate vs. danazol in the treatment of endometriosis. (Submitted)
9. Gordon, K., Williams, R.F., Danforth, D.R. and Hodgen, G.D. (1990). Induction of a prolonged hypoestrogenic status in intact primates by Antide (nal-lys): a long-acting GnRH antagonist. Presented at the 37th *Annual Meeting of the Society for Gynecologic Investigation*, March 21–24, St. Louis, Missouri
10. DeCherney, A.H. (1985). The leader of the band is tired. *Fertil. Steril.*, **35**, 521–523
11. Interceed (TC7) Adhesion Barrier Study Group (1989). Prevention of postsurgical adhesions by Interceed (TC7), an absorbable adhesion barrier: a prospective, randomized multicenter clinical study. *Fertil. Steril.*, **51**, 933–938
12. Dunn, R.C., Steinleitner, A.J. and Lambert, H. (1989). Synergistic effect of calcium channel blockade and recombinant tissue plasminogen activator to prevent adhesions via a continuous intraperitoneal pump. Presented at the *45th Annual Meeting of the American Fertility Society*, November 13–16, San Francisco
13. Steinleitner, A., Kazensky, C. and Lambert, H. (1990). Prevention of primary posttraumatic adhesion formation by analogs of the neuroendocrine-immunomodulatory peptides substance P (SP) and somatostatin (SMS). Presented at the *37th Annual Meeting of the Society for Gynecologic Investigation*, March 21–24, St. Louis, Missouri
14. Wheeler, J.M. and Malinak, L.R. (1981). Postoperative danazol therapy in infertility patients with severe endometriosis. *Fertil. Steril.*, **36**, 460–464
15. Wheeler, J.M., Maccato, M.L. and Malinak, L.R. (1985). Postoperative danazol: pregnancy rates in women with endometriosis treated by combined conservative surgical therapy/immediate postoperative danazol. Presented at the *41st Annual Meeting of the American Fertility Society*, September 28–30, Chicago
16. Murphy, A.A., Green, W.R., Bobbie, D. and Rock, J.A. (1986). Unsuspected endometriosis documented by scanning electron microscopy in visually normal peritoneum. *Fertil. Steril.*, **46**, 522–526
17. Stripling, M.C., Martin, D.C., Chatman, D.L., VanderZwaag, R. and Poston, W.M. (1988). Subtle appearance of pelvic endometriosis. *Fertil. Steril.*, **49**, 427–431
18. The American Fertility Society (1985). Revised American Fertility Society classification of endometriosis. *Fertil. Steril.*, **43**, 351–352
19. Semm, K. (1987). *Operative manual for endoscopic abdominal surgery.* (Chicago: Year Book Medical Publishers)
20. Linsky, C. and Bardi, J.A. (1990). Personal communication.
21. Maccatto, M.L., Wheeler, J.M. and Malinak, L.R. (1985). The timing of laparoscopy to laparotomy in the surgical treatment of female infertility. Presented at the *33rd Annual Clinical Meeting of the American College of Obstetricians and Gynecologists.* May 20–24, Washington, D.C.
22. Malinak, L.R. and Wheeler, J.M. (1987). Presacral neurectomy. In Garcia, C.-R., Mikata, J.J. and Rosenblum, N. (eds.) *Current Therapy in Surgical Gynecology*, pp. 70–91. (Toronto: BC Decker)
23. Wheeler, J.M. and Malinak, L.R. (1990). Combined medical and surgical therapy for endometriosis. *Prog. Clin. Biol. Res.*, **323**, 281–288
24. Wheeler, J.M. and Malinak, L.R. (1987). Computer graphic pelvic mapping, second-look laparoscopy, and the distinction of recurrent vs. persistent endometriosis. Presented at the *43rd Annual Meeting of the American Fertility Society*, September 28–30, Reno, Nevada

11
Laser laparoscopy in the treatment of endometriosis

C. J. G. Sutton

During the past two decades we have witnessed considerable technical progress in infertility surgery. Microsurgical techniques introduced new concepts in surgical operations and engendered a respect for the delicate reproductive structures. The main aim of these procedures was to reduce the incidence of tubal and ovarian adhesions by careful tissue handling, the avoidance of surface desiccation and meticulous haemostasis[1,2]. Recent research has suggested that a reduction in peritoneal mesothelial plasminogen activator activity (PAA) in the presence of trauma, infection or tissue ischaemia is the likely pathway in postsurgical adhesion formation[3,4,5]. Any surgical insult is associated with trauma but the biological interaction between lasers and living tissue minimizes this. Infection is less likely with laparoscopy than laparotomy and the ischaemia produced by surgical knots is avoided by the use of lasers. The advent of operative laparoscopic techniques has replaced the need for open surgery in many patients[6].

This chapter traces the history and development of laser laparoscopy and explains why laser laparoscopy represents an advance in the surgical treatment of endometriosis.

THE HISTORY AND DEVELOPMENT OF LASER LAPAROSCOPY

In the 1950s Arthur Schawlow and Charles Townes co-authored a paper explaining how stimulated emission could be used to generate and amplify visible light. It took a further ten years until the first working laser, a ruby laser, was produced by Theodore Maiman in 1960. The first surgical laser was used to photocoagulate retinal lesions. It was replaced in ophthalmology in the mid-1960s by the argon laser because of its more useful absorption properties. The neodymium:YAG laser was developed in 1961 for photo-coagulation of large tumours and like the argon laser its emissions could be passed down flexible endoscopes for the control of bleeding from peptic ulcers. The carbon dioxide (CO_2) laser, probably the most widely used laser in gynaecology, was developed in 1964 by Patel and his colleagues working at Bell Laboratories in California for use in the communications industry.

The first reported use of the CO_2 laser via a laparoscope came from Professor Bruhat and his team working at the Polyclinique in Clermont-Ferrand, France[7]. Having pioneered this new form of surgical treatment they turned their attention to advanced operative laparoscopic techniques using electrodiathermy, and have only recently renewed their interest in laser surgery[8]. Meanwhile, other centres started experimenting with laser laparo-scopy and prototype instruments and techniques were developed independ-ently in Israel[9], the United States[10,11], the United Kingdom[12] and Belgium[13]. One of the disadvantages of the CO_2 laser energy is that, until recently, it could only be passed down rigid systems that are rather cumbersome. Professor William Keye, working at the University of Utah, investigated an argon laser that could be aimed and fired through flexible fibre-optic fibres. He performed initial animal experiments and then used it on a series of patients with endometriosis[14].

The neodymium:YAG laser had already been used endoscopically for endometrial ablation via the hysteroscope[15], where the relatively deep penetration and the ability to function in a fluid medium was a distinct advantage. The introduction of artificial sapphire tips allowed the laser energy to focus at a point source and produced a type of laser scalpel, at the same time retaining the advantage of flexible fibres and the ability to work in haemorrhagic areas. This is a valuable surgical property, since energy at this wavelength is not absorbed by blood whereas the CO_2 laser is rendered virtually ineffective in the presence of haemorrhage[16,17].

The latest flexible-fibre laser to be developed has been the potassium–titanyl phosphate laser (KTP/532). With a wavelength of 532 nm it is a frequency-doubled Nd:YAG laser in which the KTP laser beam is generated by optically pumping Nd:YAG laser energy through a crystal of KTP. Laser energy at this wavelength has the same tissue effect as the argon laser but is associated with greater power and appears to be more effective when used laparoscopically. This laser was introduced by James Daniell in Nashville, Tennessee, who also introduced CO_2 laser laparoscopy to North America[18,19].

Newer lasers have been developed that provide greater precision but do not confer any great advantage for the treatment of endometriosis. An excimer laser is so precise that it can create serial notches in a human hair but unfortunately there is no thermal effect and when it is used laparoscopically there is inevitably small-vessel haemorrhage that cannot be stemmed by the laser energy. Before discussing the technical aspects and results of treatment with these different lasers, it is important to be certain that an accurate diagnosis is made at the initial laparoscopy.

DIAGNOSTIC LAPAROSCOPY AND STAGING

The major advantage of laser laparoscopy in endometriosis lies in the ability to provide treatment at the same time as the diagnosis is made. It is important, therefore, to obtain informed consent to proceed to laser treatment from all patients who are having a diagnostic laparoscopy for pelvic pain or infertility. In our hospital the lasers and ancillary equipment are ready for immediate use at all diagnostic laparoscopies.

The diagnosis of endometriosis carries significant implications for any woman[20] and it is therefore important that the assessment laparoscopy should be performed by a gynaecologist who is aware of the various manifestations of active disease rather than by someone who is merely looking for haemosiderin deposits on the peritoneal surface, which often represent burnt out or inactive disease. There appears to be a relationship between the colour and the age of the endometrial implants and, indeed, even with the age of the patient; the non-haemorrhagic lesions are more usually found in young women and the black deposits laden with haemosiderin are more common in the older patients[21]. These non-pigmented lesions include white opacified peritoneum resembling vesicles or 'sago-grains', red flame-like telangiectatic lesions, and glandular lesions resembling endometrium at hysteroscopy. Jansen and Russell[22] showed that many of these macroscopic appearances are associated with active endometriosis by demonstrating endometrial glands and stroma on histological inspection of peritoneal biopsies in 67–81% of cases. Other lesions such as subovarian adhesions, yellow-brown peritoneal patches and circular peritoneal defects had endometriosis in half of the biopsies[22].

A systematic and careful inspection of the peritoneal surfaces of the pelvis and abdomen should be made employing a double-puncture technique with an aspiration cannula inserted suprapubically in the midline. This is used to remove the serosanguinous fluid, usually laden with prostanoids and macrophages, that is characteristically present in women with active endometriosis[23,24,25]. Unless this fluid is removed, it is impossible to inspect the cul de sac adequately and for this reason a double-puncture approach is mandatory. A probe or grasping forceps is used to elevate the ovary to check for subovarian adhesions and the presence of endometriosis in the ovarian fossa or on the posterior surface of the ovary. If an ovarian endometrioma is suspected, needle aspiration should be performed to test for the presence of thick chocolate fluid.

All these lesions and vascular appearances should be carefully marked on a rubber stamp diagram of the pelvis, supplemented, if the equipment is available, by a polaroid photograph from a still camera or a video printer. Ideally the diagnostic laparoscopy and any operative procedures performed at laparoscopy should be recorded on videotape, since this is the only reliable way to monitor the response to treatment at any subsequent second-look laparoscopy. An attempt should be made to grade the severity of the disease using the Revised American Fertility Society Scale[26]. The clinician must be aware that the attainment of a high numerical grade on a scoring system does not necessarily correlate with the degree of pain experienced by the patient. Recent studies have shown that the pain in endometriosis is linked to prostaglandin metabolism, particularly prostaglandin F[27]. Even small lesions are capable of producing large amounts of prostaglandin F, which may account for the finding that patients with mild or moderate disease on the AFS scale can often have more pain than those with extensive disease.

ADVANTAGES OF LASER LAPAROSCOPY

The CO_2 laser is a long-wavelength (10.6 μm) invisible-light laser that produces only excitational and rotational energy in tissue, which results in rapid boiling of cell contents (vaporization). The laser is concentrated at a fine focal point and the high-energy impact produces steam that explodes the intracellular water, resulting in cell debris rising out of the wound that then ignites in the laser beam and is carried off as smoke (the laser plume). Water in the tissue adjacent to the impact zone absorbs any remaining laser energy and therefore acts as an insulator and limits the zone of cellular damage to 300–500 μm and the extent of thermal necrosis to only 100 μm[28]. The unique characteristics of this wavelength make this laser ideal for precise incision of human tissue because the thermal effect inherent in the laser–tissue interaction results in sealing of small blood vessels, lessening the problems associated with capillary oozing.

Before the advent of lasers, the only method available for the endoscopic removal of endometriosis was by laparoscopic scissors, heating the endometrial implants to 120°C for 20 seconds with an endocoagulator[29], or destroying them by the passage of an electric current. Although there is certainly a place for removal of endometriotic implants by laparoscopic scissor excision or diathermy coagulation, the former is rather haemorrhagic and the latter rather imprecise, and it is difficult to be certain that the entire lesion has been removed. Although laparoscopic diathermy is an established treatment, it is important to realize that it has no proven efficacy and it is potentially dangerous. The confidential enquiry of the Royal College of Obstetricians and Gynaecologists of the UK drew attention to the hazards of electro-diathermy burns to the bowel[29] and this is particularly important in endometriosis since the implants are often adjacent to viscera and other easily damaged structures, including the ureter[30,31].

These techniques inevitably result in bleeding or are so imprecise that there is destruction of surrounding tissue with subsequent fibrosis and scarring, a result that is undesirable in surgery that aims to ensure future fertility. In contrast, the CO_2 laser has the advantage of being able to precisely vaporize implants of endometriosis and, since all the tissue debris is evacuated as smoke in the laser plume, there is minimal fibrosis or scar tissue formation and laser wounds heal with virtually no contracture or anatomical distortion[32]. These characteristics make the CO_2 laser particularly suitable for the vaporization of endometriosis and its associated adhesions, especially in patients who are infertile or who may wish to have children in future. Endometrial implants in hazardous situations, such as the bowel, bladder or ureter, can also be vaporized as long as the surgeon is careful and is aware of the depth of penetration of the laser in different tissues and adjusts the power density accordingly. With good eye–hand coordination and careful irrigation of charred material, it is possible to limit the depth of vaporization to as little as 0.1 mm[33].

CO_2 LASER LAPAROSCOPY — TECHNICAL ASPECTS

The laser

We have a 60-W NIIC IR 103 GB laser (Sigmacon, UK) that remains in the operating department. This laser will deliver 50–55 W to the tissue and has a superpulse mode with six preselected settings. In practice we rarely need more than 30 W for laparoscopic work but superpulse, although not essential, is useful for incising thick adhesions.

Video equipment

The facility to monitor and record the operation on video is an essential component of laser laparoscopy. It allows the assistant to provide effective help with the irrigation and retraction probes and also enables the nurses to anticipate instrument needs and the technician to help with maintenance of pneumoperitoneum and smoke evacuation. If the procedure is unduly long it allows the surgeon to operate by looking at the television monitor, thus preventing considerable back strain due to the stooped and twisted position that has to be adopted when peering down a laparoscope.

Laser delivery systems

The technique of laser laparoscopy depends on whether a single- or double-puncture technique is employed and this in turn depends on the preference of the individual operator. With the single-puncture technique the laser energy passes down the operating channel of an angled laparoscope and the beam is finely focused by a micromanipulator joystick using the thumb of the right hand. The advantage of this technique lies in the fact that the path of the laser beam is exactly the same as the operator's line of vision down the laparoscope. It also gives the surgeon greater freedom to manipulate irrigators, retractors and back-stops with less need to rely on an assistant to perform these tasks. The disadvantage, however, with the long focal length inherent in such a system, is that the laser channel has to be rather large to prevent the beam from reflecting off the side walls and this means an inevitable sacrifice in the amount of cross-sectional area that is available for the light fibres and optics. Thus, although a single-puncture laser laparoscope is 14 mm in diameter, the visibility is poor compared to a conventional laparoscope and in this kind of surgery this is of paramount importance. In addition it is necessary to put the tip of the laparoscope quite close to the target tissue, with the result that tissue debris splashes back on the lens, further obscuring the view. For these reasons I prefer the double-puncture technique.

Once the initial assessment has been performed the operator should plan the incisions in such a way that the laser energy is delivered as near as possible to a 90° angle of incidence to the implants that are to be vaporized in order to avoid reflection off the shiny peritoneal surface. Sometimes this is not possible and if the angle of incidence is too low it is necessary to use a laser probe with a mirror set into the distal end at an angle of 45° so that the laser beam exits at 90° to the longitudinal axis of the probe. A third portal probe for suction and irrigation is usually placed suprapubically in the midline and great care must be taken in the placement of these probes to avoid them hitting against each other during endoscopic manoeuvres.

One of the criticisms levelled against CO_2 laser laparoscopy is that the equipment is too cumbersome when compared with the fibre laser delivery systems. Some of the commercially available second-puncture probes are unnecessarily long and this, together with the constant need to adjust the focus with the joystick, makes them unwieldy and difficult to use. We have therefore designed a much shorter probe only 230 mm long that screws into a fixed-focus zinc arsenide lens on the end of the laser arm, thereby focusing the laser energy 10 mm beyond the distal end of the probe (Rocket Ltd., London, UK).

Ancillary equipment
CO_2 laser laparoscopy generates a great deal of smoke as tissue is vaporized and this can interfere with visibility and lead to loss of laser power due to diffraction from the particles suspended in the laser plume. During our procedures we use the gas insufflators on high flow with a smoke evacuation system operated by the laser technician, who has to steer a difficult compromise between overdistension with possibly serious consequences on cardiopulmonary dynamics[34] and overzealous smoke evacuation, when the anterior parietal peritoneum falls down on the operator leading to loss of vision and allowing bowel loops to approximate to laser craters, which may still be hot. It is also essential to have a suction/irrigation probe that will flush the tissues with heparinized Ringer's lactate solution to cool the tissues and get rid of carbon deposits and at the flick of a switch suck out the irrigant fluid and debris and act as a secondary exhaust for venting smoke. Although the flexible-fibre lasers will operate in the presence of blood, the CO_2 laser will only stop small-vessel haemorrhage, since the laser energy at that wavelength is absorbed in the presence of a large amount of blood. It is therefore essential to have equipment available that can be used in the presence of uncontrollable bleeding.

CO_2 LAPAROSCOPY — PRACTICAL ASPECTS

There are two basic methods of treating peritoneal endometriosis with the CO_2 laser at laparoscopy: direct vaporization or laser excisional biopsy of the involved peritoneum.

Direct vaporization
This technique involves vaporizing all visible or palpable implants until all the haemosiderin is released and continuing until the retroperitoneal fat starts to bubble. The area circumferentially adjacent to the implants should also be vaporized and all injected blood vessels that are running into the lesions regardless of whether the lesions themselves are pigmented or non-pigmented in nature. The removal of a wide area of peritoneum to an adequate depth is the secret of the successful eradication of the disease. This is illustrated in Figures 11.1, 11.2 and 11.3 which show an area of cul-de-sac obliteration before treatment (Figure 11.1), immediately after treatment (Figure 11.2), and

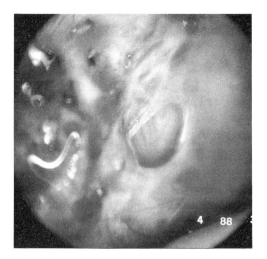

Figure 11.1 Area of endometriosis in cul de sac

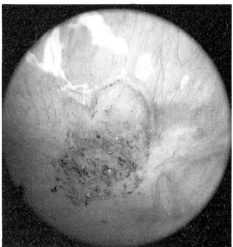

Figure 11.2 Same area as in Figure 11.1 treated with CO_2 laser

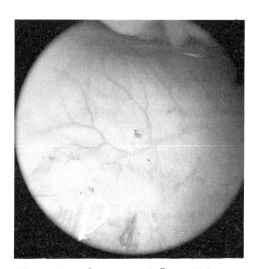

Figure 11.3 Same area as in Figure 11.2, 6 weeks later

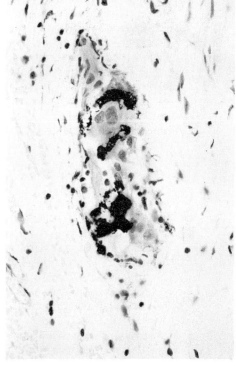

Figure 11.4 Biopsy 6 weeks after Figure 11.2. Carbon and giant cells. No endometrial glands or stroma

6 weeks later (Figure 11.3). The residual dark spots are carbon deposits and should not be confused with recurrent endometriosis. Biopsy of these deposits (Figure 11.4) shows carbon granules surrounded by foreign body giant cells but no inflammatory reaction and no endometrial glands or stroma. These deposits are the result of charring as cell contents are vaporized and every attempt should be made to remove them with a jet of isotonic irrigating fluid under pressure using an aquapurator inserted through a suprapubic midline incision.

We use heparinized Hartmann's solution to remove charred tissue and cell debris and the sequence of alternate irrigation and vaporization proceeds until all the endometriotic tissue is removed. It is particularly important to get rid of all palpable nodules and it is helpful to have an assistant with his or her fingers deep in the vaginal fornices to indicate the site of these nodules and at the same time ensuring that they have been completely vaporized. Unless vaporization continues until all endometriotic tissue has been removed, the patient will almost certainly present with recurrent disease.

We have performed second-look procedures on patients and in only one instance was there recurrence of disease at a previously treated site. It is safe to use the laser anywhere in the pelvis as long as the surgeon is aware of the underlying structures and adjusts the power density and speed of transit of the beam accordingly. Deep nodular deposits on the pelvic side walls or uterosacral ligaments can be vaporized at about 35 W in continuous mode (power density 18 000 W/cm^2 with a spot size of 0.5 mm) but over large blood vessels, the ureter, and particularly over bowel, 5−10 W and rapid movement of the beam, often employing repeated pulses, is safer. After each transit the lesion should be flushed with a jet of fluid to check the depth in relation to the underlying structure. With experience, lesions can be vaporized even on the bowel and ureter to an accuracy of 100 μm[33], but direct vaporization in dangerous areas should only be performed once considerable experience in these techniques has been acquired. I would certainly not advocate this until the laser laparoscopist has performed at least 100 cases.

Laser excisional biopsy
The area of peritoneum involved in endometriosis is circumscribed by a laser cut using high power in superpulse mode to provide high peak powers for effective cutting. A plane is then developed beneath the peritoneum by aquadissection using a jet of irrigant fluid under pressure. The entire endometriotic implant or nodule is then excised by a combination of laser vaporization, laparoscopic scissors, biopsy forceps and grasping forceps. The specimen is submitted to the pathologist to prepare sections for histology and to assess the depth of the lesion and completeness of removal in much the same way as a laser excisional cone biopsy of the cervix is processed.

In a recent study[35] 61% of the patients had clinically recognized lesions penetrating deeper than 2 mm, 43% had lesions penetrating deeper than 3 mm, and 25% had lesions penetrating deeper than 5 mm; some even went as deep as 15 mm. Thus, laser vaporization to 5 mm would have missed the full depth of endometriotic lesions in one-quarter of the patients. This technique has much to recommend it and the injection of irrigation fluid between a vital structure such as the bowel or ureter and the peritoneum adds a further dimension to safety since the interstitial fluid will absorb much of the laser energy. It should also be commended because it provides material for histological study to correlate with a variety of surface appearances, thus enhancing the scientific study of the pathology of endometriosis[22,36,37].

EFFICACY AND SAFETY OF CARBON DIOXIDE LASER LAPAROSCOPY

Carbon dioxide laser laparoscopy has been developed over the past decade and although only practised in a few centres in Europe it is much more popular in North America, where it is rapidly becoming the surgical method of choice for endometriosis. We started using this technique at St Luke's Hospital, Guildford, in October 1982 and have treated over 750 patients. The time in hospital is relatively short and complications are few and usually minor and are usually those associated with diagnostic laparoscopy — wound haematomas, puncture of blood vessels with trochars, and surgical emphysema. So far we have had no injury or morbidity due to the effects of intraperitoneal laser energy and most patients have been able to resume full activity after 48 hours. Many thousands of these procedures have been performed worldwide and a review of the world literature presents an impressive safety record, although it is fair to point out that most published series are the gathered results of acknowledged experts and only time will tell whether the procedure remains safe in the hands of the ordinary gynaecologist. The technique requires considerable patience, which must be combined with a certain boldness as well as manual dexterity and excellent hand–eye coordination. Some surgeons, even after an exasperating attempt to teach them, 'remain as maladroit as a beetle on its back'[38].

The true efficacy of laser laparoscopy is more difficult to establish because there are many uncontrolled, retrospective or poorly designed studies. In assessing the results of treatment it is a useful exercise to examine the success in alleviating each of the four cardinal symptoms of endometriosis — infertility, pelvic pain, dysmenorrhoea and dyspareunia — and then to examine the difficult area of advanced disease with cul-de-sac obliteration.

LASER LAPAROSCOPY FOR INFERTILITY

Before deciding whether any technique designed to eradicate endometriosis is effective in enhancing fertility it is essential to examine the background fertility rate and the effect of certain non-invasive techniques that can best be described as expectant management. Some authors have suggested that the relationship of mild disease to infertility is casual rather than causal[39] and a review of the literature suggests that a relatively high pregnancy rate may be expected in mild endometriosis, although the monthly fecundity rate is much less than that of the general population[40–43]. The real problem in assessing treatment efficacy in mild or minimal endometriosis is to try to establish whether any treatment regimen has a clear advantage over the mere act of dilating the cervix, passing dye through the tubes, and aspirating the yellow serosanguinous fluid laden with macrophages and prostanoids, from the pouch of Douglas[6,24,44]. Utilizing these simple techniques one can expect an overall pregnancy rate in women with mild endometriosis of 50.3% (range 30.6–72.4%) with a fecundity rate of 0.050–1.111[41–43,45,46]. It must be stressed, however, that these studies referred to mild disease only and the only report of expectant management in moderate disease gave a corrected pregnancy rate of 25% and no conceptions at all in patients with severe disease[41]. Before laser laparoscopy can be established as an effective treatment in endometriosis-associated infertility it is essential to conduct a randomized, double-blind, prospective study comparing expectant management with laser laparoscopy in the various stages of the disease. At the present time we are engaged in such a study in Guildford, although it is extremely difficult to recruit patients who are prepared to give informed consent to expectant management when they have often deliberately come to a centre that specializes in endoscopic laser surgery.

We have recently published the results of a longitudinal study over a 5-year period between 1982 and 1987 with women who have been followed up between 1 and 6 years[47]. In the Guildford series there were 56 patients with endometriosis as the only abnormal factor implicated in their infertility which ranged from 6 months to 10 years. Forty-five (80%) of these patients have become pregnant following laser laparoscopy, without adjuvant drug therapy, the majority (73%) within 8 months of the procedure, and 69% of the pregnancies ended in a successful outcome. These good results reflect the impact of this form of therapy on a typical female population presenting to a District General Hospital without sophisticated infertility services. As knowledge of our work has been disseminated, we are now inevitably attracting secondary and tertiary referrals, which is reflected in a small but definite deterioration in the success rate. Our recent update including women treated up to October 1988 shows a reduction of the pregnancy rate to 60% (75% for those with endometriosis alone) (Figure 11.5). The procedure–pregnancy interval and the relationship of the outcome to the severity of the disease are shown in Tables 11.1 and 11.2.

Our data compare favourably with results from the United States[10,37,48–51] and Europe[8,13,52]. The results of these retrospective studies are shown in Table 11.3. The only prospective study of laser laparoscopy in the literature followed one group of 64 patients treated by carbon dioxide laser laparoscopy and another control group of 44 patients who received a variety of medical treatments or laparoscopic electrocoagulation of endometrial implants[53]. This was not a fully randomized study since the allocation depended to some extent on the hospital where they were treated and on the year when they were entered into the study. The laser group achieved pregnancy at a higher overall rate and also had shorter post-treatment intervals. Using life-table analysis, the monthly fecundity rate for the laser group was 6.7% and for the control group was 4.5%.

The problem of therapeutic approaches to endometriosis-associated infertility has been exhaustively reviewed by Olive and Haney[40] and Sutton[54]. Danazol is probably the most widely prescribed drug for this condition and

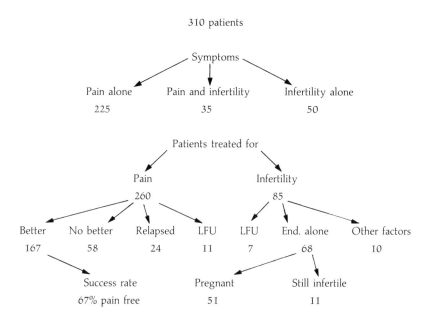

Figure 11.5 Results of laser laparoscopy in patients with endometriosis treated from October 1982 to October 1989 and followed between 1 and 7 years. Pregnancy rate (endometriosis alone) 75%. Pregnancy rate (all factors) 60%. Successful outcome (all pregnancies) 67%. Successful outcome (excluding TOPs) 74%

Table 11.1 Guildford Laser Laparoscopy Project, Oct. 1982–Oct. 1987. Procedure–pregnancy interval

Number of months	Pregnancies (number)	Percentage
0–8	33	73
8–12	7	16
12–16	4	9
> 18	1	2

From ref. 47

is associated with a pregnancy rate of 36.9% (range 0–60%). The LHRH analogues are associated with similar pregnancy rates[54,60] but both these drugs produce unpleasant side-effects and suffer from the disadvantage that the woman has to delay attempts at conception for 6–9 months. The great advantage of laser vaporization of endometriosis at the time of initial laparoscopy is that it allows the patient to attempt conception without delay.

Table 11.2 Guildford Laser Laparoscopy Project. Oct. 1982–Oct. 1987. Severity of endometriosis related to pregnancies

Stage	AFS score	No. of patients followed up	Patients with other factors	Pregnancies	(%)
Minimal	I	19	3	15	94
Mild	II	26	1	17	68
Moderate	III	16	3	11	85
Severe	IV	2	0	2	100
Total		63	7	45	
Other factors: Oligospermia: 6; cervical fibroid: 1 Endometriosis alone: 56					

From ref. 47

Table 11.3 Results of laser laparoscopy for endometriosis

Authors	Patients (number)	Pregnancies		Viability (%)
		Number	%	
Daniell (1985)	40	20	50	—
Feste (1985)	29	21	72	—
Davis (1986)	65	37	—	57
Nezhat (1986)	102	62	61	51
Donnez (1987)	70	40	—	57
Sutton[a] (1990)	56	45	80	69
Feste[a] (1989)	64	52	81	—

[a]Endometriosis alone, no other infertility factors.

An added advantage is that it appears to be the most effective treatment for patients with advanced disease where expectant management and drug therapy are associated with very poor results.

LASER LAPAROSCOPY FOR ADVANCED DISEASE

One of the most interesting developments in laser laparoscopy in recent years has been the growing tendency to extend the technique. At first treatment was limited to early-stage disease and patients with advanced disease had conservative surgery with a pre- or postoperative course of medical therapy[61]. With increasing experience and the realization that high pregnancy rates can be achieved with laparoscopic surgery even with the gross anatomical distortion of Stage IV disease, there is now a tendency to use laser laparoscopy as first-line therapy. Nezhat has produced impressive results with this technique and life-table analysis gives comparable results for all stages of endometriosis. Martin and Olive[62], using laser laparoscopy without adjunctive drug therapy, had fecundity rates for mild and moderate disease of 3.33% and 2.51% respectively, but for severe disease the rate was 5.79%[40]. Similar results have been reported from European centres ranging from 40% to 53%[52,8,47].

LASER LAPAROSCOPY FOR PELVIC PAIN

Most reports on laser laparoscopy for endometriosis deal exclusively with infertility, where success is relatively easy to measure, rather than with pelvic pain, which is much the most common symptom but far more difficult to assess in terms of treatment efficacy. There have been no prospective studies on treatment of pelvic pain, although there has been for both infertility[20] and dysmenorrhoea[63]. We have recently published our data over a 5-year period of treatment between October 1982 and October 1987, most of which cases were followed up between 1 and 5 years[47]. We have just updated these figures and of the 260 patients complaining of pelvic pain due to endometriosis, 167 (67%) claimed the pain was better. Eleven patients were lost to follow-up, 58 were no better, and a further 24 had a relapse of their symptoms between 6 and 18 months following the original laser treatment. Only one patient claimed she had been made worse.

Thirty-three patients who had not improved underwent second-look laparoscopy prior to starting on medical therapy. Just over half the patients had no evidence of endometriosis at all but 18 patients had formed endometriosis at different sites. There was no evidence of endometriosis at the sites previously lasered. This was macroscopically obvious from the appearance of inactive charcoal deposits beneath the peritoneum but in those in whom we took a peritoneal biopsy histological examination confirmed the absence of endometrial glands or stroma and also the absence of any inflammatory response. Obviously this group of patients require medical therapy to prevent further recurrence of the disease but the choice of medical therapy is by no means easy. Danazol, probably the most widely prescribed drug for endometriosis, has proved effective in reducing the majority of implants; nevertheless, a significant persistence or recurrence rate has been noted. Published data suggest a recurrence rate of from 29% to 30%, which is actually higher than that found following laser laparoscopy[64–66]. In addition, it is neither wise nor practical to take danazol or LHRH analogues for longer than 6 months, not only because of the well-documented side effects[67] but also because of the adverse changes in serum lipids with danazol[68,69] and the loss of bone calcium and trabecular density with LHRH analogues[70].

In view of the above problems we tend to treat recurrent endometriosis following laser laparoscopy with continuous progestogen therapy, usually in the form of Provera (Upjohn) at a relatively high dose of 50 mg daily or as an injection of Depo-Provera 50 mg weekly or 100 mg every fortnight. These drugs act by causing initial decidualization of endometrial tissue with eventual atrophy and seem to be the drugs of choice when endometriosis occurs after laser vaporization and there is a need for long-term suppressive therapy.

LASER LAPAROSCOPY FOR DYSMENORRHOEA DUE TO ENDOMETRIOSIS

Women with endometriosis often complain of congestive dysmenorrhoea, which usually precedes the period by a few days and is often partially relieved or, at least, changes in character once the bleeding starts. Dysmenorrhoea is particularly likely to be present when there are deposits of endometriosis on or within the uterosacral ligaments. This is because the sensory parasympathetic fibres to the cervix and the sensory sympathetic fibres to the corpus traverse the cervical division of the Lee–Frankenhauser plexus, which lies in, under and around the attachments of the uterosacral ligaments to the cervix[71]. For many years the operation of presacral neurectomy was employed for patients with intractable dysmenorrhoea but yielded disappointing results with failure rates around 11–15% in primary dysmenorrhoea and 25–40% in secondary dysmenorrhoea associated with endometriosis[72–74]. In 1952 White[75] pointed out that the nerve supply to the cervix is not usually interrupted by the presacral neurectomy procedure and then in 1963 Joseph Doyle described the procedure of paracervical uterine denervation that bears his name[76]. The operation was performed abdominally or vaginally. The results were impressive, with complete pain relief in 63 out of 73 cases (86%), and the results were equally good for primary or secondary dysmenorrhoea. The development of potent non-steroidal anti-inflammatory agents and ovulation suppressants may have reduced the demand for relatively drastic surgical intervention. Interest in Doyle's work has recently been revived with the development of surgical lasers that can be used endoscopically and will perform much the same tissue effect without the need for major surgery[47,77].

LAPAROSCOPIC UTERINE NERVE ABLATION (LUNA)

Technique

The pelvis is carefully inspected to identify the course of the ureters, which can sometimes lie close to the uterosacral ligaments. Usually they lie 1–2 cm laterally; they should be visualized and the characteristic peristaltic movement beneath the peritoneum noted and their positions checked by 'palpation' with a blunt probe. The operator should also beware of the presence of thin-walled veins that course immediately lateral to the uterosacral ligaments and should be very careful to laser medially rather than laterally because if these vessels are punctured, particularly by the CO_2 laser, the bleeding can be profuse and difficult to stop. For this reason, haemostatic clips, diathermy or an endocoagulator should be immediately available and the operator must be proficient in the use of such ancillary equipment before he undertakes laparoscopic uterine neurectomy. This is a potentially serious complication and apparently two deaths have been reported from this complication in the United States; for this reason some laser laparoscopists prefer to use flexible-fibre lasers for this procedure[78].

Once the operator has noted the potential hazards, the uterosacral ligaments are encouraged to 'stand-out' by the assistant pressing on the posterior aspect of the cervix with a blunt probe introduced through the suprapubic trochar. The laser is set at a relatively high power density between 10 000 and 15 000 W/cm^2 and the uterosacral ligaments are vaporized near their point of attachment to the posterolateral aspect of the cervix. It is best to use continuous mode since the associated charring tends to seal small vessels, whereas superpulse, although it incises the ligaments more efficiently, invariably results in more bleeding. The idea of the procedure is to destroy the sensory nerve fibres and their adjacent ganglia as they leave the uterus and because of the divergence of these fibres in the uterosacral ligaments they should be vaporized as close to the cervix as possible. A crater about 1 cm in diameter is vaporized and although we initially went down to a depth of 1 cm we now continue vaporizing for just as long as the fibres appear to be parting. The end-point is usually quite obvious but the laser surgeon should resist the impulse to vaporize deeper, since one often encounters quite large blood vessels in the base of the uterosacral ligaments. It is relatively easy to laser down to the correct depth when the uterosacral ligaments are well formed but sometimes their limits are poorly defined and the procedure is less than satisfactory simply because it is difficult to be sure that the area vaporized is in the same location as the uterine nerve fibres. A further refinement is to superficially laser the posterior aspects of the cervix between the insertion of the uterosacral ligaments to interrupt nerve fibres crossing to the contralateral side[78].

Results

During the past 5 years we have treated 126 patients with laser uterine nerve ablation (LUNA) laparoscopically[47]. Twenty-six had primary dysmenorrhoea and 100 had secondary dysmenorrhoea associated with endometriosis. In this latter group all the peritoneal implants of endometriosis were vaporized at the same session as the uterine nerve ablation. We did not include patients with secondary dysmenorrhoea due to other causes such as fibroids, adenomyosis or pelvic congestion. Patients were seen 4 months and 1 year after treatment.

In the endometriosis group, 6 patients were lost to follow-up but 81 (86%) reported an improvement in symptoms even though 26 (32%) of them had a partial (unilateral) neurectomy. In 3 patients the symptoms returned at 6 months to 1 year following the procedure. No patients were made worse but 13 reported no improvement and, interestingly, 9 of these had incomplete or partial neurectomies due to poor formation of the ligaments resulting in difficulty in localizing and vaporizing the nerve bundles (Table 11.4). There were no serious complications in this group of patients and all were treated on a day-case or overnight-stay basis. Troublesome bleeding was encountered in two patients requiring endocoagulation or haemostatic clips and the insertion of a suction drain in the pelvis for several hours postoperatively. Feste has recently reported on a larger series from Houston[11]. He performed laser neurectomy on 196 patients with intractable dysmenorrhoea who had

Table 11.4 LUNA results with carbon dioxide laser

	LFU	Improved	Same	Worse
Endometriosis				
100 patients	6	81 (86%)	13	—
Primary dysmenorrhoea				
26 patients	4	16 (73%)	6	—
Total				
126 patients	10	97 (84%)	19	—

From Sutton, C.J.G. (1989). In Donnez, J. (ed.) *Laser Operative Laparoscopy and Hysteroscopy.* (Leuven: Nauwelaerts)

failed to respond to traditional therapy. In the 124 patients that he managed to follow up, the failure rate was only 12.9%.

In order to increase objectivity we used a linear analogue pain scale before the procedure and 4 months afterwards to try to assess the response to the treatment. The initial score was an average of 9.2 (out of 10) and post-treatment the average among the successful patients was 3.4. It is important to warn the patients that the first period following LUNA may still be painful, possibly owing to oedema around the nerve fibres during the healing process after laser surgery. It is also important to counsel patients that the procedure may not necessarily alleviate this distressing symptom[19]. There is probably a large component of psychological overlay in this group who do not improve. At the present time we are conducting a study to try to identify patients with psychological problems in advance, because they react badly to surgical interference.

The only study in the literature to have addressed itself to these psychological problems is that of Lichten and Bombard[63] and it is one of the few randomized prospective double-blind studies in the entire field of operative laparoscopy. A relatively homogeneous group of women were selected who had severe or incapacitating dysmenorrhoea, who had no demonstrable pelvic pathology at laparoscopy, and who were unresponsive to NSAIDs and oral contraceptives prescribed concurrently. Coexisting psychiatric illness was evaluated with the Minnesota Multiphasic Personality Inventory and those with an abnormal psychological profile were excluded from the study. The remaining 21 patients were randomized to uterine nerve ablation or control group at the time of the diagnostic laparoscopy. Neither the patient nor the clinical psychologist who conducted the interview at follow-up was aware of the group to which the patient had been randomized. No patient in the control group reported relief from dysmenorrhoea, whereas 9 of the 11 patients (81%) who had LUNA reported almost complete relief at 3 months and 5 of them had continued relief from dysmenorrhoea 1 year after surgery.

There is a great need for further studies of this type before we can fully recommend this type of surgery. All that we can conclude from our study is that the operation appears to be effective and safe in experienced hands. It is also interesting to note that our success rate with endometriosis-associated dysmenorrhoea (86%) is almost exactly the same as that obtained by Feste[11] (87%) even though, at that time, neither of the surgeons was aware of the technique or laser power used by the other. It is also of interest that the success rate is almost identical to that achieved by Doyle at laparotomy in 1963[76] (86.8%).

CO_2 LASER LAPAROSCOPY AND DYSPAREUNIA

Patients with endometriosis complaining of deep dyspareunia are usually found to have active telangiectatic or vesicular implants in the cul de sac or deposits in the uterosacral ligaments that are responsible for the nodular feeling when such patients are examined vaginally. When using the carbon dioxide laser to eradicate these nodules it is important to continue vaporization at a relatively high power density until no further haemosiderin is released and until the assistant confirms that no further nodules are palpable on vaginal and rectal examination.

Sometimes adhesions are present between the rectum and the posterior aspect of the cervix and this is often responsible for dyspareunia. It is important to rid the cul de sac of all adhesions and implants in order to alleviate discomfort during intercourse. Care must be taken when using the laser over the rectum itself and the power density should be reduced and, until considerable experience has been amassed, the laser should be used in a pulsed mode with repeated irrigation to remove the charcoal and assess the depth of destruction in relationship to the anatomy of the rectal wall. With experience the beam can be used in continuous mode with rapid hand movement to prevent penetration of the rectal mucosa. In patients with complete obliteration of the cul de sac it is necessary to use the laser to open up a plane of cleavage between the cervix and the rectum and to use aquadissection to extend this. These techniques of advanced operative laparoscopy have been pioneered by Harry Reich[79].

In our retrospective study we did not specifically enquire about dyspareunia in our analysis of the results, although our impression is that most patients with active disease in the posterior fornix have benefited from laser treatment. Donnez reported on a series of 100 patients who have been followed for more than a year after laser uterine nerve ablation. He found that most patients complaining of dyspareunia experienced relief from this symptom following the operation. We have noticed that, even in the absence of visible endometriosis, patients with very taut uterosacral ligaments seem to complain of dyspareunia that is relieved by the simple act of dividing the ligaments with the laser.

CONCLUSION

Before the introduction of danazol in the early 1970s the mainstay of treatment for endometriosis was relatively aggressive and mutilating surgery usually reserved for severe disease often associated with ovarian endometri-omas. Because it represented a new therapeutic approach to the problem, danazol was greeted with considerable enthusiasm and in spite of the fact that some of the earlier claims regarding its efficacy were exaggerated it is still the most widely prescribed drug for this disease.

The introduction and widespread acceptance of laparoscopy for the diagnosis and follow-up of endometriosis has led to increasing skill and proficiency with this instrument and it was only a matter of time before gynaecological surgeons started to use it for various operative techniques beyond mere tubal occlusion. Electrodiathermy, initially used for female sterilization, had been associated with a number of accidental bowel injuries and the search for an alternative energy source coincided with new developments in medical laser technology. The carbon dioxide laser used down the laparoscope provided a precise, easily controlled, no-touch technique for the cytoreduction of endometriosis and, with skill and experience, could be used in hazardous situations on the bowel, ureter and bladder because of its ability to vaporize tissue to an accuracy of 100 μm without causing tissue necrosis to adjacent healthy tissue.

The past decade has seen the separate development of these techniques in several centres throughout Europe and North America and, although most of the pioneering laser surgeons were working independently, and initially unaware of each other, the striking fact to emerge is the similar results achieved and the impressive safety record in treating several thousand cases in published series. That, however is where the statement ends. All reported series, my own included, have been entirely retrospective and no attempt at all has been made to actually prove that this form of treatment is more efficacious than drug therapy or mere expectant management. At the moment, laser laparoscopy is popular with patients, particularly the infertile, because it allows them to attempt conception without delay rather than embark on a long course of drug therapy with its attendant side-effects. It is now incumbent on those surgeons advocating laser laparoscopic surgery to actually prove that it works by the proper application of well-designed, double-blind prospective clinical trials.

The future lies in the development of less cumbersome delivery systems and the development of tunable-wavelength lasers to allow surgeons to use different lasers in varying clinical situations during the same procedure. For instance, during a lengthy laparoscopic operation one might discover deposits of endometriosis on the bowel or peritubal adhesions interfering with ovum pick-up, where the precision of the CO_2 laser is essential, but in the same patient a large endometrioma may require a visible-light laser with the ability to operate around corners inside the cyst capsule and to photocoagulate tissue in the presence of the haemosiderin-laden fluid and blood. At the moment, certain laser laparoscopists are behaving like feuding warlords, each defending a certain type of laser against all comers, whereas in reality the ability to tune the wavelength at the flick of a switch would be a great breakthrough.

Another future development is the application of photodynamic therapy to endometriosis. Professor Keye and his co-workers at the University of Utah and the University of Adelaide have performed some elegant animal experiments with impeccable scientific methodology whereby they have shown that photosensitizers such as haematoporphyrin derivatives can be selectively taken up by experimentally induced endometrial deposits and can be effectively destroyed by a pulse laser, in this case a gold vapour laser. In their experiments there was no damage to healthy adjacent tissue and the scene is now set for trials on patients, but unfortunately it is likely that there will be considerable problems with skin photosensitization to sunlight. Nevertheless, it is an exciting prospect that could allow total eradication of endometriosis, including the deep peritoneal deposits that are hidden from the view of the laparoscopic surgeon.

All this lies in the future: for the present all we can say is that operative laparoscopy with different lasers appears to be an effective cytoreductive technique in treating endometriosis. It certainly does not work in all cases and a proportion of patients will present with ongoing or recurrent disease, often in other sites. These patients are candidates for long-term medical suppressive therapy. The majority, however, are helped by laser surgery and it has the great advantage that treatment can be performed at the same time as the diagnosis is made at the initial laparoscopy without any increase in the morbidity or length of hospital stay.

REFERENCES

1. Winston, R.M. (1980). Microsurgery of the fallopian tube: From fantasy to reality. *Fertil. Steril.*, **34**, 521
2. Gomel, V. (1983). *Microsurgery in Female Infertility*. Boston: Little, Brown
3. Buckman, R.F., Woods, M., Sargent, L. and Gervin, A.S. (1976). A unifying pathogenic mechanism in the aetiology of intraperitoneal adhesions. *J. Surg. Res.*, **20**, 1–5
4. Raftery, A.T. (1981). Effect of peritoneal trauma on peritoneal fibrinolytic activity and intraperitoneal adhesion formation. An experimental study in the rat. *Eur. Surg. Res.*, **13**, 397–401
5. Menzies, D. and Ellis, H. (1989). Intra-abdominal adhesions and their prevention by topical tissue plasminogen activator. *J. R. Soc. Med.*, **82**, 534–535
6. DeCherney, A.H., Kort, H., Barner, J.B. *et al.* (1980). Increased pregnancy rate with oil soluble hysterosalpingography dye. *Fertil. Steril.*, **33**, 407
7. Bruhat, M., Mages, C. and Manhes, H. (1979). Use of CO_2 laser via laparoscopy. In Kaplan, I. (ed.) *Laser Surgery III*. Proceedings of the Third Congress of the International Society for Laser Surgery, pp. 275–276. Tel Aviv: International Society for Laser Surgery
8. Bruhat, M.A., Wattiez, A., Mage, G., Pouly, J.L. and Canis, M. (1989). CO_2 laser laparoscopy. In Sutton, C.J.G. (ed.) *Laser Surgery*. Baillière's Clinical Obstetrics and Gynaecology, Vol. 3, No. 3, pp. 487–497
9. Tadir, Y., Kaplan, I. and Zuckerman, Z. (1981). A second puncture probe for laser laparoscopy. In Atsumi, K. and Nimsakul, N. (eds.) *Laser Surgery IV*, pp. 25–26. Proceedings of the Fourth Congress of the International Society for Laser Surgery
10. Daniell, J.F. (1984). Laser laparoscopy for endometriosis. *Colposc. Gynaecol. Laser Surg.*, **1**, 185–192
11. Feste, J.R. (1989). *Proceedings of the 2nd World Congress of Gynecologic Endoscopy*. Basel: Karger Publications
12. Sutton, C.J.G. (1986). Initial experience with carbon dioxide laser laparoscopy. *Lasers Med. Sci.*, **1**, 25–31
13. Donnez, J. (1987). Carbon dioxide laser laparoscopy in infertile women with endometriosis and women with adnexal adhesions. *Fertil. Steril.*, **48**(3), 390–394
14. Keye, W.R. and Dixon, J. (1983). Photocoagulation of endometriosis by the Argon laser through the laparoscope. *Obstet. Gynecol.*, **62**(3), 383–386
15. Goldrath, M.H., Fuller, T.A. and Segal, S. (1981). Laser vaporization of endometrium for the treatment of menorraghia. *Am. J. Obstet. Gynecol.*, **104**, 14
16. Lomano, J.M. (1987). Nd:YAG laser ablation of early pelvic endometriosis: a report of 61 cases. *Laser Surg. Med.*, **7**, 56–60
17. Corson, S.L. (1990). Laparoscopic applications of the Nd:YAG laser. In Sutton, C. (ed.) *Lasers in Gynaecology*. London: Chapman and Hall
18. Daniell, J.F., Miller, W. and Tosh, R. (1986). Initial evaluation of the use of the potassium-titanyl-phosphate (KTP-532) laser in gynaecologic laparoscopy. *Fertil. Steril.*, **46**(3), 373–377
19. Daniell, J.F. (1990). Advanced operative laser laparoscopy. In Sutton, C. (ed.) *Lasers in Gynaecology*. London: Chapman and Hall
20. Redwine, D.B. (1987). Age-related evolution in colour appearance of endometriosis. *Fertil. Steril.*, **48**(6), 1062
21. Thomas, E.J. and Cooke, I.D. (1987). Successful treatment of endometriosis: does it benefit infertile women? *Br. Med. J.*, **294**, 1117–1119
22. Jansen, R. and Russell, P. (1986). Nonpigmented endometriosis: Clinical, laparoscopic and pathologic definition. *Am. J. Obstet. Gynecol.*, **155**, 1154–1159

23. Khoo, S.K., Brodie, A. and Mackay, E.V. (1986). Peritoneal fluid biochemistry in infertile women with mild pelvic endometriosis: prognostic value of prostaglandin F2 alpha concentrations to subsequent pregnancy. *Aust. N.Z. J. Obstet. Gynaecol.*, **26**, 210–215

24. Haney, A.F., Misukonis, M.A. and Weinberg, J.B. (1983). Macrophages and infertility: Oviductal macrophages as potential mediators of infertility. *Fertil. Steril.*, **39**, 310

25. Halme, J., Becker, S. and Haskill, S. (1987). Altered maturation and function of peritoneal macrophages: possible role in pathogenesis of endometriosis. *Am. J. Obstet. Gynecol.*, **156**, 783–789

26. American Fertility Society (1985). Classification of endometriosis. *Fertil. Steril.*, **43**, 351–352

27. Vernon, M.W., Beard, J.S., Graves, K. and Wilson, E.A. (1986). Classification of endometriotic implants by morphologic appearance and capacity to synthesise prostaglandin F. *Fertil. Steril.*, **46**, 801–806

28. Bellina, J.H., Hemmings, R., Voros, I.J. and Ross, L.F. (1984). Carbon dioxide laser and electrosurgical wound study with an animal model. A comparison of tissue damage and healing patterns in peritoneal tissue. *Am. J. Obstet. Gynecol.*, **148**, 327

29a. Chamberlain, G.V.P. and Carron-Brown, J. (1982). *Gynaecological Laparoscopy.* The report of the working party of the confidential enquiry into gynaecological laparoscopy. Royal College of Obstetricians and Gynaecologists, London

29b. Semm, K. and Mettler, L. (1980). Technical progress in pelvic surgery via operative laparoscopy. *Am. J. Obstet. Gynaecol.*, **138**, 121–127

30. Cheng, V.S. (1976). Ureteral injury resulting from laparoscopic fulguration of endometriosis implants. *Am. J. Obstet. Gynecol.*, **126**, 1045–1046

31. Sutton, C.J.G. (1974). Limitations of laparoscopic ovarian biopsy. *Br. J. Obstet. Gynaecol.*, **81**, 317–320

32. Allen, J.M., Stein, D.S. and Shingleton, H.M. (1983). Regeneration of cervical epithelium after laser vaporization. *Obstet. Gynecol.*, **62**, 700–704

33. Wilson, E.A. (1988). Surgical therapy for endometriosis. *Clin. Obstet. Gynaecol.*, **31**(4), 857–865

34. Kershaw, E. and Van Boven, M.J. (1990). Fluid and gas hazards during operative hysteroscopy and laparoscopy. In Sutton, C.J.G. (ed.) *Lasers in Gynaecology.* London: Chapman and Hall

35. Martin, D.C., Hubert, G.D. and Levy, B.S. (1989). Depth of infiltration of endometriosis. *J. Gynecol. Surg.*, **5**, 55–60

36. Stripling, M.C., Martin, D.C., Chatman, D.L., Vander Zwaag, R. and Poston, W.M. (1988). Subtle appearance of endometriosis. *Fertil. Steril.*, **49**, 427

37. Martin, D.C. (1985). CO_2 laser laparoscopy for the treatment of endometriosis associated with infertility. *J. Reprod. Med.*, **30**(5), 409–412

38. Baggish, M.S. (1989). Editorial. Telescope and stab: The new wave surgery. *J. Gynecol. Surg.*, **5**(2), 131–132

39. Lilford, R.J. and Dalton, M.E. (1987). Effectiveness of treatment for infertility. *Br. Med. J.*, **295**, 6591

40. Olive, D.L. and Haney, A.F. (1986). Endometriosis-associated infertility: a critical review of therapeutic approaches. *Obstet. Gynecol. Surv.*, **41**, 538–555

41. Olive, D.L., Stohs, G.F., Metzger, D.A. *et al.* (1985). Expectant management and hydrotubations in the treatment of endometriosis associated infertility. *Fertil. Steril.*, **44**, 35

42. Portuondo, J.A., Echanojauregui, A.D., Herran, C. *et al.* (1983). Early conception in patients with untreated mild endometriosis. *Fertil. Steril.*, **39**, 22

43. Schenken, R.S. and Malinak, L.R. (1982). Conservative surgery vs. expectant management for the infertile patient with mild endometriosis. *Fertil. Steril.*, **37**, 183

44. Stillman, R.J. and Miller, L.C. (1984). Diethylstilboestrol exposure in utero and endometriosis in infertile females. *Fertil. Steril.*, **41**, 369

45. Garcia, C.R. and David, S.S. (1977). Pelvic endometriosis: infertility and pelvic pain. *Am. J. Obstet. Gynecol.*, **129**, 740

46. Seibel, M.M., Berber, M.J., Weinstein, F.G. and Taymor, M.L. (1982). The effectiveness of danazol on subsequent fertility in minimal endometriosis. *Fertil. Steril.*, **38**, 534–537

47. Sutton, C.J.G. and Hill, D. (1990). Laser laparoscopy in the treatment of endometriosis.

A 5-year study. *Br. J. Obstet. Gynaecol.*, **97**, 901–905

48. Nezhat, C., Crowgey, S.R. and Garrison, C.P. (1986). Surgical treatment of endometriosis via laser laparoscopy. *Fertil. Steril.*, **45**(6), 778–783

49. Davis, G.D. (1986). Management of endometriosis and its associated adhesions with the carbon dioxide laser laparoscope. *Obstet. Gynecol.*, **68**, 422–425

50. Nezhat, C. (1989). Videolaseroscopy for the treatment of endometriosis. In Studd, J.W.W. (ed.) *Progress in Obstetrics and Gynaecology*, Vol. 6, Ch. 19, pp. 293–303. (Edinburgh: Churchill Livingstone)

51. Gast, M.J., Tobler, R., Strickler, R.C., Odem, R. and Pineda, J. (1988). Laser vaporization of endometriosis in an infertile population: the role of complicating factors. *Fertil. Steril.*, **49**, 32–36

52. Donnez, J., Nisolle, M., Wayembergh, M., Clerckx, F. and Casanas-Roux, F. (1989). CO_2 laser laparoscopy in peritoneal endometriosis and on ovarian endometrial cyst. In Donnez, J. (ed.) *Operative Laparoscopy and Hysteroscopy*, Ch. 4, pp. 53–78 (Leuven: Nauwelaerts)

53. Adamson, G.D., Lu, J. and Subak, L.L. (1988). *Fertil. Steril.*, **50**(5), 704–710

54. Sutton, C.J.G. (1990). The treatment of endometriosis. In Studd, J.W.W. (ed.) *Progress in Obstetrics and Gynaecology*, Vol. 8, pp. 293–313 (Edinburgh: Churchill Livingstone)

55. Audebert, A.J., Larne-Charlus, S. and Emperaire, T.C. (1979). Danazol — endometriosis and infertility: A review of 62 patients treated with danazol. *Postgrad. Med. J.*, **55** (suppl.), 10

56. Chalmers, J.A. and Shervington, P.C. (1979). Follow up of patients with endometriosis treated with danazol. *Postgrad. Med. J.*, **55** (suppl. 5), 44

57. Guzick, D.S. and Rock, J.A. (1983). A comparison of Danazol and conservative surgery for the treatment of infertility due to mild to moderate endometriosis. *Fertil. Steril.*, **40**, 580–584

58. Buttram, V.C., Reiter, R.C. and Ward, S. (1985). Treatment of endometriosis with danazol: report of a six year prospective study. *Fertil. Steril.*, **43**, 353–360

59. Jelley, R. and Magill, P.J. (1986). The effect of LHRH agonist therapy in the treatment of endometriosis (English experience). *Prog. Clin. Biol. Res.*, **225**, 227–238

60. Shaw, R.W. (1988). LHRH analogues in the treatment of endometriosis — comparative results with other treatments. *Baillière's Clinical Obstetrics and Gynaecology*, vol. 2, no. 3

61. Rock, J.A., Guzick, D.S. and Sengos, C. (1981). The conservative surgical treatment of endometriosis: Evaluation of pregnancy success with respect to the extent of disease as categorized using contemporary classification systems. *Fertil. Steril.*, **35**, 131

62. Martin, D.C. and Olive, D.L. (1986). Cited in Olive and Haney. Endometriosis-associated infertility. A critical review of therapeutic approaches. *Obstet. Gynecol. Surg.*, **41**(9), 538–555

63. Lichten, E.M. and Bombard, J. (1987). Surgical treatment of dysmenorrhoea with laparoscopic uterine nerve ablation. *J. Reprod. Med.*, **32**, 37–42

64. Dmowski, W.P. and Cohen, M.R. (1978). Antigonadotropin (danazol) in the treatment of endometriosis: Evaluation of post-treatment fertility and three-year follow-up data. *Am. J. Obstet. Gynecol.*, **130**, 41–47

65. Greenblatt, R.B. and Tzingounis, V. (1979). Danazol treatment of endometriosis: Long term follow-up. *Fertil. Steril.*, **32**, 518–524

66. Puleo, J.G. and Hammond, C.B. (1983). Conservative treatment of endometriosis externa: The effects of danazol therapy. *Fertil. Steril.*, **40**, 164–166

67. Jelly, R.J. (1987). Multicentre open comparative study of buserilin and danazol in the treatment of endometriosis. *Br. J. Clin. Prac. Suppl.*, **48**, 64–68

68. Fahraeus, L., Larsson-Cohn, U., Ljungberg, S. and Wallentin, L. (1984). Profound alterations of the lipo-protein metabolism during danazol treatment in premenopausal women. *Fertil. Steril.*, **42**, 52–57

69. Booker, M.W., Lewis, B. and Whitehead, M.I. (1986). A comparison of the changes in plasma lipids and lipoproteins during therapy with danazol and gestrione for endometriosis. *Proceedings of the 42nd Annual Meeting of the American Fertility Society, Birmingham*

70. Matta, W.H. *et al.* (1987). Hypogonadism induced by LHRH agonist analogues: effects of bone density in premenopausal women. *Br. Med. J.*, **294**, 1523–1524

71. Campbell, R.M. (1950). Anatomy and physiology of sacro-uterine ligaments. *Am. J. Obstet. Gynecol.*, **59**, 1–5

72. Tucker, A.W. (1947). Evaluation of presacral neurectomy in treatment of dysmenorrhoea. *Am. J. Obstet. Gynecol.*, **53**, 226
73. Ingersoll, F. and Meigs, J.V. (1948). Presacral neurectomy for dysmenorrhoea. *N. Engl. J. Med.*, **238**, 357
74. Polan, M.L. and DeCherney, A. (1980). Pre-sacral neurectomy for pelvic pain in infertility. *Fertil. Steril.*, **34**, 557
75. White, J.C. (1952). Conduction of visceral pain. *N. Engl. J. Med.*, **246**, 686
76. Doyle, J.B. and Des Rosiers, J.J. (1963). Paracervical uterine denervation for relief of pelvic pain. *Clin. Obstet. Gynecol.*, **6**, 742–753
77. Daniell, J.F. and Feste, J. (1985). Laser laparoscopy. In Keye, W.R. (ed.) *Laser Surgery in Gynaecology and Obstetrics*, Ch. 11, pp. 147–165. Boston, Mass.: G.K. Hall
78. Daniell, J.F. (1989). Fibreoptic laser laparoscopy. In Sutton, C.J.G. (ed.) *Laparoscopic Surgery*, Baillière's Clinical Obstetrics and Gynaecology, Vol. 3, No. 3, Ch. 6, pp. 545–562
79. Reich, H. (1989). New techniques in advanced operative laparoscopy. In Sutton, C.J.G. (ed.) *Laparoscopic Surgery*. Baillière's Clinical Obstetrics and Gynaecology, Vol. 3, No. 3, pp. 655–681

12
Gestogens and anti-gestogens as treatment of endometriosis

E. J. Thomas and L. Mettler

INTRODUCTION

Since the 1970s the main thrust of drug research and development in endometriosis has been with danazol and latterly the LHRH analogues. The role of these drugs is explored in detail elsewhere in this book and there is no doubt about their efficacy. However, these developments have tended to overshadow the use of progestagens and anti-gestagens in treatment of the disease and yet both these types of compounds are also effective. They undoubtedly have an important therapeutic role both as first- and second-line drugs. The purpose of this chapter is to describe the place of these drugs in the treatment of endometriosis. We shall begin by describing gestagens, then move on to anti-gestagens as exemplified by the new compound, gestrinone (Roussel – UCLAF, Paris).

PROGESTAGENS

Combination of oestrogens and progestagens

Although there is conflicting evidence about the theory, it has long been considered that pregnancy improves endometriosis. Kistner[1] hypothesized that it was the hormonal changes of pregnancy that induced this improvement, basing this on observations of softening of endometriosis found at caesarean section and histological evidence of decidual transformation with areas of necrobiosis in the tissue[2]. He therefore devised a combination of oral oestrogen and progestagen that simulated pregnancy as a new treatment of endometriosis. He used a variety of combinations of two synthetic oestrogens and two progestagens on 12 patients for between 2 and 7 months and called the treatment 'pseudopregnancy'. Nine patients improved subjectively and objectively during the treatment period. Endometrial biopsy in all patients showed a decidual reaction. There was only one patient who was operated upon during treatment and biopsies of endometriosis from the ovary and uterosacral ligaments showed decidual transformation and focal necrosis. These studies were extended and larger numbers of patients were recruited[3] and further favourable results were reported. Andrews et al.[4] verified the clinical efficacy of the pseudopregnancy regime and also reported the decidual transformation, necrosis and leukocyte infiltration in the biopsies of endometriosis taken during treatment. Other studies also reported success with the pseudopregnancy regimes[5-8] using a combination of various oral oestrogens and progestagens. A combination of twice-weekly injections of 250 mg of α-hydroxyprogesterone caproate and 5 mg of oestradiol valerate for between 2 and 10 months led to resolution of symptoms in most[9]. It is interesting that this author found that courses of less than 3 months were not as effective and that ovarian cysts did not respond to the treatment. There appears to be only one comparative study of pseudopregnancy with danazol which uses a consistent regimen[10,11]. These studies showed that danazol was consistently better than the pseudopregnancy in alleviating symptoms and that it caused significantly fewer side-effects.

It is interesting to observe that the last two studies were published in the late 1970s and yet are the first to compare pseudopregnancy with other medical treatments. By then the use of progestagens alone had become established and the pseudopregnancy regime had fallen out of favour, even in the United States where it had been introduced. This is presumably because the side-effects were unacceptable, although published evidence for this is sparse. On reading the original papers it also becomes apparent that the authors considered that it was the progestagen that was the effective hormone. This is even reflected in the titles, where treatments are described as 'progestin-induced pseudopregnancy'[4] or 'effects of new synthetic progestins'[12] even though combination with an oestrogen was used in all cases. There would appear to be virtually no place for a combination of oestrogen and progesterone for the treatment of endometriosis in modern practice, not least because of the unacceptable risks of high doses of oestrogen. Progestagens, however, have an established place in treatment that has somewhat decreased lately because of danazol and the LHRH agonists. The next part of this chapter will examine that role and the rationale for their use in detail.

Progestagens

When considering the use of progestagens in the treatment of endometriosis in 1990 it is important not only to review the various compounds that have been investigated but also to consider what is currently available on prescription. The main progestagens investigated in the past without combination with oestrogen are medroxyprogesterone acetate, lynestrenol, norethynodrel, dydrogesterone and norethisterone. The current British formulary lists only medroxyprogesterone acetate, dydrogesterone and norethisterone as synthetic progestagens for the treatment of endometriosis. The situation is different in Europe and the United States but there will be limitations in each country over which progestagen can be prescribed. Before each synthetic progestagen is reviewed separately, it should be noted that there appear to be no reports of using progesterone itself in the treatment of endometriosis. Presumably this is because formerly it had to be given by injection, which was unacceptable for a long-term treatment. As there are now pessaries available, it may be instructive to see whether they are efficacious in the doses available.

Norethynodrel
This appears to be the first progestagen investigated, with three publications appearing in 1961[13-15] investigating its effect on endometriosis. In the two clinical publications[13,14], daily doses of between 40 and 100 mg were used. Subjective or objective improvement was reported in the majority of patients in each publication. Riva et al.[13] re-evaluated 81 of 123 patients with endometriosis by either laparotomy or culdoscopy and found a regression rate of 78% after an average duration of therapy of 6 months. There is consistency between the publications in the histological changes reported in endometriosis biopsied during treatment. There appears to be initial stromal oedema followed by inflammatory cell infiltration, degeneration and necrosis. This is very similar to the changes reported in the combined regimes and suggests that it is the progestagen that is the therapeutic mechanism. Further reports of the efficacy of this progestagen were published in the 1960s[16-18]. The studies reported the expected side-effects of nausea, oedema, weight gain and breast engorgement.

Lynestrenol
Lynestrenol, 5 mg daily, was first reported as successful when used for up to 9 months in three patients[19]. They extended this to 10 patients and reported that the treatment was successful[20]. They also showed histologically that the endometriosis atrophied, which they concluded was a result of the hypo-oestrogenic state. Timonen and Johansson investigated the effects in 20 patients[21] and reported that the treatment had failed in 8 and that breakthrough bleeding was a significant side-effect. More recently, Mettler has reported treatment with lynestrenol[22,23] and this will be discussed in more detail in the section reviewing comparative trials.

Medroxyprogesterone acetate (MPA)
Gunning and Moyer[24] reported the use of medroxyprogesterone acetate (Depo-Provera) in combination with oestrogen in 13 patients. Two other patients received MPA alone, which relieved their symptoms. The expected progestogenic side-effects were described but these were not severe. Three recent open studies have described the efficacy of MPA in the treatment of endometriosis. Moghissi and Boyce[25] treated 35 women with objectively proven endometriosis with 30 mg of MPA daily for 90 days. There was

subjective and objective improvement in all patients and recurrence was reported in only three. Roland et al.[26] used the same treatment regime on 24 patients and again reported that all the patients improved, although elimination of the disease was disappointing. Most recently Luciano et al.[27], in the most comprehensive study, investigated the efficacy of 50 mg MPA for 4 months. This dose was used in an attempt to overcome the breakthrough bleeding that had occurred in the two previous studies. All the patients had a pre- and post-treatment laparoscopy at which the disease was staged using the American Fertility Society classification[28]. The mean score dropped from 18 to 6 with treatment. They showed that MPA suppressed LH and oestradiol secretion. Significant progestogenic side-effects were reported but the patients appeared to accept this, with only one withdrawing and that for an unrelated reason. A comparative trial with danazol showed MPA to have equal efficacy[29] and this will be described in more detail later.

Dydrogesterone
In the early 1960s two small studies treated 9 and 14 patients respectively with dydrogesterone and clinical improvement was reported in the majority in both[30,31]. Johnston[32] described 45 patients with proven endometriosis who were treated with 5 mg of dydrogesterone twice daily for up to 9 months. Of the 32 patients who had a repeat culdoscopy, 30 were described as being cured of the disease. Of these, 21 had a normal pelvis and 9 had regression of endometriosis. Throughout treatment the menstrual cycles remained regular in all patients and no breakthrough bleeding was reported.

Norethisterone
Norethisterone has been used widely in the treatment of dysfunctional uterine bleeding but there is very little published evidence of its efficacy in endometriosis. Grant[33] used 10 or 15 mg daily from day 5 to day 25 of the menstrual cycle in 83 patients of whom 67 had the diagnosis made at laparotomy or culdoscopy. He reported clinical and objective improvement in 85% of the patients. There was a low incidence of side-effects. He extended the number of patients and the results were comparable to that previously reported[34].

Comparative trials

As mentioned previously, there would only appear to be two comparative studies of progestagens against any other treatments. Mettler and Semm have compared lynestrenol (10 mg daily), danazol (600 mg daily), gestrinone (2.5 mg, 5 mg, 7.5 mg or 10 mg weekly) in combination with pre- and post-treatment laparoscopy at which endometriotic nodules were diathermied and reconstructive surgery was performed. With combination therapy such as this it is difficult to separate the effect of medical therapy from surgical. The percentage of patients with complete resolution of the disease was 73% with gestrinone ($n = 30$), 55% with danazol ($n = 31$) and 48% with lynestrenol ($n = 33$). With the numbers of patients involved, the confidence limits of

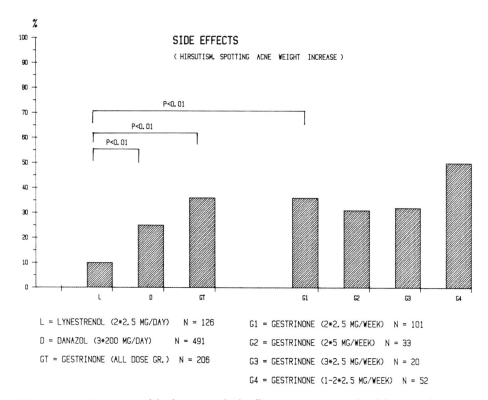

Figure 12.1 Comparison of the frequency of side-effects in patients treated with lynestrenol, danazol and gestrinone

these observations overlap and it is difficult to conclude that there is a major difference between gestrinone and the other two. Analysis of the side-effects as shown in Figure 12.1 shows that lynestrenol was significantly better tolerated than either danazol ($p < 0.01$) or gestrinone at any dose ($p < 0.01$). However, as Figure 12.2 shows, 25% of women treated with lynestrenol had a recurrence of symptoms in a 2-year follow-up compared with only 9% in the danazol group ($p < 0.01$) and 17.5% in the gestrinone group ($p < 0.01$). These studies show that lynestrenol compares satisfactorily with either gestrinone or danazol, although some anxiety must be expressed about the recurrence rate.

Telimaa *et al.*[29] compared danazol 600 mg daily to MPA 100 mg daily and matched placebo in a randomized prospective study. The placebo response is discussed elsewhere in this book. This study is interesting in that the second laparoscopy was delayed until 6 months after the end of treatment, thus overcoming the problems highlighted by Evers[35]. Unfortunately, some patients also received electrocoagulation at the initial laparoscopy. However, there

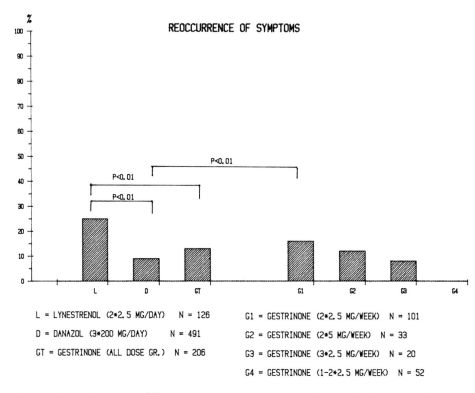

Figure 12.2 Comparison of the recurrence of symptoms in patients treated with lynestrenol, danazol and gestrinone

was total or partial resolution of the peritoneal implants in 60% of the patients receiving danazol ($n = 18$) and 63% of those prescribed MPA ($n = 16$). The patients in the danazol group had significantly higher incidences of acne and muscle cramps than either MPA or placebo. Patients on MPA had a higher incidence of oedema. They concluded that MPA represents an acceptable alternative to danazol.

Conclusion

Whilst this is not a completely comprehensive review of all the published literature about progestagen therapy, it has analysed most of the major studies. The main conclusion from this is that progestagens are an effective treatment of endometriosis and although they do cause side-effects, these are comparable to or less than those of currently available medication. It is instructive that the original experimental work in castrated monkeys[36] showed that oestrogen and progesterone maintained the experimental endometriosis and so it can be surmised that these beneficial effects in humans are a pharmacological phenomenon related to the dose of progestagen used. Progestagens are considerably cheaper than either danazol or the LHRH agonists and it is interesting to question why they are used so infrequently. There appear to be a number of reasons. Firstly, many of the publications are over 25 years old and do not fulfil the criteria that would apply for a peer-reviewed paper in 1990. This does not reduce their importance but does mean that their conclusions can be questioned. Secondly, there are a wide variety of progestagens investigated and they have been used at varying doses for very varying periods of time. No logic appears to be given for a particular choice of drug, dosage or treatment period except perhaps to lessen side-effects. Thirdly, there is a paucity of papers with objective evidence of a treatment effect determined surgically by either laparoscopy or laparotomy. Fourthly, there has been a tendency to mix both medical and surgical therapy in recent work. This is a very interesting area but can lessen the perception of the impact of the medical therapy.

There are two other possibilities. In the 1970s there was a major shift to danazol, first in the United States and then worldwide. It may be that general clinical opinion was that danazol was more effective and that this has just not been published. There is also a large body of good work demonstrating the efficacy of danazol. The other factor is that the manufacturers of the progestagens do not appear to have marketed their drugs strongly for the treatment of endometriosis. Clinicians are influenced in their choice by the presentation of evidence of drug efficacy and it may be that this was more effectively done with danazol.

Whatever the reasons, there is good argument for the role of progestagens in the treatment of endometriosis to be re-evaluated. Although there are anxieties about their effects on lipid metabolism[37], they are cheap and effective agents that are well established and their problems well known. What is needed are properly designed comparative studies using specific progestagens at specific doses so that their efficacy can be unequivocally demonstrated. Even without these, it is reasonable for clinicians to use these agents as either first- or second-line therapy.

ANTI-GESTAGENS

There are two anti-gestagens available for clinical or trial use, both manufactured by Roussel-UCLAF. Mefepristone (RU-486) has not been formerly evaluated in endometriosis. Gestrinone (R-2323) has been evaluated in open and controlled studies and this part of the chapter will concentrate on this.

Gestrinone (R-2323, Roussel-UCLAF, France) is a trienic steroid with an ethyl group in position 13. Its chemical formula is 13β-17α-ethinyl-17-hydroxygona-4,9,11-trien-3-one and its molecular structure is shown in Figure 12.3. Investigations in rats[38,39] have shown that it exhibits (a) low oestrogenic and androgenic activity, (b) moderate anti-oestrogenic activity, (c) marked

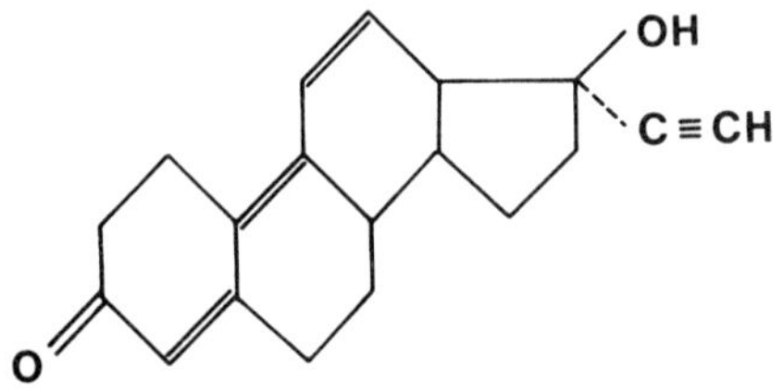

Figure 12.3 The molecular structure of gestrinone

pituitary inhibition, (d) marked anti-progesterone activity. In these animals the endometrial response to exogenous progesterone, its capacity to undergo decidual transformation and the implantation of the embryo were all inhibited by the administration of gestrinone. The precise mechanism of the action of the drug is not elucidated. It is thought that it may act directly on 3β-hydroxydehydrogenase, which catalyses the conversion of pregnenolone to progesterone and therefore may have a luteolytic effect[40]. It has been shown to interact with progesterone receptors and hence displays potent anti-progesterone activity[41,42]. *In vitro* and *in vivo* experiments in rats have demonstrated that it inhibits basal LH concentrations and the pituitary sensivitity to LHRH[43]. This is mediated through direct interaction with several classes of hypothalamic–pituitary steroid receptors[42].

In the human it is probable that gestrinone exerts its effect through a number of mechanisms. It is an androgen, a progestagen and an anti-progestagen. It alters plasma testosterone, plasma LH and plasma oestradiol concentrations. It significantly reduces the plasma concentration of sex hormone binding globulin (SHBG), which causes a lowering of total plasma testosterone concentration but an increase in free plasma testosterone[44,45]. These features were seen in a randomized placebo-controlled trial of gestrinone for 6 months in the treatment of endometriosis[46]. Figure 12.4 shows the decrease in total plasma testosterone so that by month 6 the mean concentration in the placebo group was 1.7 nmol/l whilst it was 1.2 nmol/l in the gestrinone group ($p < 0.05$). Figure 12.5 shows the decrease in SHBG so that by month 6 the mean concentration of SHBG was 63 nmol/l in the placebo group compared to 9 nmol/l in the gestrinone group ($p < 0.001$). Figure 12.6 shows the changes in the free plasma testosterone concentration. The percentage free plasma testosterone was calculated using the formula: $\log(\%$ free testosterone$) = \log 8.52 - 0.44 \log$ SHBG concentration[47]. The percentage free testosterone was then multiplied by the total plasma concentration to calculate the actual free concentration. By month 6 the concentration was 0.024 nmol/l in the placebo group and 0.042 in the gestrinone group ($p < 0.01$). Whether this change in concentration is important biologically is unknown and it cannot be presumed that this is a therapeutic mechanism of the drug's action, although that is a possibility. These data have been verified by other investigators[48–50]. Dowsett *et al.*[48] reported that the suppression of SHBG was greater in danazol than gestrinone and this

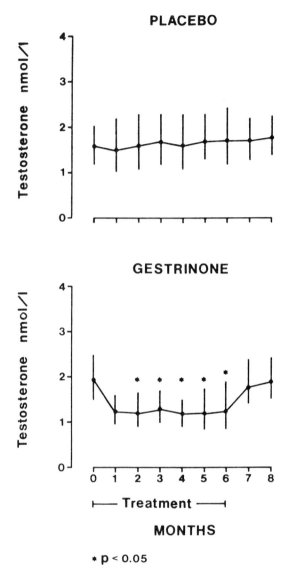

Figure 12.4 Geometric mean and 68% confidence limits of plasma testosterone concentrations in the placebo ($n = 14$) and gestrinone ($n = 15$) groups before, during and after treatment

could be explained by ethisterone, a major metabolite of danazol, competing for SHBG-binding sites.

Thomas and Cooke[46] showed that there was no consistent lowering of plasma LH concentration but that there was less variability in the data (Figure 12.7). This is consistent with an obliteration of the mid-cycle LH surge, which has been reported by other investigators[51]. There was no change in plasma

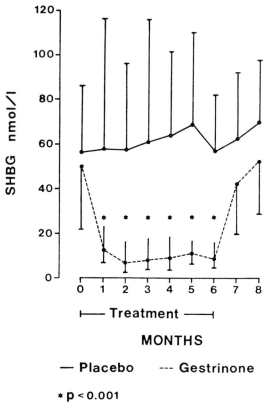

SHBG nmol/l

MONTHS

— Placebo   --- Gestrinone

* p < 0.001

Figure 12.5 Geometric mean and 68% confidence limits of plasma SHBG concentrations in the placebo ($n = 14$) and gestrinone ($n = 15$) groups before, during and after treatment

FSH concentration. Plasma oestradiol concentration was significantly lower in the gestrinone group compared to placebo (Figure 12.8). By month 6 the mean oestradiol concentration was 280 pmol/l in the placebo group compared with 134 pmol/l in the gestrinone group ($p < 0.001$). This decrease in oestradiol may occur secondarily to the changes in gonadotrophin secretion or as a direct effect of the drug on ovarian steroidogenesis. It is possible that this hypo-oestrogenic state is a mechanism of the drug's action.

Various workers have investigated the effect of the drug directly on the endometrium. Analysis of endometrial biopsies in the luteal phase of cycles during which it had been administered as a contraceptive at mid-cycle showed there to be a low progestogenic effect[41]. *In vitro*, gestrinone has been shown to have no effect on oestradiol dehydrogenase activity[52]. The same group showed that gestrinone bound to many types of steroid receptors and postulated that its greater affinity to the oestrogen receptor in comparison with the others may be a therapeutic mechanism. It does not appear to have a direct effect on endometrial proliferation *in vitro* in comparison to danazol[53]. However, there is good evidence that it will alter endometrial histology *in*

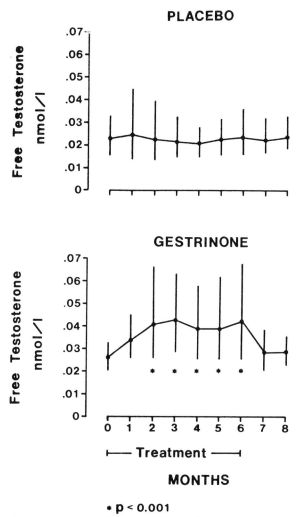

Figure 12.6 Geometric mean and 68% confidence limits of plasma free testosterone concentrations in the placebo ($n = 14$) and gestrinone ($n = 15$) groups before, during and after treatment

vivo. Brosens *et al.*[54] showed that 2 months therapy with 1.25 mg daily of gestrinone induced cellular activation and degeneration of endometriotic implants. They also showed involutionary changes in endometriotic foci after treatment that resembled a progesterone withdrawal effect[55]. These data support the hypothesis that the drug may be disrupting both the steroid signals and their interpretation by the endometrium. Very interestingly these changes were not seen in endometriosis removed from ovaries, which suggests either that this is a different disease or that its vascular supply is so different from endometriotic implants that it is not exposed to the drug. The implication

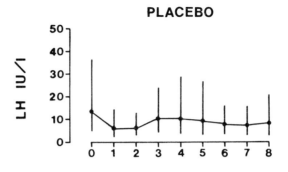

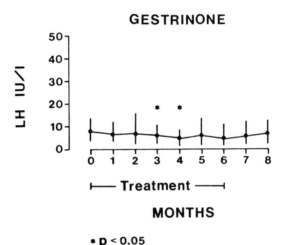

⋆ p < 0.05

Figure 12.7 Geometric mean and 68% confidence limits of plasma LH concentrations in the placebo ($n = 17$) and gestrinone ($n = 20$) groups before, during and after treatment

of this is that it may be more appropriate to treat ovarian endometriosis by surgery.

The drug can be administered either intravenously or orally and is bound to albumin. Its most important metabolic pathway is hydroxylation that creates four metabolites whose biological activity is similar to but less than that of gestrinone. Excretion of the drug occurs in bile and urine. After a 2.5 mg oral dose the mean time to peak plasma concentration was 2.1 hours and the mean elimination half-life was 27.3 hours. Plasma levels at 3 and 7 days after a single oral administration are 5% and 3% of the maximum drug concentration respectively[56,57]. These pharmacodynamic properties mean that the administration of gestrinone every third day is adequate to maintain the drug in plasma without the risk of accumulation. Until recently the recommended dose has been 2.5 mg orally twice weekly. A recent publication has reported equal clinical efficacy with a dose of 1.25 mg twice weekly

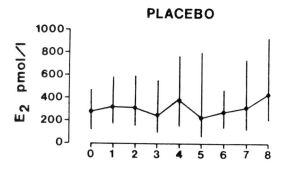

PLACEBO

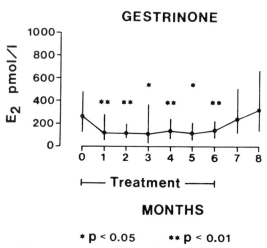

GESTRINONE

├── **Treatment** ──┤

MONTHS

* p < 0.05   ** p < 0.01

Figure 12.8   Geometric mean and 68% confidence limits of plasma oestradiol (E_2) concentrations in the placebo ($n = 17$) and gestrinone ($n = 20$) groups before, during and after treatment

compared to 2.5 mg, and if this is verified then that may become the recommended dose[58].

The clinical effect of administration is to suppress ovulation, which results in amenorrhoea or oligomenorrhoea. Administration of 5 mg orally rendered each of 20 women amenorrhoeic[59]. At a dosage of 2.5 mg twice weekly it induced amenorrhoea in 50% and 58% of women respectively[23,60]. Its main side-effects are androgenic, either related to the inherent androgenicity of the drug or as a result of raising the concentration of the free plasma testosterone. In an uncontrolled trial 71% of patients complained of seborrhoea, 65% of acne, 29% of breast hypotrophy, 9% of hirsutism and 9% of hair loss[60]. Fifty per cent of the patients complained of androgenic side-effects in a study by Mettler and Semm[23]. It is interesting, however, that in the only double-blind, placebo-controlled trial of gestrinone[46] no increase in side-effects was seen in the treatment group. This could be due to the small number of patients in the study, but the percentage of side-effects reported in the placebo group was high. Recently there has been a report of the use of gestrinone vaginally[61]. Patients treated by the vaginal route reported less androgenic side-effects than those treated orally. They also showed a lower weight gain. There was no difference in the efficacy of the treatment whatever the route of administration.

Because gestrinone inhibits ovulation, studies were performed to investigate its efficacy as a contraceptive. Analysis of its use in mid-cycle in 1362 cycles in Haitian women demonstrated it to be effective[62]. In 138 treatment cycles of 5 mg of gestrinone once a week in 28 subjects there were no pregnancies[63]. A larger study of 800 patients using the same dose demonstrated an overall pregnancy rate of 4.6 per 100 woman-years[64]. This failure rate is too high for the drug to be recommended as a safe contraceptive. The drug has also been shown to decrease the volume of fibroids during treatment[65].

The capacity of gestrinone to induce amenorrhoea led to the exploration of the possibility that it could be an effective treatment of endometriosis by causing a pseudomenopause. Coutinho[59] treated 20 patients with laparoscopically diagnosed endometriosis with 5 mg twice weekly for between 4 and 8 months. The symptoms resolved in all patients by the third month and of the nine women who wished to conceive, five had done so within a year. A further 15 were administered 2.5 mg twice weekly and four of them had conceived within a year of therapy[60]. One of the authors performed the first study in which efficacy was described by pre- and post-treatment laparoscopy[23]. At the initial procedure the endometriosis was cauterized and then gestrinone was prescribed at a dose of 5 mg twice weekly for 6 months. There was marked improvement or disappearance of the disease in 21 out of 24 patients. The other author performed the first placebo-controlled trial of the drug[46]. Infertile patients with asymptomatic endometriosis were randomly allocated to receive either 2.5 mg of gestrinone orally twice weekly or matched placebo for 24 weeks. The endometriosis was scored using the original AFS score[66] at the first laparoscopy and then re-evaluated at a second laparoscopy in the final week of treatment. Gestrinone appeared to eradicate the disease more than placebo, although this did not reach statistical significance ($p < 0.06$). It significantly improved endometriosis in comparison with placebo ($p < 0.02$). In detail, 15 out of the 18 patients on gestrinone improved in comparison with only 5 out of the 17 on placebo. This study also described the natural history of the disease and this is addressed elsewhere in this book. Only one comparative study with danazol has been reported[67]. Thirty-nine patients were randomly allocated to receive either danazol or gestrinone as treatment of their endometriosis. The initial doses were gestrinone 2.5 mg twice weekly or danazol 600 mg danazol daily and these were increased until all the patients became amenorrhoeic. Those patients with pain showed marked improvement in both groups. Only 16 patients had a second laparoscopy, 7 in the gestrinone and 9 in the danazol group. These showed significant reduction in the disease with no significant differences between the therapies. Danazol showed a higher frequency of side-effects than gestrinone. A large multicentre trial of gestrinone against danazol has been performed in the United Kingdom and the data are being analysed.

In conclusion, gestrinone is an effective and safe treatment for endometriosis that appears to be an alternative to danazol. Larger studies are needed to document whether it has a more acceptable profile of side-effects, but if this proves to be the case then it represents a significant new therapy. The LHRH analogues have significant side-effects and gestrinone may represent an alternative to them. Gestrinone is not only an acceptable first-line treatment but also can be used if other therapies prove ineffective or have unacceptable side-effects.

GENERAL CONCLUSION

Both the progestagens and the anti-progestagens are effective therapies for endometriosis. The progestagens are a cheap and safe treatment whose use could be increased. Gestrinone is a new compound that has yet to receive a licence in many countries but may well represent an alternative to danazol.

REFERENCES

1. Kistner, R.W. (1958). The use of newer progestins in the treatment of endometriosis. *Am. J. Obstet. Gynecol.*, **75**, 264–278
2. Kistner, R.W. (1965). Current status of the hormonal treatment of endometriosis. *Clin. Obstet. Gynecol.*, **9**, 271–292
3. Kistner, R.W. (1959). Treatment of endometriosis by inducing pseudo-pregnancy with ovarian hormones. *Fertil. Steril.*, **10**, 539–554
4. Andrews, M.C., Andrews, W.C. and Strauss, M.D. (1959). Effects of progestin-induced pseudopregnancy on endometriosis: Clinical and microscopic studies. *Am. J. Obstet. Gynecol.*, **78**, 776–785
5. Thomassen, H. and Berthelsen, H.G. (1966). Treatment of endometriosis with progestogens. *Dan. Med. Bull.*, **13**, 33–35
6. Chalmers, J.A. (1962). Treatment of endometriosis with Anovlar. *J. Obstet. Gynaecol. Br. Commonw.*, **69**, 801–803
7. Ostergaard, E. (1965). The oral progestational and anti-ovulatory properties of megestrol acetate and its therapeutic use in gynaecological disorders. *J. Obstet. Gynaecol. Br. Commonw.*, **72**, 45–58
8. Kourides, I.A. and Kistner, R.W. (1968). Three new synthetic progestins in the treatment of endometriosis. *Obstet. Gynecol.*, **31**, 821–828
9. Thomas, H.H. (1960). Conservative treatment of endometriosis. Use of long-acting ovarian steroid hormones. *Obstet. Gynecol.*, **15**, 498–503
10. Noble, A.D. and Letchworth, A.T. (1979). Medical treatment of endometriosis: a comparative trial. *Postgrad. Med. J.*, **55** (suppl. 5), 37–39
11. Noble, A.D. and Letchworth, A.T. (1980). Treatment of endometriosis: A study of medical management. *Br. J. Obstet. Gynaecol.*, **87**, 726–729
12. Kistner, R.W. (1965). The effects of new synthetic progestogens on endometriosis in the human female. *Fertil. Steril.*, **16**, 61–80
13. Riva, H.L., Wilson, J.H. and Kawaski, D.M. (1961). Effect of norethynodrel on endometriosis. *Am. J. Obstet. Gynecol.*, **82**, 109–118
14. Lebherz, T.B. and Fobes, C.D. (1961). Management of endometriosis with nor-progesterone. *Am. J. Obstet. Gynecol.*, **83**, 102–110
15. Dito, W.R. and Batsakis, J.G. (1961). Norethynodrel-treated endometriosis: A morphologic and histochemical study. *Obstet. Gynecol.*, **18**, 1–12
16. Riva, H.L., Kawaski, D.M. and Messinger, A.J. (1962). Further experience with norethynodrel in treatment of endometriosis. *Obstet. Gynecol.*, **19**, 111–117
17. Williams, B.P.F. (1962). Conservative treatment of endometriosis with progestin therapy. *Am. J. Obstet. Gynecol.*, **83**, 715–719

18. Williams, B.F.P. (1967). Conservative management of endometriosis: Follow-up observations of progestin therapy. *Obstet. Gynecol.*, **30**, 76–82

19. Soiva, K. and Castren, O. (1963). The conservative treatment of endometriosis with lynestrenol. *Ann. Chir. Gynaecol. Fenn.*, **52**, 376–382

20. Soiva, K. and Castren, O. (1964). Clinical observations on the effect of lynestrenol on endometriosis and ovarian function. *Int. J. Fertil.*, **9**, 253–255

21. Timonen, S. and Johansson, C.-J. (1968). Endometriosis treated with lynestrenol. *Ann. Chir. Gynaecol. Fenn.*, **57**, 144–147

22. Mettler, L. (1987). Vergleich der medikamentosen Behandlung der Endometriosis genitalis externa mit Gestrinon, Lynestrenol und Danazol in Rahmen-Stufen-Behandlung. *Fertilitat*, **3**, 133–139

23. Mettler, L. and Semm, K. (1984). 3-Step therapy of genital endometriosis in cases of human infertility with lynestrenol, danazol or gestrinone administration with the 2nd step. In Raynaud, J.P., Ojasso, T. and Martini, L. (eds.) *Medical Management of Endometriosis*, pp. 233–247. (New York: Raven Press)

24. Gunning, J.E. and Moyer, D. (1967). The effect of medroxyprogesterone acetate on endometriosis in the human female. *Fertil. Steril.*, **18**, 759–774

25. Moghissi, K.S. and Boyce, C.R. (1976). Management of endometriosis with oral medroxyprogesterone acetate. *Obstet. Gynecol.*, **47**, 265–267

26. Roland, M., Leisten, D. and Kane, R. (1976). Endometriosis therapy with medroxyprogesterone acetate. *J. Reprod. Med.*, **17**, 249–252

27. Luciano, A.A., Turksoy, R.N. and Carleo, J. (1988). Evaluation of oral medroxyprogsterone acetate in the treatment of endometriosis. *Obstet. Gynecol.*, **72**, 323–327

28. American Fertility Society. (1985). Revised American Fertility Society classification for endometriosis. *Fertil. Steril.*, **43**, 351–352

29. Telimmaa, S., Puolakka, J., Ronnberg, L. and Kauppila, A. (1987). Placebo-controlled comparison of danazol and high-dose medroxyprogesterone acetate in the treatment of endometriosis. *Gynecol. Endocrinol.*, **1**, 13–23

30. Aydar, C.K. and Greenblatt, R.B. (1964). 6-Dehydro-retroprogesterone (Duphaston) an interesting progesterone-like compound. *Int. J. Fertil.*, **9**, 585–95

31. Backer, M.H. (1962). Isopregnenone (Duphaston): A new progestational agent. *Obstet. Gynecol.*, **19**, 724–729

32. Johnston, W.I.H. (1976). Dydrogesterone and endometriosis. *Br. J. Obstet. Gynaecol.*, **83**, 77–80

33. Grant, A. (1961). The non-surgical treatment of endometriosis by progestagens. *Med. J. Aust.*, **48**, 936–938

34. Grant, A. (1963). An evaluation of the conservative treatment of endometriosis. *Aust. N.Z. Obstet. Gynaecol.*, **3**, 162–167

35. Evers, J. (1987). The second look laparoscopy for the evaluation of the results of medical treatment of endometriosis should not be performed during ovarian suppression. *Fertil. Steril.*, **47**, 502–504

36. Scott, R.B. and Wharton, L.R. (1957). The effect of estrone and progesterone on the growth of experimental endometriosis in rhesus monkey. *Am. J. Obstet. Gynecol.*, **74**, 852–863

37. Teichmann, A.T., Cremer, P., Wieland, H., Kuhn, W. and Seidel, D. (1988). Lipid metabolic changes during hormonal treatment of endometriosis. *Maturitas*, **10**, 27–33

38. Sakiz, E. and Azadian-Boulanger, G. (1970). R-2323 — An original contraceptive compound. In *Hormonal Steroids. Proceedings of the Third International Congress*. Excerpta Medical International Congress Series, No. 219, pp. 865–871

39. Azadian-Boulanger, G., Secchi, J. and Sakiz, E. (1971). Biological study of the anti-progesterone effect of R2323. In *Recent Investigations in Reproduction*. Excerpta Medica International Congress Series, No. 278, pp. 129–133

40. Sakiz, E., Azadian-Boulanger, G. and Raynaud, J.P. (1972). Antiestrogens, antiprogesterones. In *Proceedings of the Fourth International Congress of Endocrinology*. Excerpta Medica International Congress Series, No. 273, pp. 988–994

41. Azadian-Boulanger, G., Secchi, J., Laraque, F., Raynaud, J.P. and Sakiz, E. (1976). Action of the midcycle contraceptive (R 2323) on the human endometrium. *Am. J. Obstet. Gynecol.*, **125**, 1049–1056

236

42. Moguilewsky, M. and Philibert, D. (1984). Dynamics of the receptor interactions of danazol and gestrinone in the rat: Correlation with biological activities. In Raynaud, J-P., Ojasoo, T. and Martini, L. (eds.) *Medical Management of Endometriosis*, pp. 163–181. (New York: Raven Press)

43. Proulx, L., Labrie, F., Veilleux, R. and Azadian-Boulanger, G. (1984). Actions of progestins and androgens at the hypothalamo-adenohypophyseal level in the female rat. In Raynaud, J-P., Ojasoo, T. and Martini, L. (eds.) *Medical Management of Endometriosis*, pp. 149–162. (New York: Raven Press)

44. Pugeat, M., Nicolas, B., Tournaire, J. and Forest, M.G. (1984). Interaction of gestrinone with human plasma steroid binding proteins. In Raynaud, J-P., Ojasoo, T. and Martini, L. (eds.) *Medical Management of Endometriosis*, pp. 183–192. (New York: Raven Press)

45. Kauppila, A., Isomaa, V., Ronnberg, L., Vierikko, P. and Vihko, R. (1985). Effect of gestrinone in endometriosis tissue and endometrium. *Fertil. Steril.*, **44**, 466–470

46. Thomas, E.J. and Cooke, I.D. (1987). The impact of gestrinone upon the course of asymptomatic endometriosis. *Br. Med. J.*, **294**, 272–274

47. Dowsett, M., Attree, S.L., Virdee, S.S. and Jeffcoate, S.L. (1985). Oestrogen-related changes in sex hormone binding globulin levels during normal and gonadotrophin stimulated menstrual cycles. *Clin. Endocrinol.*, **23**, 303–312

48. Dowsett, M., Forbes, K.L., Rose, G.L., Mudge, J.E. and Jeffcoate, S.L. (1986). A comparison of the effects of danazol and gestrinone on testosterone binding to sex hormone binding globulin *in vitro* and *in vivo*. *Clin. Endocrinol.*, **24**, 555–563

49. Bergquist, A., Landgren, B-M. and Diczfalusy, E. (1988). Clinical, pharmacokinetic and pharmacodynamic study of three progestagens in the treatment of endometriosis. *New Trends Gynaecol. Obstet.*, **4**, 65–84

50. Venturini, P.L., Fasce, V., Bertolini, S. *et al.* (1989). Endocrine metabolic and clinical effects of gestrinone in women with endometriosis. *Fertil. Steril.*, **52**, 589–599

51. Robyn, C., Delogne-Desnoeck, J., Bourdoux, P. and Copinschi, G. (1984). Endocrine effects of gestrinone. In Raynaud, J-P., Ojasoo, T. and Martini, L. (eds.) *Medical Management of Endometriosis*, pp. 207–222. (New York: Raven Press)

52. Kitawaki, J., Yamamoto, T. and Okada, H. (1988). Induction of estradiol dehydrogenase activity in human uterine endometrium by synthetic steroids. *J. Endocrinol. Invest.*, **11**, 351–354

53. Rose, G.L., White, J.O., Dowsett, M., Mudge, J.E. and Jeffcoate, S.L. (1988). The inhibitory effects of danazol, danazol metabolites, gestrinone and testosterone on the growth of human endometrial cells in vitro. *Fertil. Steril.*, **49**, 224–228

54. Brosens, I.A., Verleyen, A. and Cornillie, F. (1987). The morphologic effect of short-term medical therapy of endometriosis. *Am. J. Obstet. Gynecol.*, **157**, 1215–1221

55. Cornillie, F.J., Brosens, I.A., Vasquez, G. and Riphagen, I. (1986). Histologic and ultrastructural changes in human endometriotic implants treated with the antiprogesterone steroid ethylgestrienone (Gestrinone) during 2 months. *Int. J. Gynaecol. Pathol.*, **5**, 95–109

56. Raynaud, J-P., Salmon, J., Azadian-Boulanger, G., Bucourt, R. and Sakiz, E. (1973). Metabolic studies of R-2323, an original contraceptive compound. In *Abstracts, Federation International Pharmac.*, Stockholm, p. 39

57. Salmon, J., Cousty, C. and Mouren, M. (1984). Gestrinone pharmacokinetics and metabolism. In Raynaud, J-P., Ojasoo, T. and Martini, L. (eds.) *Medical Management of Endometriosis*, pp. 103–206. (New York: Raven Press)

58. Hornstein, M.D., Gleason, R.E. and Barbieri, R.L. (1990). A randomised double blind prospective trial of two doses of gestrinone in the treatment of endometriosis. *Fertil. Steril.*, **53**, 237–241

59. Coutinho, E.M. (1982). Treatment of endometriosis with gestrinone (R-2323) a synthetic antiestrogen, antiprogesterone. *Am. J. Obstet. Gynecol.*, **144**, 895–898

60. Coutinho, E.M., Husson, J.M. and Azadian-Boulanger, G. (1984). Treatment of endometriosis with gestrinone — five years experience. In Raynaud, J-P., Ojasoo, T. and Martini, L. (eds.) *Medical Management of Endometriosis*, pp. 249–261. (New York: Raven Press)

61. Coutinho, E.M. and Azadian-Boulanger, G. (1988). Treatment of endometriosis by vaginal administration of gestrinone. *Fertil. Steril.*, **49**, 418–422

62. Sakiz, E., Azadian-Boulanger, G., Laraque, F. and Raynaud, J.P. (1974). A new approach

to estrogen-free contraception based on progesterone receptor blockade by mid-cycle administration of ethyl norgestrienone. *Contraception*, **10**, 467–474

63. David, S.S., Huggins, G.R., Garcia, C-R. and Busacca, C. (1979). A synthetic steroid (R-2323) as a once a week contraceptive. *Fertil. Steril.*, **31**, 278–281

64. Deltour, G., Azadian-Boulanger, G., Nelson, J. and Sakiz, E. (1984). Tolerance and contraceptive efficacy of gestrinone in 800 patients in the United States from 1974 to 1978. In Raynaud, J-P., Ojasoo, T. and Martini, L. (eds.) *Medical Management of Endometriosis*, pp. 223–232. (New York: Raven Press)

65. Coutinho, E.M. and Goncalves, M.T. (1989). Long-term treatment of leiomyomas with gestrinone. *Fertil. Steril.*, **51**, 939–946

66. American Fertility Society (1979). Classification of endometriosis. *Fertil. Steril.*, **32**, 633

67. Fedele, L., Bianchi, S., Viezzoli, T., Arcaini, L. and Candiani, G.B. (1989). Gestrinone versus danazol in the treatment of endometriosis. *Fertil. Steril.*, **51**, 781–785

13
The use of danazol as a treatment of endometriosis

R. L. Barbieri

During the past 50 years, the medical management of endometriosis has evolved from a primitive clinical art utilizing agents with poor specificity, to a scientific endeavour utilizing pharmacological compounds that are highly specific in their molecular actions and extensively studied in randomized clinical trials. The first medical regimens developed to treat endometriosis utilized high-dose testosterone propionate[1] or high-dose diethylstilboesterol[2]. These regimens were moderately effective in the treatment of endometriosis, but they were associated with major unwanted side-effects, such as virilization in the case of testosterone proprionate therapy[1]. In the late 1950s Kistner introduced progestin-only[3] and pseudopregnancy[4] regimens for the treatment of endometriosis. These regimens remained the standard medical therapy until danazol (Figure 13.1) was approved for use in 1976. This chapter will review the clinical pharmacology of danazol, including its mode of action and its therapeutic applications.

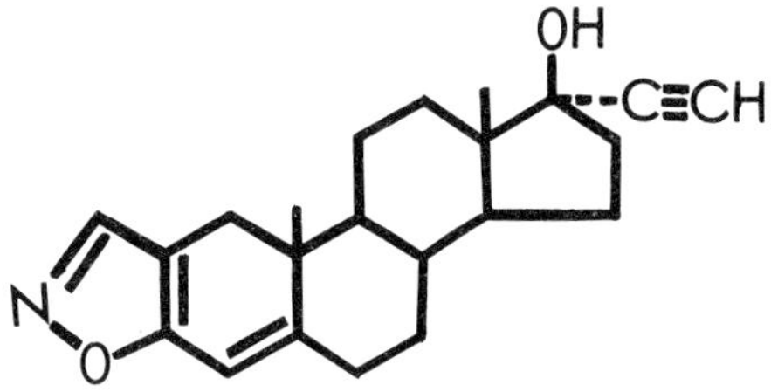

Figure 13.1 Chemical structure of danazol

239

DANAZOL: MECHANISM OF ACTION

A central dogma in pharmacology is that most drugs produce therapeutic effects by interacting with specific classes of proteins, thereby modifying the properties of these proteins. Within the framework of this central dogma, the pharmacology of danazol is best understood by a detailed analysis of all the proteins with which danazol can interact. Current laboratory evidence indicates that danazol can interact with three major classes of proteins: (1) enzymes of steroidogenesis, (2) intracellular steroid receptors, and (3) circulating steroid-binding proteins[5]. The effects of danazol on each of these classes of proteins will be reviewed below.

Danazol and enzymes of steroidogenesis

Enzymes of steroidogenesis can be divided into two major groups: steroid monooxygenases and steroid oxidoreductases. The steroid monooxygenase group includes cholesterol side-chain cleavage enzyme, 17α-hydroxylase, 17,20-lyase, 11-hydroxylase, 21-hydroxylase and aromatase. The steroid oxidoreductase group includes the 17-ketosteroid oxidoreductase and the 3β-hydroxysteroid dehydrogenase isomerase. Danazol has been demonstrated to inhibit the function of all these enzymes of steroidogenesis by binding at the steroid substrate binding site[5–7].

The steroid monooxygenases are enzyme complexes that consist of phospholipid, an NADPH cytochrome c reductase and a cytochrome P450 enzyme system that mediates terminal electron transfer and catalyses the insertion of oxygen into the steroid. The cytochrome P450 protein contains at least two important binding sites: a haem ion that captures molecular oxygen for the hydroxylation reaction and a steroid substrate binding site. When a steroid binds to the steroid substrate binding site, allosteric changes in the cytochrome P450 protein occur, and the electrons in the outer orbitals of the haem ion move into higher-energy orbitals. This causes the cytochrome P450 to change its spectrophotometric properties. The spectrophotometric changes caused by the binding of a steroid to the steroid substrate binding site is called a Type I cytochrome P450 difference spectrum (Figure 13.2). The effects of drugs on cytochrome P450 systems can often be determined by observing the effect of the drug on the spectrophotometric properties of the enzyme.

Spectrophotometric studies have demonstrated that danazol induces Type I cytochrome P450 difference spectra when added to the following cytochrome P450 enzyme systems: (1) 17α-hydroxylase, (2) 17,20-lyase, (3) 11β-hydroxylase and (4) 21-hydroxylase[6,7] (Figure 13.2). The observation that danazol produces a Type I cytochrome P450 binding spectrum suggests that danazol binds directly to the steroid binding site on the enzyme system. By binding to the substrate site, danazol prevents the access of substrate to the enzyme and thereby inhibits enzyme function. By analysing the relationship between the concentration of danazol added to the enzyme preparation and the magnitude of the spectral changes, an estimation of the affinity of danazol for the steroid binding site on the cytochrome P450 was determined. This

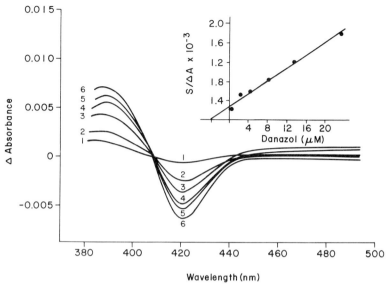

Figure 13.2 Danazol binding to 17-hydroxylase cytochrome P450. Danazol was added to a preparation of rat testis microsomal cytochrome P450, and the spectral changes were measured. The addition of danazol to the rat testis microsomes caused an increase in absorbance at 390 nm and a decrease in absorbance at 420 nm. Concentration of danazol: (1) 0.4 μM; (2) 2.4 μM; (3) 4.4 μM; (4) 8.4 μM; (5) 13.5 μM; (6) 23.5 μM. Inset: Hanes plot of danazol binding to cytochrome P450. $K_s = 4.8 \mu$M. In the inset S is substrate concentration and ΔA is the change in absorbance. From Barbieri, R.L., Canick, J.A. and Ryan, K.J. Danazol inhibits steroidogenesis in rat testis in vitro. *Endocrinology*, **101**, 1676–1682. Copyright the Endocrine Society

value is the spectral dissociation constant (K_s). The smaller the spectral dissociation constant, the higher the affinity of the steroid for the enzyme. Table 13.1 lists the K_s values for danazol to steroid monooxygenases.

In addition to spectral techniques, classical enzyme techniques have been used to evaluate the effects of danazol on steroidogenesis. Danazol has been

Table 13.1 Spectral dissociation constants (K_s) and Michaelis–Menten inhibition constants (K_i) for danazol interaction with enzymes of steroidogenesis

Enzyme	K_s (μM)	
17α-Hydroxylase	4.8	
21-Hydroxylase	5	
11β-Hydroxylase	1	

Enzyme	K_i (μM)	Type of inhibition
Cholesterol side-chain cleavage	20	Unknown
3β- HSD	5.8	Competitive
17α-Hydroxylase	2.4	Competitive
17,20-Lyase	1.9	Competitive
17-Ketosteroid reductase	4.4	Competitive
21-Hydroxylase	0.8	Competitive
11β-Hydroxylase	3.0	Competitive

reported to decrease the velocity of multiple steroidogenic enzymes including: (1) cholesterol side-chain cleavage, (2) 3β-hydroxysteroid dehydrogenase-isomerase, (3) 17α-hydroxylase, (4) 17-ketosteroid oxidoreductase, (5) 11β-hydroxylase and (6) 21-hydroxylase[6-9]. The Michaelis–Menten inhibition constants for danazol inhibition of these enzymes are listed in Table 13.1. Using classical Michaelis–Menten techniques, danazol has been demonstrated to competitively inhibit all these enzymes. Competitive inhibition implies that the addition of an infinite amount of substrate to the enzyme preparation will completely overcome any inhibition produced by danazol.

To estimate the quantitative effects of danazol *in vivo*, four biochemical values must be known: (1) the affinity of danazol for the enzyme, (2) the affinity of the natural substrate for the enzyme, (3) the concentration of danazol in the organ containing the enzyme, and (4) the concentration of the substrate in the organ containing the enzyme[10,11]. Using these four biochemical values, an estimate can be made of the enzyme inhibition caused by danazol. Such calculations are presented in Table 13.2. In women taking 600 mg of danazol daily, the circulating concentration of danazol is in the range of 2 μM[12]. This value was assumed to be the intraorgan concentration of danazol. The calculations in Table 13.2 suggest that danazol has no significant direct effect on the aromatase enzyme system *in vivo*. The model used to calculate the values in Table 13.2 suggests that danazol would produce a 5% inhibition of the 3β-HSD, the 17α-hydroxylase and the 17,20-lyase *in vivo*. Danazol is predicted to inhibit the 21-hydroxylase, 11β-hydroxylase and 17-ketosteroid reductase by approximately 20% *in vivo*. Steroidogenesis involves multiple, linked sequential reactions. Consequently, it is difficult to utilize these quantitative estimates to predict the *in vivo* effects of danazol on steroidogenesis in organs such as the adrenal. However, recent clinical investigations demonstrate that danazol inhibits adrenal, ovarian and testicular steroidogenesis *in vivo*.

Steingold and colleagues[13] reported two experiments that suggest that danazol inhibits ovarian steroidogenesis *in vivo*. In the first experiment, women were assigned to receive injections of human menopausal gonadotropins (hMG) alone, or hMG plus danazol. Danazol produced a 50% decrease in

Table 13.2 Calculated effects of danazol on enzymes of steroidogenesis. Danazol concentration assumed to be 2 μM

Enzyme	Substrate K_m (mM)[a]	Intraorgan substrate concentration (μM)	Danazol inhibition constant K_I (μM)[b]	Percentage calculated in vivo inhibition by danazol
3β-HSD	0.3	2.0	5.8	4.3
17-Hydroxylase	0.09	2.4	2.4	2.9
17,20-Lyase	0.12	3.0	1.9	3.9
Aromatase	0.23	1.5	> 100	0
21-Hydroxylase	0.94	3.0	0.8	37
11-Hydroxylase	1.27	2.0	3	21
17-Ketosteroid reductase	1.0	1.5	4.4	15

[a]K_m – Michaelis–Menten constant
[b]K_I – Michaelis inhibition constant

oestradiol response to the hMG. This study demonstrates that danazol blocks the effects of gonadotropins on the ovary by a direct ovarian action. This human study is consistent with the findings of Asch and colleagues[14] that, in the monkey, danazol blocked the effects of hCG on progesterone secretion by a direct action on the corpus luteum. In a second study, Steingold and colleagues[13] assigned women to receive dexamethasone alone, or dexamethasone plus danazol. Treatment with danazol resulted in a large increase in pregnenolone and a decrease in 17-hydroxypregnenolone, suggesting that danazol directly inhibited the 17α-hydroxylase reaction. The fact that the abnormal ratio of circulating pregnenolone to 17-hydroxypregnenolone was present during dexamethasone treatment suggests that danazol produced these changes by a direct effect on the ovary.

The most complete study of the effects of danazol on adrenal steroidogenesis was performed by Stillman and colleagues[12]. They evaluated the effects of danazol treatment on adrenal steroid response to an ACTH challenge. Five healthy, normally menstruating women were studied on the sixth day of two consecutive menstrual cycles, once as a pretreatment control and again after the administration of 600 mg of danazol daily for 6 days. While taking danazol, baseline levels of progesterone, dehydroepiandrosterone and androstenedione were elevated, whereas baseline levels of LH, FSH and ACTH were not significantly changed. As compared with pre-danazol control values, the response to ACTH after danazol administration was greater for pregnenolone and 11-deoxycortisol and smaller for progesterone and cortisol. These results are consistent with the inhibition by danazol of adrenal 17α-hydroxylase, 3β-hydroxysteroid dehydrogenase-isomerase and 11β-hydroxylase enzymes.

Reyniak and Gurpide[15] evaluated the effects of danazol on testicular steroidogenesis in three XY individuals with a defect in the androgen receptor system. Administration of danazol to these individuals resulted in no change in circulating LH and FSH. However, the administration of danazol resulted in marked decreases in circulating testosterone. These investigators also demonstrated that the magnitude of the decrease in circulating testosterone was dependent on the amount of danazol administered. These studies suggest that danazol directly inhibits testicular synthesis of testosterone *in vivo*. Taken together, these studies suggest that danazol inhibits the production of oestradiol, progesterone and testosterone by a direct action on organs of steroidogenesis.

Danazol and intracellular steroid receptors

Steroid hormones produce biological effects in steroid responsive tissues ('end organs') by binding to intranuclear steroid receptors and thereby altering the rate of transcription of tissue-specific genes. Naturally occurring steroids demonstrate a great deal of specificity in their interaction with receptors. For example, oestradiol binds well to the oestradiol receptor, but does not significantly interact with androgen or progesterone receptors. In contrast, synthetic steroids are often less specific in their receptor-binding profiles and can bind to multiple classes of receptors. In the first systematic screening of the interaction of danazol with steroid-binding proteins, our laboratory demonstrated that danazol could bind to intracellular androgen, progesterone, glucocorticoid and oestrogen receptors[16] (Figure 13.3). The affinity of danazol for each of these receptors is listed in Table 13.3. These values suggest that danazol has high affinity for the androgen receptor, moderate affinity for the progesterone and glucocorticoid receptors and poor affinity for the oestrogen receptor. Chamness and colleagues[17] and Tamaya and colleagues[18] have published similar results.

The interaction of a steroid with an intracellular steroid receptor system can result in three possible outcomes. The steroid can act as an agonist, antagonist or mixed agonist–antagonist. In most androgen receptor bioassays,

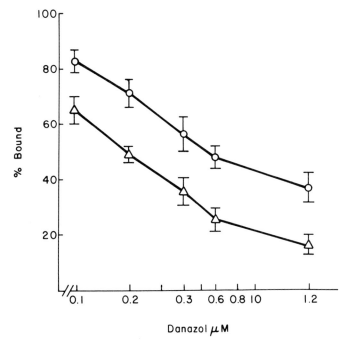

Figure 13.3 Semilogarithmic plot of danazol displacement of [³H]dihydrotestosterone from the 8 S androgen receptor of rat prostate cytosol. △, 2 nM dihydrotestosterone; ○, 7 nM dihydrotestosterone. Apparent inhibition constant (K_i) for danazol = 0.09 μM. (From Barbieri, R.L., Lee, H. and Ryan, K.J. (1979). Danazol binding to rat androgen, glucocorticoid, progesterone, and estrogen receptors: correlation with biologic activity. *Fertil. Steril.*, **31**, 182. Reproduced with the permission of the publisher, the American Fertility Society

Table 13.3 Binding of danazol to testosterone, progesterone, glucocorticoid and oestrogen receptors

Receptor system	Binding affinity (nM)	Biological effect
Testosterone	90	Agonist
Progesterone	6,000	Agonist–antagonist
Glucocorticoid	5,000	? Agonist
Estrogen	80,000	Agonist

for example bioassays of prostate growth, danazol is an androgen agonist. In progesterone bioassays, danazol can act as an agonist or antagonist. The biological effects of danazol on glucocorticoid and oestrogen receptor systems have not been extensively studied, but danazol appears to be an agonist in both receptor systems (Table 13.3).

In summary, danazol is an androgen and glucocorticoid agonist, and mixed agonist–antagonist with respect to the progesterone receptor system. Danazol's very poor affinity for the oestrogen receptor suggests that danazol has minimal biological effects with regard to this system. However, at very high concentrations, danazol is an oestrogen agonist. Steroid receptors play an important role in regulating cell function in a large number of tissues. Table 13.4. summarizes the biological effects of danazol in a number of major tissues.

Danazol and circulating steroid binding proteins

In addition to binding to intracellular steroid receptors, danazol also interacts with circulating steroid hormone binding globulins. Danazol has been reported to displace testosterone from sex-hormone binding globulin (SHBG)[19] and cortisol from corticosteroid binding globulin (CBG). Of these two interactions, danazol binding to SHBG is clinically more important. In premenopausal women, circulating testosterone is distributed in three phases: 1% is free, 39% is bound to albumin, and 60% is bound to SHBG. In women taking danazol, the circulating testosterone is distributed as follows: 3% is free, 79% is bound to albumin, and 18% is bound to SHBG[20]. The ability of danazol to increase circulating free testosterone suggests that part of its androgenic effects may be due to the displacement of testosterone and dihydrotestosterone from SHBG.

Metabolites of danazol

Danazol appears to interact with multiple classes of proteins, including enzymes of steroidogenesis, intracellular steroid receptors and steroid binding

Table 13.4 Biological effects of danazol mediated through intracellular steroid receptors

Tissue	Receptor	Biological effect
Hypothalamus–Pituitary	Androgen agonist Progestin agonist Oestrogen agonist	Decrease GnRH, LH and FSH secretion
Endometrium	Androgen agonist Progestin agonist–antagonist	Atrophy endometrial glands and stroma
Ovarian follicle	Androgen agonist	Disruption of follicular growth
Central metabolism	Androgen agonist	Decrease HDL-cholesterol, increase LDL-cholesterol, insulin resistance
Immune system	Glucocorticoid agonist Progestin agonist	Suppression of immune function

proteins. To further complicate the pharmacology of danazol, danazol is metabolized to over 60 metabolites, some of which are biologically active[21]. For example, one of the major metabolites of danazol is ethinyltestosterone[21]. This steroid is a progestin and a weak androgen[22]. Ethinyltestosterone inhibits pituitary secretion of LH and FSH. Conceivably, some of the 'antigonadotropic' properties of danazol are due to one of its metabolites, ethinyltestosterone. Ethinyltestosterone is the only metabolite of danazol that has been extensively studied. The endocrine pharmacology of the other metabolites of danazol is not well understood. Until these metabolites are better studied, the pharmacology of danazol will remain incompletely characterized.

Integrated endocrine pharmacology of danazol

The central dogma that guides the hormonal therapy of endometriosis is that steroid hormones are the major regulators of the growth and function of endometriotic tissue. Oestrogen appears to support the growth and function of endometriotic tissue. Testosterone appears to produce atrophy in endometriotic tissue. Danazol is effective in the treatment of endometriosis because it decreases ovarian oestrogen production, and because it increases the exposure of the endometriosis to androgens. Danazol decreases ovarian oestrogen production by at least two mechanisms. Danazol probably decreases GnRH pulse frequency, and LH and FSH secretion. This impedes follicular growth and oestrogen secretion. In addition, danazol also directly blocks ovarian oestrogen production by inhibiting ovarian enzymes of steroidogenesis and possibly by directly disrupting follicular growth. Danazol increases the exposure of endometriosis to androgens because danazol is inherently androgenic, and because it increases free testosterone by displacing testosterone from SHBG and by decreasing SHBG production. These integrated effects of danazol produce an anovulatory, hypo-oestrogenic–hyperandrogenic environment that inhibits the growth and function of endometriotic tissue. Unfortunately, the hypo-oestrogenic–hyperandrogenic environment produced by danazol causes a large number of undesirable symptomatic effects that many women find difficult to tolerate. These side-effects are discussed below.

CLINICAL APPLICATIONS OF DANAZOL

Although endometriosis is one of the most common gynaecological disorders, few randomized, controlled clinical trials of therapeutic regimens for this disease have been reported. Current recommendations for the treatment of endometriosis are largely derived from clinical experience and not from controlled scientific studies. In the future, results from controlled scientific studies may change our current approach to the clinical management of endometriosis. Until these scientific studies are completed, therapeutic decisions must be based on currently available clinical data, much of which is anecdotal. Patients with endometriosis usually present with one of three complaints: (1) pelvic pain, (2) an adnexal mass or (3) infertility. Each clinical presentation requires a different therapeutic approach, and these considerations are discussed in more detail below.

Initiation of danazol therapy

A widely accepted clinical rule is that hormonal therapy for endometriosis should not be started until the diagnosis of endometriosis has been confirmed by a surgical procedure, such as laparoscopy or laparotomy. It is important that danazol is not administered to a pregnant woman. Female pseudohermaphroditism is common in females born to mothers treated with danazol during the first and second trimesters of pregnancy[23]. To help ensure that danazol is not administered to a pregnant woman, danazol therapy should be initiated after completion of a normal menses, and women receiving danazol should use a barrier contraceptive.

Danazol: dose response

Danazol, like most drugs, produces biological effects that are dose dependent. For example, at doses of 400 mg or 800 mg per day danazol inhibits ovulation in more than 95% of women[24]. However, at doses under 200 mg per day, many women still ovulate. Since danazol is teratogenic, common sense indicates that a dose sufficient to inhibit ovulation be administered. Consequently, we will seldom prescribe doses of danazol of less than 400 mg per day. Three groups of investigators have reported the results of phase II dose–response trials. Dmowski and colleagues[25] randomized 27 women with endometriosis to receive 100 mg, 200 mg, 400 mg or 600 mg of danazol per day for 6 months. Using a pre- and post-therapy surgical scoring system, they observed a 40% improvement in endometriosis in women receiving 100 mg or 200 mg per day, and a 74% improvement in women receiving 400 mg or 600 mg per day. Moore and colleagues[26] randomized 38 women with endometriosis to receive 100 mg, 200 mg, 400 mg or 600 mg of danazol per day for 6 months. Stage I and II endometriosis responded well to doses of less than 400 mg per day, but Stages III and IV endometriosis required larger doses of danazol. These findings are similar to those of Biberoglou and Behrman[27].

These dose–response results suggest the following treatment regimens. Owing to cost considerations, and a desire to minimize side-effects, we start patients with Stage I or II endometriosis on 400 mg per day of danazol. Patients with Stage III or IV endometriosis are started on 600 mg or 800 mg per day, and after a good clinical response has occurred, the danazol dose is slowly tapered to 400 mg per day.

Danazol: length of therapy

Most clinical trials investigating the efficacy of danazol in the treatment of endometriosis have evaluated 26-week therapy regimens[5]. This therapy interval is relatively arbitrary, and can be altered to the specific therapeutic goals of each patient. For example, in the patient with advanced endometriosis and infertility who is scheduled for a conservative laparotomy, a 12-week preoperative course of danazol might be appropriate. In our experience, 12 weeks of preoperative danazol produces near maximal regression of endometriosis. Longer courses of preoperative therapy do not usually produce additional, clinically significant regression of the endometriosis. For the patient with painful endometriosis who does not desire fertility, and who is adamantly opposed to surgery, a 52- to 78-week course of danazol is reasonable if side-effects are carefully monitored.

Danazol and pelvic pain

As noted above, women with endometriosis typically present with one of three problems: (1) pelvic pain, (2) adnexal mass, and (3) infertility. Multiple studies strongly suggest that hormonal therapy for patients with endometriosis and pelvic pain completely or partially improves the pain in more than 85% of treated patients[5,28,29]. This high success rate makes pelvic pain one of the major indications for hormonal treatment of endometriosis. Women with endometriosis can present with three types of pain: (1) dysmenorrhoea, (2) dyspareunia and (3) pain not occurring with menses. Barbieri and colleagues[29] examined the effects of 800 mg of danazol per day on these types of pain in 100 women with endometriosis. In these women, 75% had complete relief of dysmenorrhoea, 62% had complete relief of dyspareunia and 59% had relief from pain not associated with menses[29]. As noted above, clinical trials have demonstrated that danazol at doses of 100 mg or 200 mg per day can provide some relief of pelvic pain[25–27]. However, since ovulation can occur at these doses, we seldom recommend utilization of these very low-dose regimens. Although hormonal therapy for pelvic pain due to endometriosis is typically successful, discontinuation of the hormonal therapy usually results in a recurrence of the pelvic pain within 12 months. Retreatment will usually result in regression of the pain.

Adnexal mass

Most persistent, large ($>$ 4 cm) ovarian masses need to be surgically removed. Surgical removal of the mass is simultaneously diagnostic and therapeutic. In general, hormonal therapy of endometriomas is ineffective. In the best of circumstances, the hormonal therapy may result in a 50% decrease in the diameter of the mass, but the endometrioma will return to pre-treatment size after hormone therapy is discontinued. In addition, in the absence of a pathological diagnosis, it is impossible to know whether the adnexal mass is truly an endometrioma. We have seen women diagnosed as having an endometrioma who were proved to have a mature cystic teratoma or ovarian carcinoma at pathological analysis of the surgical specimen. The surgical removal of an endometrioma should be followed by a long-term therapeutic plan. The majority of young women who have had an endometrioma surgically removed have had a recurrence of their endometriosis within 5 years[29]. For some young patients, long-term hormonal therapy may be necessary to prevent the repetitive recurrence of endometriomas.

Danazol and infertility

There is no strong scientific evidence to support the hypothesis that Stage I or Stage II endometriosis causes infertility. Given this fact it is not surprising that there are no controlled clinical trials that demonstrate that the treatment of Stage I or Stage II endometriosis improves fecundibility. Seibel and colleagues[30,31] were the first to report the results of a randomized, controlled trial to assess the effects of danazol on fertility in women with Stage I endometriosis. Women with laparoscopically proven Stage I endometriosis were randomized postoperatively to receive danazol or no treatment. Thirteen of 37 (35%) danazol-treated women and 17 of 36 (47%) control women became pregnant[31]. This study demonstrates that danazol therapy did not improve fecundibility in women with Stage I endometriosis.

Given the paucity of scientific evidence, the use of hormonal or surgical therapy for the treatment of infertility associated with mild or moderate endometriosis is a clinical decision to be made jointly by the doctor and patient after all alternatives have been explored. Stage III and IV endometriosis probably does cause infertility. In cases of infertility associated with Stage III or IV endometriosis, surgical therapy is usually necessary to improve fecundibility. In our experience, preoperative hormonal therapy makes the surgical procedure technically easier to perform.

Danazol: pre- and postoperative therapy

No experimental evidence is available to guide the clinician in choosing to use danazol pre- or postoperatively. For patients with advanced endometriosis and infertility who are planning to have a conservative laparotomy, preoperative danazol therapy may minimize the extent and difficulty of the surgery by decreasing the size and number of endometriotic implants. In addition, the resection of endometriomas is made significantly more difficult if a corpus luteum is present in the ovary. If the ovary contains both an endometrioma and a corpus luteum, resection of the endometrioma usually results in serious trauma to the corpus luteum and requires the resection of the corpus luteum. The preoperative use of danazol for 8–12 weeks ensures that no corpus luteum will be present at the time of surgery. We routinely advise preoperative hormonal therapy for women who are scheduled to have a conservative laparotomy for endometriosis. For patients with advanced endometriosis planning to have a definitive surgical procedure (bilateral salpingo-oophorectomy and hysterectomy), preoperative danazol may simplify the surgery by minimizing inflammation and facilitating the identification of surgical planes.

Use of danazol in the postoperative management of the infertile patient with endometriosis is controversial. Most conceptions following surgical therapy for endometriosis occur in the first 12 months after surgery[29].

Therefore, by using danazol for a prolonged period postoperatively, the time interval with the highest fertility potential will be passed over. Given these considerations, the postoperative use of danazol in fertility patients should be minimized to 3 months or less.

Danazol and the AFS endometriosis score

Clinical trials of hormone therapy for endometriosis are hampered by the lack of a simple, objective, non-invasive method of assessing disease activity. Most clinical trials of hormone therapy for endometriosis rely on pre- and post-treatment laparoscopy with measurement of the American Fertility Society (AFS) endometriosis score[32] to objectively assess disease activity. Henzl and colleagues[28] have reported that 6 months of danazol therapy results in a 43% decrease in the AFS endometriosis score. Other investigators have reported that GnRH agonists[28], medroxyprogesterone acetate[33], and gestrinone[34] therapy also result in an approximately 50% decrease in the AFS endometriosis score. Most of the decrease in AFS endometriosis score during danazol therapy is due to a decrease in size and number of endometriotic implants[28]. However, the 'adhesions' component of the score also decreases slightly during danazol therapy[28]. An emerging concern is that hormone therapy for endometriosis may not eradicate implants of endometriosis, but may make the implants difficult to visualize at the time of laparoscopy. The lesions may then 'regrow' rapidly after discontinuing drug therapy. Additional studies are necessary to assess AFS endometriosis scores in the post-treatment period.

Danazol: undesirable symptomatic effects

The major side-effects seen with danazol are, in decreasing order of frequency, weight gain, bloating, decreased breast size, acne, oily skin, hirsutism, headache, deepening of the voice, hot flushes, and muscle cramps[28,29]. In women receiving 800 mg per day of danazol, the weight gain averages 4 kg[28]. More than 75% of patients receiving danazol will complain of one or more undesirable symptomatic effects. Some of the side-effects are dose dependent, and can be minimized by using doses of 400 mg per day rather than 800 mg per day. The weight gain can be minimized by control of caloric intake and by starting an aerobic exercise programme prior to initiating danazol therapy. Unfortunately, many women cannot tolerate the side-effects of danazol, and they discontinue the drug. As noted above, danazol and the GnRH agonists are quantitatively similar in reducing pain due to endometriosis and in reducing the AFS endometriosis score. However, in general the side-effects associated with the GnRH agonists tend to be better tolerated by women than the side-effects of danazol. Consequently, when the GnRH agonists become widely available it is likely that they will become the agents of choice for the treatment of endometriosis.

Danazol: biochemical abnormalities

Danazol therapy can produce a large number of biochemical abnormalities. Danazol can produce mild increases in serum CPK, LDH, SGOT and SGPT[35]. Typically, these are minor, clinically insignificant alterations, but in an occasional woman the increases can be marked. Danazol increases the hepatic production of prealbumin, C1-esterase inhibitor, haptoglobin, transferrin, antithrombin III, prothrombin and plasminogen[36]. Danazol decreases the hepatic production of sex-hormone binding globulin, thyroxine-binding globulin (TBG) and pregnancy zone protein[36]. The decrease in TBG is clinically important when interpreting thyroid function tests from women receiving danazol. In women taking danazol the decrease in TBG results in a decrease in total thyroxine and an increase in the T_3 resin uptake[37]. Free thyroxine and TSH remain in the normal range. In a woman taking danazol, a decrease in total thyroxine in association with a normal TSH should not lead to a diagnosis of primary hypothyroidism.

Danazol therapy produces marked alterations in the circulating lipid profile. Danazol at doses of 600 mg per day can produce a 50% decrease in HDL-cholesterol and a 40% increase in LDL-cholesterol[38,39]. These lipid alterations resolve within 3 months of discontinuing danazol therapy. The decrease in HDL-cholesterol and the increase in LDL-cholesterol results in an atherogenic lipid profile. The clinical importance of this atherogenic lipid profile in young women of reproductive age is unknown and deserves further investigation.

Comparison of danazol and pseudopregnancy

Very few data are available that directly compare the efficacy of danazol versus a pseudopregnancy regimen in the treatment of endometriosis. The results of one small, prospective, randomized trial of danazol versus mestranol/norethynodrel were reported by Noble and Letchworth[40]. Danazol therapy resulted in symptomatic improvement in 86% of patients. In contrast, pseudopregnancy treatment resulted in symptomatic improvement in 30% of patients. Improvement in objective findings was demonstrated in 84% of patients treated with danazol compared to only 18% of patients on the pseudopregnancy regimen. Side-effects were a major problem for patients receiving both regimens.

In our practice we reserve pseudopregnancy regimens for two specific clinical situations. Pseudopregnancy appears to be specially effective in treating teenagers and young women with Stage I or II endometriosis and severe dysmenorrhoea. Our mini-pseudopregnancy regimen involves prescribing a monophasic oestrogen–progestin contraceptive pill for 105 days followed by 7 days off medication followed by 105 days of hormone administration. The second clinical situation in which pseudopregnancy is prescribed is for women with a history of recurrent endometriomas. For women with recurrent endometriomas the mini-pseudopregnancy will be prescribed for up to 5 years.

Comparison of danazol and the GnRH agonists

During the 1980s danazol was the primary hormonal agent used in the treatment of endometriosis. During the 1990s it is likely that the leading hormonal agents used to treat endometriosis will be the GnRH agonists. The development of the GnRH agonists resulted in the execution of high-quality well-designed, randomized, controlled Phase III clinical trials comparing the efficacy of the GnRH agonists versus danazol in the treatment of endometriosis. Henzl and colleagues[28] randomized 213 women with endometriosis to receive either nafarelin 400 µg per day, nafarelin 800 µg per day or danazol 800 mg per day. Placebo nasal spray and placebo tablets were used to double-blind the study. Every subject had a pre-treatment and post-treatment laparoscopy to objectively assess disease response. Over 80% of subjects in all three treatment groups had symptomatic improvement. The mean AFS endometriosis score decreased from 21.9 to 12.6 with 800 µg of nafarelin, from 20.4 to 11.7 with 400 µg of nafarelin and from 18.4 to 10.5 with 800 mg of danazol. There were no significant differences between the treatment groups with respect to symptomatic or objective responses[28].

Although the objective responses to danazol and nafarelin were similar, the side-effects of the two regimens were markedly different. Danazol therapy was associated with weight gain, hot flushes, bloating, and muscle cramps. Nafarelin treatment was associated with hot flushes, headaches, decreased libido and dry vagina. In our clinical experience, most women who have been treated with danazol and a GnRH agonist prefer the side-effects associated with the GnRH agonist. Patient preference for each drug deserves further evaluation in a randomized, cross-over trial. In the study by Henzl and colleagues[28], danazol and nafarelin differed markedly in their effects on circulating lipids. Danazol produced a 25% decrease in HDL-cholesterol and a 20% increase in LDL-cholesterol. Nafarelin at a dose of 400 µg per day produced a 20% increase in HDL-cholesterol and no change in LDL-cholesterol. These findings demonstrate that danazol produces an atherogenic lipid profile, while the GnRH agonists produce minimal changes in the lipid profile. Similar findings have been observed in a randomized clinical trial comparing buserelin versus danazol for the treatment of endometriosis[41].

Although GnRH agonist therapy for endometriosis is superior to danazol therapy with regard to most side-effect parameters, the GnRH agonists appear to produce significant trabecular bone loss that is not observed with danazol therapy. For example, Dawood and colleagues[42] reported that 6 months of GnRH agonist therapy, with buserelin 1200 µg nasally per day, resulted in a 7% decrease in trabecular bone density. Six months after completing GnRH agonist therapy the trabecular bone density was still 4% below pre-treatment values. Similar losses in trabecular bone during GnRH agonist therapy have been reported by Johansen and colleagues[43] and Matta and colleagues[44]. Interestingly, Matta and colleagues[44] reported that the bone loss was completely reversible once the GnRH agonist was discontinued. In contrast to the GnRH agonists, danazol treatment resulted in a small, non-significant increase in trabecular bone density[42]. The clinical meaning of the adverse effects of GnRH agonists on trabecular bone density remains to be characterized. It is conceivable that small losses in trabecular bone density at age 25 have little immediate clinical meaning for that woman. However, when that woman becomes 70 years old, the 4% bone loss caused by the GnRH agonist may increase the risk of vertebral fracture. It will be difficult to design a clinical trial to directly evaluate this concern.

Danazol plus GnRH agonist therapy for endometriosis

The trabecular bone loss associated with GnRH agonist therapy is probably due to the hypo-oestrogenism caused by the GnRH agonist. One possible solution to minimize the GnRH agonist-induced bone loss is to 'add-back' small amounts of oestrogen, progestin or androgen. Since danazol treatment appears to cause small increases in trabecular bone density[42], one regimen might include combining GnRH agonist treatment with low-dose danazol. A GnRH agonist-plus-danazol regimen might be additive in its ability to cause regression of endometriotic implants. These combination regimens deserve further investigation.

REFERENCES

1. Wilson, L. (1940). Action of testosterone proprionate in a case of endometriosis. *Endocrinology*, **27**, 29–34
2. Karnaky, K.J. (1948). The use of stilbesterol for endometriosis. *South. Med. J.*, **41**, 1109–1121
3. Kistner, R.W. (1958). The use of newer progestins in the treatment of endometriosis. *Am. J. Obstet. Gynecol.*, **75**, 264–278
4. Kistner, R.W. (1959). The treatment of endometriosis by inducing pseudo-pregnancy with ovarian hormones: a report of 58 cases. *Fertil. Steril.*, **10**, 539–548
5. Barbieri, R.L. and Ryan, K.J. (1981). Danazol: endocrine pharmacology and therapeutic applications. *Am. J. Obstet. Gynecol.*, **141**, 453–463
6. Barbieri, R.L., Canick, J.A. and Ryan, K.J. (1977). Danazol inhibits steroidogenesis in the rat testis in vitro. *Endocrinology*, **101**, 1676–1682
7. Barbieri, R.L., Osathanondh, R., Canick, J.A., Stillman, R.J. and Ryan, K.J. (1980). Danazol inhibits human adrenal 21- and 11-hydroxylation in vitro. *Steroids*, **35**, 251–263
8. Barbieri, R.L., Canick, J.A., Makris, A., Todd, R.B., Davies, I.J. and Ryan, K.J. (1977). Danazol inhibits steroidogenesis. *Fertil. Steril.*, **28**, 808–813
9. Barbieri, R.L., Osathanondh, R. and Ryan, K.J. (1981). Danazol inhibition of steroidogenesis in the human corpus luteum. *Obstet. Gynecol.*, **57**, 722–724
10. Dickerman, Z., Grant, D.R., Faiman, C. and Winter, J.S.D. (1984). Intra-adrenal steroid concentrations in man: zonal differences and developmental changes. *J. Clin. Endocrinol. Metab.*, **59**, 1031–1036
11. Couch, R.M., Muller, J., Perry, Y.S. and Winter, J.S.D. (1987). Kinetic analysis of inhibition of human adrenal steroidogenesis by ketoconazole. *J. Clin. Endocrinol. Metab.*, **65**, 551–554
12. Stillman, R.J., Fencl, M., Schiff, I., Barbieri, R.L. and Tulchinsky, D. (1980). Inhibition of adrenal steroidogenesis by danazol in vivo. *Fertil. Steril.*, **33**, 401–406
13. Steingold, K.A., Lu, J.K.H., Judd, H.L. and Meldrum, D.R. (1986). Danazol inhibits steroidogenesis by the human ovary in vivo. *Fertil. Steril.*, **45**, 649–654
14. Asch, R.H., Fernandez, E.O., Siler-Khodr, T.M., Bartke, A. and Pauerstein, C.J. (1980). Mechanism of induction of luteal phase defects by danazol. *Am. J. Obstet. Gynecol.*, **136**, 932–940
15. Reyniak, J.V. and Gurpide, E. (1982). Effect of danazol on gonadal steroidogenesis in patients with a complete form of testicular feminization. *Am. J. Obstet. Gynecol.*, **142**, 479–481

16. Barbieri, R.L., Lee, H. and Ryan, K.J. (1979). Danazol binding to rat androgen, glucocorticoid, progesterone and estrogen receptors: correlation with biological activity. *Fertil. Steril.*, **31**, 182–186

17. Chamness, G.C., Asch, R.H. and Pauerstein, C.J. (1980). Danazol binding and translocation of steroid receptors. *Am. J. Obstet. Gynecol.*, **136**, 426–429

18. Tamaya, T., Furuka, N., Motomyama, T., Boku, S., Ohono, Y. and Okada, N. (1978). Mechanism of antiprogestational action of synthetic steroids. *Acta Endocrinol.*, **88**, 190–198

19. Nilsson, B., Sodergard, R., Damber, M.G. and Von Schouler, B. (1982). Danazol and gestogen displacement of testosterone and influence of sex hormone binding globulin capacity. *Fertil. Steril.*, **38**, 48–53

20. Nilsson, B., Sodergard, R., Damber, M.G., Damber, J.E. and Von Schouler, B. (1983). Free testosterone levels during danazol therapy. *Fertil. Steril.*, **39**, 505–509

21. Davison, C., Banks, N. and Fritz, A. (1976). The absorption, distribution and metabolic rate of danazol in rats, monkeys and human volunteers. *Arch. Int. Pharmacodyn. Ther.*, **221**, 294–298

22. Desaulles, P.A. and Krabenbuhl, C. (1964). Comparison of the anti-fertility and sex hormone activities of sex hormones and derivatives. *Acta Endocrinol.*, **47**, 444–458

23. Duck, S.C. and Katayama, K.P. (1981). Danazol may cause female pseudohermaphroditism. *Fertil. Steril.*, **35**, 320–322

24. Dmowski, W.P., Scholer, H.F.L., Mastesh, V.V. and Greenblatt, R.B. (1971). Danazol, a synthetic steroid derivative with interesting physiologic properties. *Fertil. Steril.*, **22**, 9–18

25. Dmowski, W.P., Kaperawakis, E. and Scommegna, A. (1982). Variable effects of danazol on endometriosis at 4 low-dose levels. *Obstet. Gynecol.*, **59**, 408–415

26. Moore, E.E., Harger, J.H., Rock, J.A. and Archer, D.F. (1981). Management of pelvic endometriosis with low dose danazol. *Fertil. Steril.*, **36**, 15–20

27. Biberoglou, K.O. and Behrman, S.J. (1981). Dosage aspects of danazol therapy in endometriosis: short-term and long-term effectiveness. *Am. J. Obstet. Gynecol.*, **139**, 645–654

28. Henzl, M.R., Corson, S.L., Moghissi, K., Buttram, V.C., Berqvist, C. and Jacobson, J. (1988). Administration of nasal nafarelin as compared with oral danazol for endometriosis. *N. Engl. J. Med.*, **318**, 485–589

29. Barbieri, R.L., Evans, S. and Kistner, R.W. (1982). Danazol in the treatment of endometriosis: analysis of 100 cases with a 4-year follow-up. *Fertil. Steril.*, **37**, 737–742

30. Seibel, M.M., Berger, M.J., Weinstein, F.G. and Taymor, M.L. (1982). The effectiveness of danazol on subsequent fertility in minimal endometriosis. *Fertil. Steril.*, **38**, 534–537

31. Bayer, S.R., Seibel, M.M., Saffan, D.S. and Berger, M.J. (1988). The efficacy of danazol treatment for minimal endometriosis in an infertile population: a prospective randomized study. *J. Reprod. Med.*, **33**, 179–183

32. The American Fertility Society. (1985). Revised American Fertility Society classification of endometriosis. *Fertil. Steril.*, **43**, 351–353

33. Luciano, A.A., Turksoy, R.N. and Carleo, J. (1988). Evaluation of oral medroxyprogesterone acetate in the treatment of endometriosis. *Obstet. Gynecol.*, **72**, 323–327

34. Hornstein, M.D., Gleason, R.E. and Barbieri, R.L. (1990). A randomized double-blind prospective trial of two doses of gestrinone in the treatment of endometriosis. *Fertil. Steril.*, **53**, 237–241

35. Holt, J.P. and Keller, D. (1984). Danazol treatment increases serum enzymes. *Fertil. Steril.*, **41**, 70–72

36. Laurell, C.B. and Rannevik, G. (1979). A comparison of plasma protein changes by danazol, pregnancy and estrogens. *J. Clin. Endocrinol. Metab.*, **49**, 719–725

37. Barbieri, R.L. (1980). Danazol and thyroid function. *Ann. Intern. Med.*, **92**, 133

38. Telimaa, S., Penttila, I., Puolakka, J., Ronnberg, L. and Kauppila, A. (1989). Circulating lipid and lipoprotein concentrations during danazol and high-dose medroxyprogesterone acetate therapy of endometriosis. *Fertil. Steril.*, **52**, 31–35

39. Burry, K.A., Patton, P.E. and Illingsworth, D.R. (1989). Metabolic changes during medical treatment of endometriosis: nafarelin acetate versus danazol. *Am. J. Obstet. Gynecol.*, **160**, 1454–1459

40. Noble, A.D. and Letchworth, A.T. (1979). Medical treatment of endometriosis: a comparative trial. *Postgrad. Med. J.*, **55**, 37–41

41. Dmowski, W.P., Radwanska, E., Binor, Z., Tummon, I. and Pepping, P. (1989). Ovarian suppression induced with buserelin or danazol in the management of endometriosis: a randomized comparative study. *Fertil. Steril.*, **51**, 395–400

42. Dawood, M.Y., Lewis, V. and Ramos, J. (1989). Cortical and trabecular bone mineral content in women with endometriosis: effect of gonadotropin releasing hormone agonist and danazol. *Fertil. Steril.*, **52**, 21–26

43. Johansen, J.S., Riis, B.J., Hassager, C., Moen, M., Jacobson, J. and Christiansen, C. (1988). The effect of a gonadotropin releasing hormone analog (nafarelin) on bone metabolism. *J. Clin. Endocrinol. Metab.*, **67**, 701–706

44. Matta, W.H., Shaw, R.W., Hesp, R. and Evans, R. (1988). Reversible trabecular bone density loss following induced hypoestrogenism with the GnRH analog, buserelin, in premenopausal women. *Clin. Endocrinol.*, **29**, 45–51

14
GnRH analogues in the treatment of endometriosis – rationale and efficacy

R. W. Shaw

INTRODUCTION

Endometriosis in the reproductive years has its peak incidence between 30 and 45 years as the continued growth of endometriotic tissue is dependent upon oestrogen. As has been outlined in other chapters in this book, the treatment of endometriosis depends upon the site, extent, symptoms of the disease, the patient's age and her childbearing expectations. Thus treatment is tailored to individual needs. It may be broadly surgically based or a medical approach.

With regard to medical treatments there are a number of endocrine and pharmacological approaches being utilized. These include continuous combined oral contraceptive preparations; progestogens alone; danazol or gestrinone. Although efficacious, the above treatment modalities are associated with side-effects in a variable proportion of patients in varying degrees of severity that are intolerable for some patients and result in failure of completion of the prescribed course of therapy. New and more effective treatment approaches have thus been sought and currently the possibility of selectively suppressing the ovarian secretion of steroids by repetitive administration of GnRH analogues is under investigation.

Surgical castration has so far been the most effective treatment for endometriosis. A reversible means of achieving medical castration would offer many advantages. Such an approach can be achieved by repetitive administration of luteinizing hormone-releasing hormone analogues (GnRH$_A$). The current available data published on the use of GnRH analogues in both open and more recently from randomized open, double-blind placebo controlled trials will now be reviewed in this chapter.

STRUCTURE AND MODE OF ACTION OF GnRH ANALOGUES

The structure of GnRH was identified in 1971[1]. The availability of synthetic GnRH for investigations of physiological action and clinical application has been extensively investigated. This has led to an increased knowledge of the mechanisms by which GnRH stimulates the release of LH and FSH from pituitary cells. It is apparent that the intracellular pathways through which GnRH stimulates biosynthesis and secretion of pituitary gonadotrophins and is receptor mediated and calcium dependent. A number of pathways of intracellular signalling have been implicated with regard to gonadotrophe function. These include cyclic nucleotides, phospholipids, inositol phosphates, calcium, arachidonic acid, protein kinase-C, prostaglandins and leukotrienes. In addition, the ovarian steroids oestrogen and progesterone themselves further modulate gonadotrophe function. A summary of our current understanding of GnRH mechanism of action is shown in Figure 14.1. This has been recently reviewed in detail by Clayton[2] and Kiesel and Runnebaum[3].

GnRH analogues

Because of the relatively short half-life of GnRH when administered intravenously or subcutaneously (t_1 half-life $= 3\frac{1}{2}$ min) there became a need to develop analogues of GnRH with prolonged half-lives that could be developed for application in clinical medicine. Many hundreds of GnRH analogues have been synthesized and fall into two main groups, those that are basically agonistic analogues and those that are essentially antagonists. It is the agonistic analogues that have progressed more rapidly towards introduction to clinical practice. This has been because of the resultant local side-effects at sites of injection for many of the antagonists. The experimental data on agonistic analogues demonstrated that replacements of amino acid, particularly in position 6 and 10 of the native GnRH molecule, produced a series of superactive agonistic analogues that had a reduced susceptibility to degradation by pituitary enzymes and thus a prolonged therapeutic half-life and action. In addition, the analogues demonstrated a high binding affinity for the GnRH receptor. The physiological function of the gonadotrophe is dependent on its pulsatile stimulation by GnRH, but administration of GnRH in a continuous fashion results in a very marked reduction in gonadotrophe responsiveness and a resultant suppression of gonadal function.

The high affinity of GnRH agonists for GnRH receptors and the resistance to enzymatic degradation[4] results in a number of molecular effects on the pituitary gonadotrophe. These can mainly be described by down-regulation of GnRH receptor numbers and post-receptor desensitization of the pituitary cells. Resultant endocrine effects of these actions are reviewed in detail in subsequent sections.

Formulations of GnRH analogues

GnRH analogues are available in a number of formulations (see Table 14.1). For conditions that require short-term administration a number of different

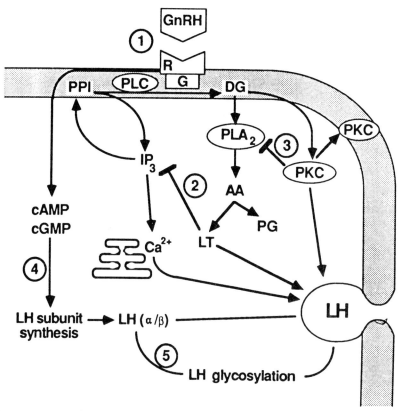

Figure 14.1 Mechanisms of GnRH action and potential sites of GnRH-induced desensitization of gonadotrophin synthesis and secretion. *Abbreviations*: GnRH = gonadotrophin-releasing hormone; R = receptor; G = GTP-binding protein; PPI = polyphosphoinositide; PLC = phospholipase C; IP_3 = inositol 1,4,5-phosphate; DG = diacylglycerol; PLA_2 = phospholipase A_2; AA = arachidonic acid; LT = leukotrines; PG = prostaglandins; PKC = protein kinase C; LH = luteinizing hormone. (From Kiesel, L. and Runnebaum, B. (1990). In Chandra, D.R. and Buttram, U.C. (eds.) *Current Concepts in Endometriosis*, p. 185. (New York: Alan R. Liss) Reproduced with permission)

Table 14.1   Formulations for GnRH analogues

Aqueous solutions
Intravaginal/buccal/rectal
Subcutaneous
Intranasal
Depot slow release formulations
   Non-degradable polymers
   Biodegradable polymers

formulations and treatment approaches may be suitable – e.g. intranasal administration, daily subcutaneous injections. However, in conditions such as endometriosis that require prolonged treatment and perhaps repetitive treatment regimes, depot formulations may offer some advantages.

Aqueous solutions

Various aqueous solutions, while ideal for acute administration for assessment of pituitary function, are unsuitable for prolonged administration. It is feasible to administer subcutaneous or intramuscular preparations on a daily basis but again for prolonged periods of treatment they have certain disadvantages for the patients.

Intranasal

Intranasal delivery systems have become popular in long treatment regimes because of their simplicity of patient use. However, problems of variation in absorption rates can be quite marked and are related to the molecular size and hydrophilic/lipophilic characteristics of the peptide and its stability. In addition, multiple daily administration is necessary, the frequency depending upon the exact analogue and its half-life.

Depots

Depot formulations with life expectancies of 1 or 3 months thus offer many attractions in long treatment protocols. A number of hydrophobic polymers and hydrogels are available as carrier vehicles for the GnRH analogues. However, many of these carriers are non-degradable and such formulations would suffer from the disadvantage that surgical retrieval of the expired depot would be necessary. The development of biodegradable polymer bases provides a much more acceptable formulation and those utilizing sustained release matrices of DL,L-lactide–glycolactide copolymers in which the GnRH agonist is homogeneously dispersed are being developed (such as that by ICI Pharmaceuticals — goserelin).

The GnRH analogues which are currently being investigated for the treatment of endometriosis are summarized in Table 14.2. They are essentially either nonapeptides or decapeptide analogues with substitution in position 6 and/or position 10 of the native structure.

Gonadotrophin and ovarian steroid hormone changes following administration of GnRH analogues

Normally GnRH is released from the hypothalamus in a series of small pulses during the follicular phase at approximately 90-minute intervals. GnRH binds

Table 14.2 Amino acid sequence of native GnRH and major agonistic analogues currently under investigation in the treatment of endometriosis

Native	1	2	3	4	5	(6)	7	8	9	(10)
GnRH	p-GLU	HIS–	TRP–	SER–	TYR–	GLY–	LEU–	ARG	PRO–	GLY-NH$_2$
Decapeptide analogues										
Nafarelin						(D-NAL)$_2$				
Tryptorelin						D-TRP				
Goserelin						D-SER(Bu^t)				AZA-GLY-NH$_2$
Nonapeptide analogues										
Buserelin						D-SER(Bu^t)				PRO-NET
Leuprolide						D-LEU				PRO-NET
Histrelin						D-HIS (Imbzl)				PRO-NET
—						D-TRP				PRO-NET

Gonadotrophin and ovarian steroid hormone changes following administration of GnRH analogues

Normally GnRH is released from the hypothalamus in a series of small pulses during the follicular phase at approximately 90-minute intervals. GnRH binds to the GnRH receptor present on the cell surface of the gonadotrophe and receptors occupied by GnRH from aggregated clumps — 'coated pits' — and the receptor complex becomes internalized from the cell surface. Internalization from the receptor complex triggers a number of series of intracellular events, ultimately resulting in the release of stores of LH and FSH and biosynthesis of new gonadotrophin to replenish stores. Producing the excess of GnRH receptors present on the pituitary cell results in allowing sufficient receptors to be available to respond to the next GnRH pulse. This process allows an orderly and systematic secretion of LH in response to each GnRH pulse.

If a GnRH analogue is given at sufficient dosage, the majority of GnRH receptors are occupied and subsequently internalized, which results in a supraphysiological release of LH and FSH, and an associated initial stimulation of gonadal steroid synthesis. Because of the delayed enzymatic breakdown of the GnRH analogues and hence their prolonged biological half-life in comparison to GnRH (between 3 and 8 hours as opposed to $3\frac{1}{2}$ minutes of native hormone) increased levels of LH and FSH baseline can be maintained for 24 hours following a single intravenous or intranasal bolus administration.

However, continued exposure of the pituitary gonadotrophe to GnRH analogues results in marked loss of LH receptors and a failure of receptor replenishment. This results in pituitary cells that have few receptors and which therefore are unable to respond to the presence of either the potent GnRH agonist or the physiological pulsed release of native GnRH from the hypothalamus. This results in the marked reduction of LH and FSH secretion from the pituitary, which becomes less responsive to GnRH-induced intracellular events. A secondary effect of this marked reduction in gonadotrophin secretion is suppression of ovarian steroid hormone production and ovarian folliculogenesis.

The acute changes in LH, FSH, oestradiol and progesterone as seen in a group of menopausal patients administered a single dose of goserelin [D-SER (tBu)^6-AzaGly^{10} LHRH] depot containing 3.6 mg goserelin on day 1 of the menstrual cycle are shown in Figure 14.2. The initial agonist induced release of LH and FSH is readily apparent with its associated increased oestrogen secretion. Administration in the early follicular phase of the cycle has no associated progesterone increase, which is noted, however, if the GnRH analogue therapy is commenced during the luteal phase of the cycle. Within a few days of continued pituitary exposure to GnRH analogues, pituitary desensitization begins to occur and FSH levels return to pre-treatment basal levels by the third day of administration, while LH basal levels are reached within 7–10 days. Thereafter, LH and FSH remain at or below baseline early follicular phase levels until the depot ceases to release GnRH analogue. Following cessation of release of the analogue, FSH and LH levels begin to increase with the return of ovarian steroidogenesis, subsequent ovulation and resumption of menstruation.

Continuous administration of GnRH analogues thus achieves a reversible

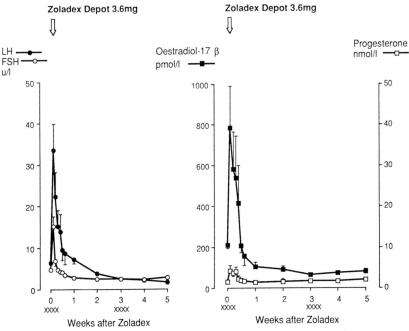

Figure 14.2 Action of GnRH analogue Zoladex on gonadotrophin and ovarian steroid levels in eight premenopausal women receiving a single 3.6 mg depot intramuscularly. XX = Menstruation. From Shaw, R.W. (1988). *Clin. Obstet. Gynaecol.*, **2**, 666. Reproduced with permission

and quite marked suppression of the pituitary ovarian axis with resultant normo- or hypogonadotrophic hypogonadism.

EARLY STUDIES IN THE USE OF GnRH ANALOGUES IN THE TREATMENT OF ENDOMETRIOSIS

The first report of GnRH analogue use in patients with endometriosis was from Meldrum *et al.*[5], with publication on a series of five women treated with D-TRP[6] PRO[9] Net LHRH administered subcutaneously from day 2 of the cycle. This study primarily assessed endocrine responses in these patients and compared these with a group of 12 women who had undergone surgical oophorectomy. At the end of 1 month of treatment with GnRH analogues, serum levels of FSH had decreased below basal levels whilst serum levels of LH were slightly elevated. Four of the five women's serum 17β-oestradiol concentrations had reached castrate levels. These levels were maintained to the end of the treatment period and, even though it was short, four patients reported an improvement or even disappearance of their symptoms related to endometriosis. The study concluded that a prolonged course of treatment might have similar beneficial effects and promoted similar investigations of patients with endometriosis. Many studies have now been published investigating these aspects.

The first definitive report of an attempt to treat patients with endometriosis using a GnRH analogue came from our own group[6]. Six patients were studied during a 6-month treatment period utilizing the GnRH analogue D-SER(tBU)[6] PRO[9] Net LHRH (buserelin). In this study the GnRH analogue was administered intranasally at a dose of 200 μg three times daily in five subjects and in one subject at a single daily dose of 400 μg. The patient receiving the single daily dose of 400 μg continued to complain of symptoms, mainly abdominal pain, and was found to have an endometrioma that increased in size. Treatment was therefore discontinued after 3 months and the patient underwent surgical treatment. The remaining five patients completed the 6 months' course of therapy and at repeat laparoscopy endometriotic deposits had been either completely eliminated or markedly resolved in all cases. Detailed studies of urinary levels of total oestrogens and pregnanediol confirmed that ovulation had been suppressed throughout treatment with the 600-μg dose with an occasional increase in oestrogen secretion being noted, presumably as the result of some resumption of follicular activity. In some patients these episodes were followed by a slight withdrawal bleed. In other patients suppression of oestrogen secretion was achieved, with amenorrhoea persisting throughout therapy. There were no reported significant side-effects in this group of patients although some experienced hot flushes. Histological examination of the endometrium at the end of the 6-month treatment phase showed that three patients had poorly proliferative or atrophic endometrium, and in two patients the endometrium was consistent with late proliferative development. This paper confirmed the value of the use of GnRH analogues in subjects with endometriosis in relieving symptoms and inducing regression of endometriotic deposits, pointing the way for more definitive studies. It also emphhasized the caution that would be needed in the presence of ovarian endometriomata.

One year later, Lemay et al.[7] reported a series of 10 women treated over a similar period of time with the same GnRH analogue, buserelin. These women were administered buserelin twice daily by subcutaneous injection 200 μg for 5 days, then given 400 μg intranasally three times per day for between 25 and 31 weeks. On this regimen, gonadotrophin levels following initial administration showed that serum FSH returned to basal levels on the third day of treatment, while serum LH took some weeks to return to basal levels. Serum 17β-oestradiol on the 30th day of treatment decreased below early follicular phase level and tended generally to decrease for the next few weeks to reach the post-menopausal range. During the first month of treatment some vaginal bleeding, commonly seen as episodes of spotting, was reported in all the 10 women, occurring between 12 and 20 days of commencing therapy. Systematic relief of dyspareunia and abdominal pain were reported as improved or completely relieved within 2 months of commencing therapy. At repeat laparoscopy at the end of treatment, resorption of endometriotic lesions to a major degree was observed in all patients. Endometrial biopsies taken at the end of treatment showed atrophic or only weak proliferative endometrium and a return to spontaneous menstruation occurred within a mean of 45 days of ceasing treatment.

During this study more extensive side-effects were reported, primarily related to those induced by oestrogen deficiency, namely hot flushes and dryness of the vagina. The administered dose of buserelin in the study[7], i.e. 1200 μg intranasally daily, was twice that given in our original pilot study[6]. The increase in incidence of side-effects probably resulted from a greater degree of suppression of 17β-oestradiol.

A further study comparing the effects of different doses of GnRH analogue was reported in 1986[8], when patients were administered buserelin either 200 μg three times daily intranasally, or 300 μg three times daily for a period of 6 months. Both doses reduced circulating 17β-oestradiol to mean levels in many instances within the post-menopausal range. It was noted, however, that patients on the lower dose (200 μg three times daily intranasally) showed a base level of follicular activity with rises in oestrogen level from time to time. This was infrequently observed on the higher dose (300 μg three times daily). Hot flushes in the subjects receiving 300 μg three times daily were reported more commonly and to a more severe degree than in those on 200 μg three times daily. Other side-effects, associated with reduced circulating oestrogen were vaginal dryness, superficial dyspareunia and loss of libido, but these were not experienced by all.

With regard to symptomatic relief in this study, 11 of the 18 women had mild to moderate dysmenorrhoea prior to treatment. Six months after treatment, one remained unchanged, 5 had improved and 5 had no dys-menorrhoea. All had no pain whilst on therapy. Six women complained of deep dyspareunia pre-treatment and after 3 months of therapy all but one reported relief of this symptom[8]. In all patients improvement of the American Fertility Society (AFS) score was achieved with a reduction of AFS staging. In 13 of the 18 patients classified as AFS stage 1 or 2 prior to treatment, 12 patients had complete resolution of visible deposits at the end of 6 months' treatment. The remaining 5 patients had more advanced AFS stages with the presence of adhesions. These adhesions remained unchanged during treatment, although complete or partial resolution of endometriotic deposits was achieved, thus improving AFS classification. The study failed to show any apparent difference between the two doses of buserelin studied. This may merely reflect the small number of patients in the study.

A number of other GnRH analogues have been utilized in the treatment of endometriosis, with reports of their effect in the literature. Schrioch et al.[9] reported the effects of the analogue, nafarelin — (D-NAL$_2$)[6]-LHRH in 8 patients receiving 400 μg 12-hourly. All patients reported complete relief of pain. At second-look laparoscopy performed at the end of 6 months' treatment, 7 of 8 of the women showed complete resolution of active endometriotic deposits in 5 and a small active implant in the Pouch of Douglas remained only in the sixth patient. The seventh patient had a large ovarian endometrioma that decreased slightly in response to treatment but persisted throughout therapy.

This report compares well with the buserelin studies already described[6-8]. Of the women who complained of hot flushes, these were severe enough in three women to result in the dose of nafarelin being decreased to 200 μg twice daily. When the dose of analogue was reduced it was noted that oestradiol levels transiently rose in one of these three women, but subsequently decreased to similar levels despite maintenance of the lower dose of analogue. Other listed side-effects were vaginal dryness, transient mild headaches and mild transient depression. In one patient, leukopenia developed but there was no cause found for this and it was thought perhaps to be unrelated to drug usage.

Another GnRH analogue (Imbzl-D-HIS[6] PRO[9] LHRH) administered as a daily injection of 100 μg in the treatment of 16 patients has been reported[10]. This dosage administration induced near-castrate levels of oestrogen achieved during the greater part of treatment. Two of the 16 patients treated, however, ceased therapy after 10 and 22 weeks respectively because of emotional side-effects. By the end of 2 months' treatment all women complained of hot flushes and 11 of the 16 women complained of vaginal dryness. Greater suppression of serum FSH was achieved than LH but in all patients this fell below basal parameters following the first month of treatment.

From our own observation in studies using a depot preparation of GnRH analogue [D-SER(tBU)[6] AZAGLY[10] - LHRH), goserelin, 3.6 mg administered monthly, there was a low incidence of breakthrough bleeding[11] comparing favourably with intranasally administered preparations where a significant incidence of breakthrough bleeding has been reported by several workers[7,12]. A state of hypogonadotrophic hypogonadism was achieved with the goserelin depot as well as a more profound and consistent suppression of FSH and LH than that seen with the intranasally administered preparations. This perhaps reflects the mode of administration, with consistent release of GnRH analogue from the depot as opposed to intermittent exposure of the pituitary gonadotrophes with the intranasal spray preparations. Depot preparations also result in a more profound suppression of serum oestradiol levels (see Figure 14.3). The more consistent suppression of oestradiol resulted in hot flushes developing in virtually every patient, varying in both frequency and severity throughout the treatment period but peaking at some 12 weeks after commencement of therapy. Also there appeared to be a correlation between patients who experienced increased frequency of flushes also experiencing the most severe form of flushing[13].

These initial studies were open, with small numbers of patients treated in one centre. However, recently an international multicentre trial has been reported comparing buserelin 900 μg per day intranasally in 275 patients in an open label non-comparative study[14]. The study reported that in 95% of all patients serum oestradiol levels were significantly suppressed during the treatment period. An improvement in the implants according to AFS classification occurred in 80% of patients with no change in 9% and progression in 11%. There was a discontinuation of treatment in 9% of patients, half of these ceased therapy because of side-effects experienced. During therapy, dysmenorrhoea, pelvic pain and dyspareunia improved considerably.

All of these studies have been uncontrolled, non-randomized, initial assessments of the value of GnRH analogue treatment for endometriosis. While they have confirmed the drugs' efficacy, comparative studies are necessary to compare GnRH analogues with other established medical treatments with regard to efficacy, patient tolerance and recurrence. A number

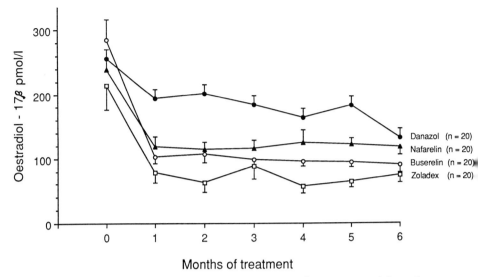

Figure 14.3 Serum 17β-oestradiol values in various groups of patients treated for endometriosis with danazol 200 mg three times daily, nafarelin 200 μg twice daily intranasally, buserelin 400 μg three times daily intranasally or Zoladex depot 3.6 mg monthly for 6 months. ●, Danazol (n = 20). ▲, Nafarelin (n = 20). ○, Buserelin (n = 20). □, Zoladex (n = 20). From Shaw, R.W. (1988). *Clin. Obstet. Gynaecol.*, **2**, 670. Reproduced with permission

of open randomized, or double-blind placebo studies have now been initiated as large multicentre studies and results are becoming available in the literature for review. Danazol is currently the most effective medical treatment for endometriosis but some patients have unpleasant and intense side-effects. It is therefore with danazol that most of the comparisons of GnRH analogues have been performed.

RESULTS OF COMPARATIVE RANDOMIZED TRIALS

In a study reported by Matta and Shaw[15] (as part of a large multicentre study), 61 patients were recruited and randomized between danazol (20 patients) and buserelin (41 patients). At the end of the 6-month study period, 5 patients had been excluded from the trial — 4 for failure to regularly attend follow-up and one for declining her second laparoscopy. During this study patients were reviewed monthly and at each visit assessments of symptoms, side-effects of therapy and endocrine measurements of LH, FSH and oestradiol were made. Those taking buserelin received 400 μg 8-hourly, and those receiving danazol were administered a dose of 400 mg to 800 mg daily, the dose being adjusted according to the severity of the disease and side-effects experienced according to the manufacturer's recommendations. Follow-up was then for a further 6 months post-treatment.

In this study significant hypo-oestrogenism was achieved in both groups but was more marked and more consistent in the buserelin group. The overall cure rate — complete resolution of deposits — was 82% for buserelin and

72% for danazol. This was based on staging the disease by deposits and not taking into account adhesions. In this study it was noted that there was no significant change in the AFS score on adhesions. There was significant improvement in the staging of the disease in both groups treated and a significant and sustained improvement in symptoms in both groups. The percentage of patients with no symptoms at the end of 6 months' therapy and after at least 3 months' follow-up, and the main symptoms of dyspareunia, dysmenorrhoea, pelvic pain and rectal bleeding are shown in Figure 14.4. Patients with cyclical rectal bleeding were infrequent in either treatment group and no conclusions are drawn from these symptom data.

No patients dropped out of the study because of side-effects but it seems that danazol-treated patients reported more problems. The patients on buserelin reported a sense of well-being on therapy, increased energy levels and increased libido. Some patients on buserelin complained of dry vagina, headaches, hot flushes and vaginal bleeding. The incidence of side-effects in danazol and buserelin is shown in Table 14.3.

Jelley reported a similar study[12] but compared a dose of 900 μg buserelin (300 μg three times daily intranasally) with a dose of danazol 600 mg daily. In this study there was excellent compliance and a 7-month treatment period was used. Sixty per cent of patients were relieved of symptoms and 75% no longer had deep dyspareunia at the end of treatment. At the second laparoscopy there was a marked decrease in AFS score in both groups but with no significant difference between the two treatment arms. The danazol-treated patients menstruated more promptly after cessation of treatment but there were no patients with prolonged amenorrhoea after either treatment. Hot flushes and dryness of the vagina were more prevalent in the buserelin group, while seborrhoea or hirsutism were not seen in the buserelin group but were seen in the danazol group. Gastrointestinal side-effects were more common in the danazol group, while headaches were more frequent on buserelin treatment. Jelley[12] found that 20% of patients being given 900 μg buserelin still continued to have episodes of vaginal bleeding and in these individuals it was noted that endometriotic lesions reduced favourably in

Table 14.3 Principal side-effects reported by patients receiving either buserelin or danazol for 6 months

Dose	Buserelin 400 μg t.d.s. intranasally	Danazol 600–800 mg daily orally
Number of patients	39	18
Symptoms		
Hot flushes	74%	22%
Headaches	20%	39%
Vaginal dryness	23%	5.5%
Superficial dyspareunia	5.2%	Nil
Breakthrough bleeding	23%	55%
Reduced breast size	2.6%	5.5%
Weight gain (> 3 kg)	Nil	66%
Acne/oily skin	Nil	39%
Mild hirsutism	Nil	18%

From Matta and Shaw (1986)[8]

spite of oestradiol levels not being reduced to menopausal levels in all of these patients throughout the treatment period. In 1988 Lemay et al.[16] reported an initial analysis of the multicentre HRPI buserelin protocol 310 study group results. This showed comparable results to our own initial subgroup in that study[15]. More extensive analysis of these data has now been reported[17]. Having undergone baseline evaluation, patients enrolled in the study were assigned to one of two drug treatment groups according to randomization schedules. They were randomized to receive buserelin or danazol in the ratio of 2:1 respectively within each investigating centre. Once randomized to buserelin, the patient had a choice of receiving the drug by intranasal insufflation 400 μg three times daily (149 patients) or by daily subcutaneous injection 200 μg (60 patients). Thirty-one patients were allocated to danazol with a starting dose of 400 mg daily, 35 patients to 600 mg daily, and 57 to 800 mg. There was an alteration of danazol dosage during treatment in 17 patients with an increase of 400 to 600 mg, or 600 to 800 mg daily. In one patient an initial dose of 800 mg daily was reduced. These drug regimens resulted in significant reduction in serum oestradiol levels after 1 month of treatment. There was no further decrease until the fifth month of treatment, where levels were slightly lower. The mean reduction in circulating oestradiol was not sufficiently different between the two drugs; however, serum oestradiol levels were always lower in the buserelin group than in the danazol group. In the HRPI trial[17] incidences of intermenstrual pelvic pain and dyspareunia were 61.5% and 53.5% in the buserelin group, 58.5% and 42.6% in the danazol group on admission. In both treatment groups there was gradual alleviation of these symptoms during the treatment period but no significant difference between the two drugs.

Improvement of revised AFS scores which for this study are available for the second laparoscopy in 176 patients treated with buserelin and 84 with danazol. Based on laparoscopy the baseline scores are somewhat higher in the buserelin group than in the danazol group but the mean scores at the end of treatment are similar for the two groups, thus indicating a slightly greater reduction in the mean values for implants and adhesions in the total score for buserelin than danazol. The mean reduction of implant in total scores was highly significant ($p < 0.001$) with both drugs. The occurrence of side-effects with both drug regimens as alluded to earlier in the text was reported in this study. Menopausal symptoms of hot flushes, vaginal dryness and decreased libido were more common in the buserelin-treated patients than in those on danazol, whereas anabolic symptoms (weight gain, myalgia, oedema) and androgenic symptoms (acne, hirsutism, alopecia, breast atrophy) were more common in the danazol-treated group. Symptoms attributable to CNS — headaches, emotional stability, nervous depression — were commonly reported in both treatment regimes. Preliminary evaluation of ongoing follow-up on the data base indicates that the frequency of pregnancies is supposed to be equivalent on the two types of drug used. Initial rates have so far not been reported and it may well be that a larger sample of patients over a longer period of time is required to properly assess the numerous factors implicated in fertility.

A large multicentre study compared the effects of nafarelin (D-Nal$_2$[6] LHRH) with danazol by Henzl and co-workers in 1988[19]. In this large multicentre comparative trial, the effects of either 400 μg or 800 μg of nafarelin intranasally were compared with danazol 800 mg daily. Placebo nasal sprays or tablets were used in this double-blind study. More than 80% of patients in each treatment group had improved AFS scores at the post-treatment laparoscopy. The mean scores decreased from 21.9 to 12.6 with 800 μg nafarelin, from 20.4 to 11.7 with 400 μg nafarelin, and from 18.4 to 10.5 in the danazol-treated groups. These decreases in revised AFS scores are statistically significant, although there is no statistical difference between the various treatment regimens. Symptomatic relief was excellent on all treatments and similar pregnancy rates have been found in each treatment group on cessation of therapy in those wishing to conceive, an overall rate of approximately 59%.

Some side-effect profiles were reported, with hot flushes and decreased libido being more common in the women treated with nafarelin. The authors conclude that nafarelin is an effective treatment for endometriosis with a few side-effects but none related to the hypo-oestrogenic state it induces.

There has been one randomized comparative double-blind multicentre trial reported using a GnRH analogue depot preparation, that of lupron depot 3.75 mg monthly versus danazol 800 mg daily. In this study, 270 patients were evaluated for efficacy and analysis[19]. Both the lupron depot and danazol were in fact efficacious in reducing the extent of endometriosis. Pre-treatment revised AFS score on lupron depot was 25, and post-treatment was 15. For danazol the pre-treatment score was 22 and post-treatment was 13. Dysmenorrhoea, pelvic pain, dyspareunia and pelvic tenderness responded significantly to the lupron depot and danazol treatment. Menstruation was suppressed in all but one patient (99%) on lupron and in all but one (96%) of the danazol-treated patients. Mean oestradiol decrease from baseline in month 3 and month 6 was significantly greater for the lupron depot than for the danazol patients.

As alluded to earlier, there is increasing indication that the depot analogues can more effectively inhibit oestradiol than danazol or the intranasally administered GnRH analogues. However, whether the greater decrease in oestradiol achieved by the depot GnRH analogues is more efficacious in inducing resolution of endometriotic deposits than intranasal preparations or danazol has not yet been demonstrated.

Optimal dose of analogues

The above studies have investigated a variety of individual doses of various GnRH analogues. There have been few comparative studies of different dose regimens. In 1986 Shaw and Matta[8] offered a comparative study between either 600 μg or 900 μg daily intranasally administered buserelin. With those on the higher dose of 900 μg daily there was significantly greater suppression of serum oestradiol and an increased incidence of oestrogen deficiency side-effects as compared with the 600 μg group. However, there was no significant difference in response from patients in terms of symptomatic relief or reduction

269

in AFS staging. A similar comparative study was published by Minaguchi and co-workers[20]. They studied doses of 300 μg, 600 μg and 900 μg total daily dose of buserelin and concluded that a dose of 900 μg daily was necessary for clinical effectiveness and suppression of ovarian function, but that complete suppression may not be necessary to achieve resolution of endometriotic deposits. This latter conclusion seems to become apparent from reviewing data above in which higher doses of intranasal buserelin (1200 μg daily) or depot preparations that achieve even greater degrees of oestradiol suppression do not appear to be more effective than lower doses of intranasally administered buserelin. The optimal doses of intranasal preparations or of depot preparations have thus not yet been established and they may well differ for the varying stages of the disease.

Safety issues

The ability of GnRH analogues to induce a state of hypo- or normogonado-trophic hypogonadism and significant hypo-oestrogenism has implications in a number of metabolic processes. It can be expected that a metabolic environment in terms of hypo-oestrogenism is comparable to that in the postmenopausal woman. There could therefore be changes in serum lipoproteins and ratios in the circulation as well as alterations of bone homeostasis.

Blood biochemistry changes

Serial values of haematological clotting system, clinical chemistry electro-lytes and liver metabolism have been assessed in a number of published studies[8,14–16,18]. They are well summarized in tabular form in a paper published by Kiesel and co-workers[14], who could demonstrate no change in haemoglobin, haematocrit, erythrocytes, thrombocytes, leukocytes, or prothrombin time in patients receiving buserelin 900 μg intranasally in a large multicentre study. Likewise no changes were seen in mean values for creatinine, protein, albumin, sodium, potassium, calcium or inorganic phosphate. Liver enzymes SGOT, SGPT, and alkaline phosphatase showed no significant changes during or following treatment.

Serum lipid changes

Lipoprotein changes were assessed in a number of studies but very often only limited subfractions. However, these subfractions were analysed in depth and reported in our own group study[13,21]. In summary, these indicated that total cholesterol showed no change during the 6 months of therapy with the potent GnRH analogue goserelin, 3.6 mg depot, monthly for 6 months. However, there was a slight but insignificant increase in LDL cholesterol and a non-significant reduction in HDL. Apolipoprotein B showed an insignificant rise and apolipoprotein A_1 had a questionable increase. These lipoprotein changes did not appear to be marked and were not deemed to be atherogenic.

Alterations in bone mineral homeostasis

As GnRH analogues are so efficient in inducing a hypo-oestrogenic state, it is not surprising that alterations in calcium metabolism have been reported, with an increase in urinary calcium secretion comparable to that seen in the menopause during GnRH analogue therapy. In 1987 Matta et al.[22] studied a cohort of patients receiving buserelin 1200 μg daily intranasally and observed no changes in cortical bone loss by dual photon densitometry assessment of the forearm, but utilizing computed tomography (QCT) of the lumbar spine (vertebrae L2–L4) they reported a mean 5.6% reduction in trabecular bone density. A follow-up study has shown that this trabecular bone loss is reversible after 6 months off treatment[23] (Figure 14.4).

These results clearly demonstrated the potentially deleterious effect of GnRH analogue on bone density. Techniques such as dual photon absorptometry and computed tomography have permitted the measurement of bone density with high precision and accuracy in clinically relevant anatomical sites. The studies using QCT[24] showed similar reductions in bone density in patients who were receiving nafarelin to those published above. Studies using dual photon densitometry have shown small reductions in lumbar vertebrae density[25–27] and an increased loss of bone density in Ward's trial in the femoral neck[28].

While this decline from baseline is clinically insignificant at these levels in terms of clinical risk of fracture, the difference between pre-treatment and post-treatment levels is of significance. We would not expect any significant decrease in bone density over a 6-month period in premenopausal women of

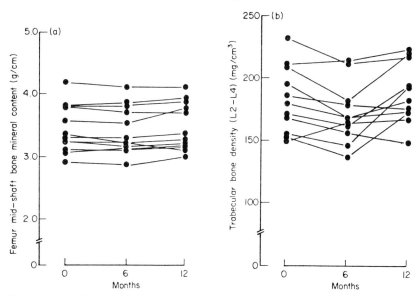

Figure 14.4 (a) Femoral cortical bone mineral content ($n = 12$) and (b) lumbar vertebral trabecular bone density ($n = 11$) in patients before treatment, after 6 months' treatment with buserelin 400 μg three times daily, and 6 months post-treatment. From Matta, W.H., Shaw, R.W., Hesp, R. and Evans, R. (1988). *Clin. Endocrinol.*, **29**, 45–51. Reproduced with permission

this age group[29]. The majority of studies to date show that bone loss in the spine caused by GnRH analogue treatment is reversed following cessation of therapy[23-25]. However, these studies are of short-acting analogues and there are no long-term data yet published on long-acting analogue depots. It can, however, be stated that the degree of transient bone loss associated with a 6-month course of therapy with GnRH agonists for endometriosis should not be detrimental to eumenorrhoeic women who had normal initial bone loss.

RECURRENCE OF ENDOMETRIOSIS AND IMPROVEMENT OF FERTILITY STATUS

Data from our own initial uncontrolled studies indicate that patients who have received buserelin can develop recurrence of the disease often within 12 months of ceasing treatment and the return of normal cycles. Recurrence in randomized trials as reported above[15] was 25% (proved at repeat laparoscopy) after a completed 12-month follow-up period. It was similar both for those receiving buserelin or danazol. Results on current rates on long-term follow-up of patients receiving analogue are as yet unpublished in the literature.

With regard to effects on patients achieving pregnancy following GnRH analogue therapy, successful conception rates range between 30% and 52% in various studies[15,17,18]. However, it would be difficult to say whether these rates are comparable to those in randomized trials achieved by danazol. A number of factors are known to influence pregnancy likelihood and outcome and data still need to accrue from long-term studies and follow-up to establish whether this form of treatment is more effective than any other.

CONCLUSIONS

Induction of a state of hypo-oestrogenism is found to be effective in the treatment of endometriosis with the continued administration of agonistic analogues of GnRH. The initial uncontrolled studies reported the efficacy of GnRH analogues in patients with mild, moderate and severe endometriosis, which have now been confirmed from a number of large multicentre, randomized open or double-blind trials comparing GnRH analogues against danazol.

The side-effects experienced from GnRH analogues are those expected from the induced state of hypo-oestrogenism — primarily hot flushes, vaginal dryness, headaches, and superficial dyspareunia — but the drug therapy is usually well tolerated by the patients. The altered observations in bone and calcium metabolism are comparable to those of the menopause — calcium loss and reversible loss of trabecular bone density. These effects may limit the duration and frequency of GnRH analogue therapy.

The valuable role of GnRH analogues in the treatment of endometriosis has now been established, and as newer formulations of these agents become available it is likely they will play an increasingly important part in the management of patients with endometriosis.

REFERENCES

1. Schally, A.V., Arimura, A., Baba, Y., Nair, R.M.G., Matsuo, H., Redding, T.W., Debdjuk, L. and White, W.F. (1971). Isolation and properties of the FSH and LH-releasing hormone. *Biochem. Biophys. Res. Commun.*, **43**, 393–399
2. Clayton, R.N. (1989). Cellular actions of gonadotrophin-releasing hormone: the receptor and beyond. In Shaw, R.W. and Marshall, J.C. (eds.) *LHRH and its Analogues — Their Use in Gynaecological Practice*, pp. 19–34. (London: Wright)
3. Kiesel, L. and Runnebaum, B. (1990). Mechanisms involved in the hormonal treatment of endometriosis. In Chandha, D.R. and Buttram, V.C. (eds.) *Current Concepts in Endometriosis*, pp. 179–196. (New York: Alan R. Liss)
4. Sandow, J. (1983). Clinical applications of LHRH and its analogues. *Clin. Endocrinol.*, **18**, 571–592
5. Meldrum, D.R., Chang, R.J., Lu, J., Vale, W., Rivier, J. and Judd, H.L. (1982). 'Medical oophorectomy' using a long-acting GnRH agonist: a possible new approach to the treatment of endometriosis. *J. Clin. Endocrinol. Metab.*, **54**, 1081–1083
6. Shaw, R.W., Fraser, H.M. and Boyle, H. (1983). Intranasal treatment with luteinizing hormone-releasing hormone agonist in women with endometriosis. *Br. Med. J.*, **287**, 1167–1169
7. Lemay, A., Maheux, R., Faure, N., Jean, C. and Fazekas, A. (1984). Reversible hypogonadism induced by a luteinizing hormone-releasing hormone (LHRH) agonist (buserelin) as a new therapeutic approach for endometriosis. *Fertil. Steril.*, **41**, 863–871
8. Shaw, R.W. and Matta, W. (1986). Reversible pituitary ovarian suppression induced by an LHRH agonist in the treatment of endometriosis: comparison of two dose regimens. *Clin. Reprod. Fertil.*, **4**, 329–336
9. Schriock, E., Monroe, S.E., Henzl, M. and Jaffe, R.B. (1985). Treatment of endometriosis with a potent agonist of gonadotrophin releasing hormone (Nafarelin). *Fertil. Steril.*, **44**, 585–588
10. Steingold, K.A., Cedars, M., Lu, J.K.H., Randle, R.N., Judd, H.L. and Meldrum, D.R. (1987). Treatment of endometriosis with a long-acting gonadotrophin-releasing hormone agonist. *Obstet. Gynecol.*, **69**, 403–411
11. Shaw, R.W. (1988). LHRH analogues in the treatment of endometriosis — comparative results with other treatments. *Clin. Obstet. Gynaecol.*, **2**, 659–675
12. Jelley, R.J. (1986). Multicentre open comparative study of buserelin and danazol in the treatment of endometriosis. *Br. J. Clin. Pract.*, **41** (suppl. 48), 64–68
13. Shaw, R.W. (1990). Goserelin-depot preparation of LHRH analogue used in the treatment of endometriosis. In Chandha, D.R. and Buttram, V.C. (eds.) *Current Concepts in Endometriosis*. (New York: Alan R. Liss)
14. Kiesel, L., Thomas, K., Tempore, A., Trabant, H., Widdra, W. and Runnebaum, B. (1989). Efficacy and safety of buserelin treatment in women with endometriosis — a multicentre open-label study. *Gynaecol. Endocrinol.*, **3** (suppl. 2), 5–19
15. Matta, W.H. and Shaw, R.W. (1986). A comparative study between buserelin and danazol in the treatment of endometriosis. *Br. J. Clin. Pract.*, **41** (suppl. 48), 69–73
16. Lemay, A. (1988). Comparison of GnRH analogues to conventional therapy in endometriosis. In *International Symposium on GnRH Analogues*, Geneva, Abstract 020
17. Dawood, M.Y., Spellacy, W.N., Dmowski, W.P., Gambrell, R.D., Greenblatt, R.B., Girard, Y., Lemay, A., Mishell, D.R., Nagamani, M., Pepperell, R.J., Shaw, R.W., Seibel, M.M., Sondheimer, S.J., Klioze, S.S., Schreider, J., Setescak, L. and Spiro, T. (1990). A comparison of the efficacy and safety of Buserelin vs Danazol in the treatment of endometriosis. In Chandha, D.R. and Buttram, V.C. (eds.) *Current Concepts in Endometriosis* (New York: Alan R. Liss)
18. Henzl, M.R., Corson, S.L., Moghissi, K., Buttram, V.C., Bergqvist, C. and Jacobson, C. (1988). Administration of nasal nafarelin as compared with oral danazol for endometriosis. *N. Engl. J. Med.*, **318**, 455–489
19. Miller, J.D. (1990). Lenprolide acetate for the treatment of endometriosis. In Chandha, D.R. and Buttram, V.C. (eds.) *Current Concepts in Endometriosis* (New York: Alan R. Liss)
20. Minaguchi, H., Vermura, T.L. and Shitzsu, K. (1989). Clinical study on finding the optimal dose of a potent LHRH agonist (Buserelin) for the treatment of endometriosis —

multicentre trial in Japan. In Rolland, R., Chandha, D.R. and Willemsen (eds.) *Gonadotrophin Down Regulation in Gynaecological Practice*, pp. 211–225. (New York: Alan R. Liss)

21. Crook, D., Gardner, R. and Worthington, M. (1989). Zoladex (ICI 118630) versus Danazol in the treatment of pelvic endometriosis: effects on plasma lipid risk factors. In Stoll, Basil A. (ed.) *Proceedings of the International Symposium on Endocrine Therapy*, pp. 157–160. (Basel: Karger) (*Hormone Research*, **32** (suppl. 1))

22. Matta, W.H., Shaw, R.W., Hesp, R. and Katz, D. (1987). Hypogonadism induced by luteinizing hormone-releasing hormone agonist analogues: effects on bone density in premenopausal women. *Br. Med. J.*, **294**, 1523–1524

23. Matta, W.H., Shaw, R.W., Hesp, R. and Evans, R. (1988). Reversible trabecular bone density loss following induced hypo-oestrogenism with the GnRH analogue Buserelin in premenopausal women. *Clin. Endocrinol.*, **29**, 45–51

24. Cann, C.E., Henzl, M., Burry, K. *et al.* (1986). Reversible bone loss is induced by GnRH agonists. In *The Endocrine Society 68th Annual Meeting*, Abstract 24

25. Devogelaer, J.P., Nagant de Deuxhcaisnes, C. and Donnez, J. (1987). LHRH analogues and bone loss. *Lancet*, **1**, 1498

26. Scharla, S.H., Minne, H.W. and Waibel, S. (1988). GnRH agonist therapy alters calcium homeostasis and reduces bone mineral content. *Acta Endocrinol.*, **117** (suppl. 287), 208

27. Tummon, I.S., Radwanska, E. and Ali, A. (1988). Bone mineral density in women with endometriosis before and during ovarian suppression with gonadotrophin-releasing hormone agonists or danazol. *Fertil. Steril.*, **49**, 792–796

28. Stevenson, J.C., Lees, B., Gardner, R. and Shaw, R.W. (1989). A comparison of the skeletal effects of Zoladex and Danazol in premenopausal women with endometriosis. In Stoll, Basil A. (ed.) *Proceedings of the International Symposium on Endocrine Therapy*, pp. 161–164. (Basel: Karger) (*Hormone Research*, **32** (suppl. 1))

29. Stevenson, J.C., Lees, B. and Davenport, M. (1988). Determinants of bone density in normal women: risk factors for future osteoporosis? *Br. Med. J.*, **298**, 924–928

15
The role of definitive surgery and hormone replacement therapy in the treatment of endometriosis

A. F. Henderson and J. W. W. Studd

INTRODUCTION

Since the first reported case of endometriosis, called an 'adenomyoma' by von Rokitansky in 1860[1], and the introduction of the term endometriosis by Blair Bell in 1922[2], the condition has continued to attract much debate concerning the correct surgical management. It is currently the second most common gynaecological surgical abnormality encountered after uterine leiomyomata. The overall incidence is estimated at between 1–2%[3,4] and 7–10.5%[5] of women during their reproductive years. Darbois[5] claims that 9% of all gynaecological surgery is undertaken for endometriosis, and American figures are higher: Jeffcoate[6] and Tyson[7] estimate that endometriosis accounts for 10–25% of surgical intervention for pain. The discrepancy between the various figures undoubtedly results from the range in severity of the condition and the difficulty in establishing a standard classification of this severity.

Endometriosis is also a major cause of morbidity in all age groups, and in younger women where infertility is an important sequela it is estimated that endometriosis accounts for 40% of all causes of female infertility[8]. Medical treatment is frequently associated with metabolic and symptomatic side-effects and has limited success in controlling symptoms due to adhesive disease or damaged pelvic organs. Furthermore, recurrence rates following such therapy are reported as 16–52% at 1 year depending on the method of diagnosis and the type of treatment[9]. There is also a residual 10–20% of patients in whom the disease fails to improve with any of the standard hormonal therapies available[10]. Conservative surgery with minimal disruption of the pelvic organs may be relevant where fertility is still of primary concern,

275

but has limited effect in controlling symptoms in the long term, and is associated with cumulative recurrence rates of 13% at 3 years and 40% at 5 years respectively[11]. When the decision has finally been taken to perform hysterectomy, ovarian tissue is still frequently preserved to prevent menopausal symptoms[12]. Even in cases where bilateral oophorectomy is performed, oestrogen therapy, if prescribed at all, is commonly given in the lowest dose available[13] often following an arbitrary postoperative delay of several months or years[14] during which time menopausal symptoms may be severe[15]. This reluctance to remove ovaries may result from the belief that conservative surgery is associated with reasonable cure rates[16-18] and carries a low risk of repeat surgery[17,18]. There may also be fears of a recurrence of the disease[13] if oestrogen therapy is provided to control subsequent menopausal symptoms and the associated long-term sequelae of a premature menopause[19].

The validity of these arguments is, however, questionable. A recent study by Thomas and Cooke[20] revealed direct evidence of progression of the disease in women in a prospective placebo-controlled study. This agrees with the earlier view of Hill[21], who reported an increase in the number and size of endometriosis deposits in all patients with time, but contradicts the generally held belief that there is no significant association between age and severity of the disease[22]. Furthermore, work from our team has shown that failure to remove the ovaries at hysterectomy is far from satisfactory in preventing a recurrence of symptoms, as over 45% of patients will require further surgery[15]. This study did not reveal any adverse effects related to oestrogen replacement therapy, a finding that has been supported by other reports[23-26].

This chapter will attempt to resolve the conflicts between the theoretical and practical approaches to the role of hysterectomy, oophorectomy and oestrogen replacement therapy in the management of endometriosis.

OESTROGENIC RESPONSIVENESS OF ENDOMETRIOTIC TISSUE

Oestrogen

The exact role of oestrogens and ovarian activity in the pathogenesis of endometriosis is complex. The clinical evidence for the oestrogen-dependent nature of endometriosis is largely based on the occurrence of the condition largely during the reproductive years of life. It is rare, but not unreported, postmenopausally. The condition often exhibits cyclical fluctuations related to the menstrual cycle and may improve in cases of prolonged amenorrhoea such as pregnancy. However, contrary to earlier work that described endometriotic deposits as being morphologically[27] and histologically[28] similar to endometrium, the nature of the hormonal response of endometriotic tissue is unpredictable, as it differs from that of endometrium in several respects.

Janne et al.[29] studied 41 patients and found oestrogen and progestin cytosol receptors in only 30% of endometriosis biopsies, and these were present at much lower concentrations than in normal endometrium. Fifty per cent of tissue contained only progestin receptors, while 20% had no detectable receptors of either type. Histological studies have shown concordant[30] and discordant[31] growth between uterine endometrium and endometriotic deposits in women with regular cycles. Only 13% of deposits have been reported to show histological changes synchronous with corresponding changes in uterine endometrium[32]. Although steroid receptors for oestrogen, progesterone and testosterone are present in most deposits, concentrations are lower than in endometrium and receptor binding state is unrelated to the menstrual cycle[33,34], which may indicate defective hormonal regulation. Similarly, no cyclical patterns are found in secretory receptor products[28,34,35] or enzymes[36] that are commonly hormone-dependent. Kauppila et al.[37] found that, among other changes, treatment with danazol or gestrinone significantly reduced the concentration of oestrogen and progesterone receptors in uterine endometrium but not in endometriotic deposits. Endometriosis thus responds differently from endometrium and may be resistant to hormonal therapy. This would partly account for the high recurrence rates after medical treatment: for example, 33% with danazol[38], 25% with GnRH analogues[39], 31% with gestrinone[40], and 42% with medroxyprogesterone acetate[41]. Undoubtedly other factors, including progression of the disease, formation of new deposits, and the inability to alter scarring and adhesive disease, also contribute to this failure to control recurrence.

The exact role of oestrogens is further questioned by other evidence. Dizerega et al.[42] reported that in castrated cynomolgus monkeys transplanted endometriotic deposits did not require oestrogen or progestogen for initiation, but required a combination of oestrogen or progestogen or both for maintenance. Endometriosis can also persist in relatively hypo-oestrogenic states such as episiotomy scars[43] and cases of primary amenorrhoea[5], and has even been reported in a case of 46XY gonadal dysgenesis[44].

Postmenopausal endometriosis

More interesting are the reported cases of postmenopausal endometriosis. The diagnosis is rarely suspected and presenting symptoms include abdominal pain, bleeding, gastrointestinal or ureteric obstruction or asymptomatic masses[45–47]. No single causative factor has been implicated, although a considerable number of subjects in most studies report a previous history of pelvic surgery, suggesting that dissemination of endometriotic tissue at operation may play a role. Abeshouse and Abeshouse[48] found that in 39 out of 56 cases of urogenital endometriosis there was a past history of pelvic surgery. Vorstman et al.[47] reported a 64-year-old woman who presented with transmural vesical endometriosis 24 years following a total abdominal hysterectomy (TAH) with no hormone replacement therapy in the intervening period. Henriksen[49] reported 37 cases of postmenopausal endometriosis out of a total of 1000 cases. Twenty-nine of these had previously undergone hysterectomy and bilateral salpingo-oophorectomy (BSO) yet active deposits of endometriosis were found in all cases. Kempers et al.[45] reported 136 cases of postmenopausal endometriosis of which 39 had 'clinically significant' microscopically proven endometriosis defined as extensive gastrointestinal tract or pelvic endometriosis, endometriotic cysts greater than 3 cm diameter,

In addition to the role played by previous surgery, it has been suggested that continuing high circulatory oestrogen levels from exogenous sources, adrenal glands or peripheral conversion, may play a role in some cases. Kempers et al.[45] base this conclusion on the fact that of the 16 patients with endometriotic deposits showing significant activity and in whom an endometrial sample was available, nine showed evidence of similar cellular activity in the form of proliferative or hyperplastic endometrial change. Ranney[16] and Punnonen et al.[50] also reported cases of endometriosis developing several years postmenopause with no history of preceding hormone therapy. Punnonen et al. suggested that extra-gonadal peripheral oestrogen production related to obesity may be implicated in 70% of their subjects. The phenomenon of continuing oestrogenic stimulus may reflect a different end-organ response in particular women, but unfortunately no record of plasma oestrogen levels is given in any of these studies to support or refute this possibility.

The role of oestrogens in the development of postmenopausal endometriosis is further refuted by other findings. There is a marked paucity of reported cases in the literature linking hormone replacement and the development of endometriosis except following the use of high-dose synthetic oestrogens such as mestranol[51] or the inappropriate use of unopposed conjugated oestrogens[52]. Prolonged high-dose synthetic oestrogen therapy with chlorotrianisene has also been linked to the development of vesical endometriosis in men[53,54]. Further conflicting evidence is provided by Djursing et al.[55], who reported a case of extensive active endometriosis in a classical hypo-oestrogenic state, and in the 136 cases reported above by Kempers et al.[45] only one had a history of previous oestrogen therapy.

Ray et al.[52] have suggested that the additional use of progestogens may provide protection against the proliferation of endometrium and the development of endometriosis. However, other reports[56] have shown that hormone replacement therapy (HRT) with cyclical progestogens, even after TAH, does not prevent the development of endometriosis, and the long-term use of progestogens may be inadvisable in postmenopausal women because of the associated deleterious effects on plasma lipids and mood.

Pregnancy and endometriosis

The effect of pregnancy on endometriosis is generally assumed to be beneficial[57,58]. It has been reported that pregnancy results in direct effects on deposits, causing growth arrest, secretory changes and necrosis[59]. Schenken et al.[60] have shown in monkeys that resolution of mild disease and objective improvement in severe disease occurs post-pregnancy. This beneficial effect may be due to the fact that progesterone levels are grossly elevated in pregnancy or due to the absence of cyclical ovarian activity and cyclical stimulation of endometriotic deposits.

However, conflicting reports suggest that the response of endometriosis to pregnancy is variable and first-trimester exacerbation and reactivation of deposits has been reported[61]. Persistent disease post-pregnancy is much commoner than regression[61,62]. Wheeler and Malinak[11] showed that after the surgical removal of all visible deposits the average time to the recurrence of symptoms was 35 months (no pregnancy), 47 months (one pregnancy) and 67 months (two or more pregnancies). Thus the gaps are those represented by the 9 months' gestational amenorrhoea of pregnancy and there is no direct effect on the deposits other than this.

Combined oral contraceptives and endometriosis

Similarly, the role of the oral contraceptive pill is generally assumed to be beneficial. A pseudopregnancy regimen using a high-dose combined oral contraceptive pill was adopted as early as 1956[63] in an attempt to mimic the hormonal milieu of pregnancy. Use of the contraceptive pill has been advocated both for the prophylaxis and the treatment of endometriosis on the basis that lighter menstrual flow would decrease the risk of retrograde flux, and that the abolition of ovulation and cyclical hormonal changes would reduce the stimulation of deposits.

In reality the role of the pill remains to be defined. Three main studies have produced conflicting results. Sensky and Liu[64] showed a decreased prevalence of endometriosis in pill users. However, Cramer et al.[65] showed contradictory findings, with a higher than expected incidence of pill use in endometriosis sufferers. Buttram[66] found that the severity of endometriosis had an inverse ratio to the length of pill use. Cramer et al.[65] also found a significantly increased risk of endometriosis with the use of high-dose pills containing more than 50 μg ethinyloestradiol. This supports the previously discussed cases using high-dose synthetic oestrogens[51,53,54], which were thought to be implicated in the development of endometriosis. The role of the low-dose pill in limiting progression of the disease or reducing recurrence is still unclear and requires further investigation.

Testosterone and endometriosis

Testosterone is also believed to exert a beneficial effect on the endometrium, but again the evidence for this is poor. Hamblen[67] used methyltestosterone to temporarily relieve the symptoms of endometriosis without affecting ovulation or the menstrual cycle. However, only minimal regressive effects on the endometrium were obtained and this may explain the transitory benefits obtained. Hammond et al.[68] report 100% recurrence after 3–6 months of therapy and 42% of patients subsequently required surgery. Salmon et al.[69] reported unacceptable side-effects in 40–100% of patients, including voice changes, hirsutism, acne, vaginitis, and clitoromegaly.

THE ROLE OF DEFINITIVE SURGERY AND OESTROGEN REPLACEMENT

The ultimate goal of treatment in endometriosis is the relief of symptoms, preferably with the minimum of side-effects. Conservative surgery is vital where preservation of fertility is still of primary concern, but the assessment of this approach has been compromised by the lack of randomized controlled trials and by the variety of measures used by surgeons to assess the therapeutic response. Recurrence rates following conservative surgery do appear to be high: Schenken and Malinak[70] reported that over 42% of women with severe endometriosis will require a second surgical procedure, while Wheeler and Malinak[11] reported cumulative recurrence rates of 15% at 3 years and 40% at 5 years. In the latter study neither age, initial staging, nor the subsequent ability to conceive significantly affected recurrence, in contrast to other studies[25,70,71].

The decision to proceed to hysterectomy is clearly the major step. This decision should be guided by three factors: firstly, the presence of severe symptoms, particularily intractable pain; secondly, the failure of other treatments; and thirdly, where the desire for pregnancy is no longer possible or of primary concern. The percentage of patients who will require such surgery is estimated at 13% by Spangler et al.[72] and 12% by Schenken and Malinak[70], but other reports suggest that these figures are an underestimate. Pratt and Williams[73] in a 5-year prospective study of 968 patients found a 50% incidence of endometriosis in women aged 15–55 years undergoing conservative surgical treatment. Fifty-five per cent of these women subsequently underwent TAH and BSO. Puolakka et al.[74], in a review of 208 women treated surgically for endometriosis, found that in the group overall, 41% underwent radical surgery, i.e. TAH $\pm$ BSO, compared to 47% who had conservative surgery. However, in those women aged 39 years or more, 83% underwent radical surgery.

Having decided to carry out definitive surgery, the next problems that arise are whether to perform a bilateral oophorectomy and whether or not oestrogen replacement should be given. Opinion is still divided on the wisdom of oophorectomy, despite the fact that the ovaries are the commonest site for deposits of endometriosis and the condition is driven largely by cyclical ovarian activity. Wheeler and Malinak[11] report only a 1–3% incidence of repeat surgery if the ovaries are retained. Wilson[17] has also suggested that normal ovarian tissue should be preserved at hysterectomy and quotes a 3% recurrence rate for persistent symptoms with this approach. He further suggests that only low-dose oestrogen therapy (0.625 mg conjugated oestrogens) should be used if oophorectomy is performed, with the addition of a progestogen should the symptoms of endometriosis recur. Ranney[18] also reports that very few women require re-operation following TAH with ovarian conservation. Unfortunately, these and other similar reports are based largely on anecdotal evidence rather than on the analysis of patient data and are thus somewhat unreliable.

Even proponents of oophorectomy at the time of hysterectomy suggest only minimal oestrogen replacement therapy because of fears over recurrence. Matta and Shaw[13] advocate TAH and BSO and removal of pelvic endometriotic deposits as the definitive procedure for endometriosis, but advise only minimal low-dose oestrogen therapy owing to the risk of recurrence of the disease in a small proportion of patients. Malinak[14] advocates the use of low-dose oestrogen only after an arbitrary postoperative delay of 3–6 months if active endometriosis is found at operation.

There is, on the contrary, much evidence that removal of ovaries is a prudent step and that the use of HRT is not associated with any adverse effects. Brosens et al.[75], in a long-term (5–9 year) follow-up study of 92 women treated conservatively for ovarian endometriosis, found that 7.6% required further surgery, mainly owing to adhesive disease. Two recent studies from our team that have specifically addressed the role of definitive surgery, oophorectomy and oestrogen therapy in endometriosis have similarly shown that the risk of repeated surgery remains until the last ovarian remnant is removed. In an initial retrospective study, Montgomery and Studd[15] studied 50 women who had previously undergone a hysterectomy for endometriosis followed by hormone replacement in the form of 50 mg oestradiol and 100 mg testosterone implants. Thirty-nine of the 50 women had no remaining ovarian tissue, while 11 women had some residual ovarian tissue at the time of commencing hormone replacement. Only 29 women had TAH and BSO as a primary procedure, while 10 of the 39 women (25.6%) had undergone two or more laparotomies to remove their ovaries for recurrent symptoms prior to commencing HRT. In a 5-year follow-up, none of the group of 39 women with no residual ovarian tissue required further surgical intervention and all achieved satisfactory control of both endometriosis and menopausal symptoms. In the group of 11 women with ovarian tissue present at the commencement of HRT, 6 women (54.5%) had already undergone two or more operations prior to commencing HRT. Five of these 11 women (45.5%) underwent repeat laparotomy while taking HRT, for the recurrence of symptoms, mainly pain, but no evidence of active disease was found at surgery in any case and the symptoms were presumed to be due to adhesions and the residual ovary syndrome. The previously high (54.5%) incidence of repeat surgery in this group was not therefore increased following commencement of HRT. Ten women in this study were not prescribed oestrogen therapy immediately post-oophorectomy and suffered severe climacteric symptoms for a mean of 2.5 years before receiving HRT. All the other women received immediate HRT with no adverse effects.

In a larger study, Henderson et al.[76] assessed 109 women with endometriosis similarly treated by hysterectomy and oestrogens. Information was obtained regarding age, parity, duration of the disease, method of diagnosis, duration and nature of medical and surgical treatments and the state of the pelvis at the final laparotomy. The women were also questioned about their attitude to hysterectomy and oophorectomy and the effect of HRT on their endometriosis and climacteric symptoms.

Implants of 50–75 mg oestradiol with 100 mg testosterone were inserted in the manner described by Thom and Studd[77]. The mean duration of treatment was 5.3 years (range 0.3–18 years). Mean oestradiol levels were 810 pmol/l (range 105–2100 pmol/l) and mean testosterone levels were 1.4 nmol/l (range 0.4–3.1 nmol/l). The mean age at the time of the study was 46.9 years and the mean duration of endometriosis was 11.4 years (Table 15.1). Medical treatment had been prescribed in 100 women for a mean duration of 6.8 years, ranging from simple analgesia to GnRH analogues (Table 15.2). Seventy of the 109 women (64.2%) had one laparotomy prior to commencing HRT, while the remaining 39 women (35.8%) had multiple operations.

Table 15.1 Endometriosis study

	Mean (years)	(Range) (years)
Age at time of study	46.9	(32–68)
Age at onset of endometriosis symptoms	32.8	(13–63)
Age at diagnosis of endometriosis	35.5	(15–67)
Age at first laparotomy	37.5	(16–64)
Age at hysterectomy	39.5	(23–67)
Age at bilateral oophorectomy (88 patients)	39.7	(23–64)

Table 15.2 Medical treatment prior to surgery

	No.	Percentage
Oral contraception	36	33
Progestogens	30	27.5
Danazol	19	17.4
Buserelin	1	0.9
Others (heat treatment, analgesics)	14	12.8
None	9	8.3

The patients formed two main groups depending on the presence of ovarian tissue. Eighty-five women (78%) had no residual ovarian tissue and the remaining 24 women (22%) had some residual tissue at the commencement of HRT. Of the 85 women with no residual tissue, 53 (63.3%) underwent TAH and BSO as the primary procedure for endometriosis. The remaining 32 women (37.6%) required two or more operations to complete the removal of ovarian tissue prior to commencing HRT (Table 15.3). Of the 24 women with ovarian tissue present, 7 (29%) underwent two or more operations prior to commencing HRT. There was thus a high incidence of repeat surgery in both groups prior to commencing HRT. As in the earlier study, during follow-up these two groups showed significant differences in outcome. The 85 women with no residual tissue were followed up for a mean of 5.3 years (range 0.5–18 years). Only one patient required a further laparotomy after commencing HRT: this was a ureteric re-implantation that followed nine previous laparotomies (none by the authors!) (Table 15.4). All the women in this group had excellent improvement in their endometriosis symptoms, particularly pelvic pain and dyspareunia, and none had appreciable climacteric symptoms.

Table 15.3 Number of laparotomies prior to commencement of HRT

No. of laparotomies	No ovarian tissue at commencement HRT		Residual ovarian tissue at commencement HRT	
1	53[a]		17	
2	18 ⎫		4 ⎫	
3	6 ⎬ 37.6%		2 ⎬ 29.2%	
> 3	8 ⎭		1 ⎭	
Total	85 (78%)		24 (22%)	

[a]TAH + BSO as primary surgical procedure

Table 15.4   No ovarian tissue at commencement of oestrogen therapy

	No. of patients	Mean age (years)	Mean duration oestrogen (years)	Laparotomies following oestrogen
One operation (TAH + BSO)	53	49.8 (31–68)	5.5 (0.5–16	0
More than one operation	32	45.7 (32–68)	5.2 (0.5–18)	1[a]

[a]Ureteric re-implantation following 9 laparotomies

The group of 24 women with residual ovarian tissue was followed up for a mean of 3.4 years (range 0.25–8 years). Six women (25%) required further surgery during this period for the apparent recurrence of endometriosis symptoms, mainly pelvic pain (Table 15.5). Four women required one further laparotomy each: two had a bilateral oophorectomy and two had division of adhesions. Two women underwent two further laparotomies each: one had subacute bowel obstruction secondary to adhesions, and one had a bilateral oophorectomy in two stages. There was no advantage to be gained by delaying HRT after oophorectomy. In the group of 85 women with no remaining ovarian tissue, 75 had immediate HRT with no adverse effects. The remaining 10 women had a mean delay of 3.5 years (range 0.5–10 years) with predictable menopausal symptoms in the interim period. These were successfully controlled with implants.

The results of this study support the view that repeated surgery is often necessary for the control of symptoms until the last ovarian remnant is removed. Furthermore, oestrogen therapy does not seem to stimulate progression or recurrence of the disease. In the group of women with no residual ovarian tissue, 32 women (37.6%) had undergone two or more operations to complete the removal of ovarian tissue prior to commencing HRT. None required intervention related to recurrent symptoms after commencing HRT. In the group of 24 women with residual ovarian tissue, the use of oestrogen therapy did not increase the risk of further surgery. The incidence of multiple surgery in this group remained high at 29.2% prior to, and 25% after commencing HRT.

Patients' attitudes to hysterectomy and oophorectomy were notably different. Only five women (4.6%) had expressed any regrets about hysterectomy at the time of the operation but none had continuing regrets at the time of the study. Only one woman (age 32, nulliparous) expressed long-

Table 15.5   Ovarian tissue at commencement of oestrogen therapy

	No. of patients	Mean age (years)	Mean duration oestrogen (years)	Laparotomies following oestrogen
One operation (TAH alone)	17	46.6 (36–55)	3.7 (0.5–8)	4
More than one operation	7	46.5 (42–54)	3.1 (0.25–6.5)	2

term retrospective regrets still present at the time of the study. However, 75 women (62.6%) had expressed regret at undergoing bilateral oophorectomy at the time of hysterectomy. This was not significantly related to parity or the number of previous operations but was significantly related to age at hysterectomy (Table 15.6). It is of interest that even one patient who eventually underwent oophorectomy after seven previous laparotomies and whose symptoms were well controlled on HRT, still expressed regret at the ultimate loss of her ovaries. There is clearly a strongly emotional, and perhaps irrational, attitude to oophorectomy in many of these women, although this does not in any way reduce the validity of the patient's response.

Further research is required to clarify the role of testosterone implants in the treatment of endometriosis. It has been suggested that the androgenic effect of testosterone may exert a suppressant effect on the condition and thus discourage progression[13]. However, testosterone has a limited role, if any, to play in altering the pathogenesis or even controlling symptoms of the disease[67,68]. Furthermore, the doses used in the original therapeutic regimens were considerably higher than in the above studies, resulting in androgenic side-effects in virtually all patients. None of the patients in our studies reported adverse effects related to testosterone therapy and mean testosterone levels remained in the therapeutic range (1.8 nmol/l). The rationale behind the use of testosterone in our patients is not to suppress the endometriosis deposits but to control the insidious symptoms of depression, fatigue and loss of libido[78,79]. These are thought to be due to the decrease in plasma testosterone levels that follows surgical oophorectomy[80] and which respond well to replacement therapy. Our research is currently investigating a further group of women who have been treated with oestrogen replacement alone, omitting testosterone. This group appears to show similar results to those on combined therapy with very little evidence of progression or recurrence of the disease.

MALIGNANT TRANSFORMATION OF ENDOMETRIOSIS

The risk of malignant transformation of endometriosis is rare, but has been well documented since the first reported case by Sampson[81], who described malignancy arising in ovarian endometriosis arising 3 years after the original diagnosis. The ovary is the site most commonly affected[82,83] and 10–15% of cases of endometrioid adenocarcinoma of the ovary arise in, or are associated with, endometriosis[83]. Extragonadal sites also occur[83,84] and about 50 cases

Table 15.6 Attitude to oophorectomy at time of hysterectomy

	No.	Mean age at hysterectomy (years)	Mean parity	No. of operations
Happy/no preference	34	41.7	1.2	2.8
Unhappy	75	37.3	1.2	2.3
Overall	109	39.5	1.2	2.5
Significance		$p < 0.01$	NS	NS

NS = not significant

Table 15.7 Malignant transformation of endometriosis with oestrogen stimulation

Report	Age (years)	Symptoms	Site	Therapy	Survival[a,b]	Features
Young and Gamble[89]	47	Bleeding	Rectovaginal septum	Pelvic exenteration	NED[a] 13 months	TAH & BSO; E + T for 14 years
Lott et al.[93]	53	Bleeding	Rectum	Rectosigmoid resection	NED 44 months	TAH & BSO; E for 15 years
Brooks and Wheeler[90]	48	Pain, mass	Pelvic	Cytoreduction Radiotherapy	NED 22 months	TAH & BSO E for 4 years
Shamsuddin et al.[91]	55	Flank pain	Vesicovaginal septum	Cytoreduction Chemotherapy Progestogen	NED 17 months	TAH & BSO; E for 14 years
Granai et al.[92]	46	Bleeding	Vagina	Pelvic radiotherapy	NED 20 months	TAH & BSO; E for 13 years
Reimnitz et al.[94]	58	Ureteric obstruction	Pelvis	Cytoreduction Progestogen	NED 11 months	TAH & BSO; E for 12 years
Reimnitz et al.[94]	47	Ureteric obstruction	Pelvis	Cytoreduction Radiotherapy Progestogen	DOD 11 months	TAH & BSO; E for 4 years
Reintoft et al.[96]	36	Mass	Rectum	TAH & LSO Radiotherapy	DOD[b] 4 months	Ovarian granulosa cell tumour
Laslahti[95]	73	Bleeding	Umbilicus	TAH & BSO	NED 24 months	Ovarian thecoma

[a]NED = No evidence of disease
[b]DOD = Died of disease

have been reported to date in the literature. These account for 25% of all cases of malignant transformation and usually involve the uterovaginal septum[82,85-89].

There have been a total of seven reported cases of extragonadal transformation of endometriosis following TAH and BSO with unopposed oestrogen therapy[89-94] (Table 15.7). A further two cases related to oestrogen-producing sex-cord stromal tumours of the ovary have also been reported[95,96]. In the former group the delay between TAH/BSO and the development of malignancy ranged from 4 to 15 years and the average duration of oestrogen therapy was 11 years. Of the nine cases in total, two had died at the time of review, giving an overall survival of 78%. However, these data must be viewed cautiously as the mean follow-up was only 29 months. Similarly, other studies of malignant transformation without the involvement of HRT have shown good survival rates, but long-term follow-up is again limited. Of 32 cases of adenocarcinoma reviewed by Brooks and Wheeler[90], there were three reported deaths, but only two women had been followed up for 4 years or more.

Some authorities have suggested the use of oestrogen and testosterone together to exert an additional suppressant effect on remaining deposits, although, as discussed above, the lack of documented evidence for the beneficial effects of testosterone suggests this is unlikely. There has also been a reported case of extragonadal adenocarcinoma developing 14 years after TAH and BSO following combined oestrogen and testosterone therapy[90].

On the basis of the currently available literature, the link between oestrogen and malignancy remains tenuous and a case of malignant transformation of endometriosis following BSO without subsequent HRT has also been reported[90]. Furthermore, the incidence of malignant transformation is too rare to warrant refusing or discontinuing oestrogens in cases of endometriosis. Indeed, if the theoretical risk of malignancy is to alter our management in any direction, it should be to reaffirm that bilateral oophorectomy is a vital part of radical surgery for endometriosis. This step alone will reduce the risk of ovarian malignancy regardless of whether oestrogen replacement therapy is used[97].

CONCLUSION

On the basis of the above evidence we strongly advocate that when the radical decision is made to perform a hysterectomy for severe and intractable endometriosis, then bilateral oophorectomy should also be performed. Immediate hormone replacement therapy should then be given in adequate doses without fear of exacerbation of the disease. Despite the apparent reluctance of most women to undergo removal of their ovaries, they can be reassured that this approach will reduce the risk of recurrent surgery and, theoretically, the risk of ovarian cancer, while providing excellent control of symptoms and preventing the long-term sequelae of the menopause.

REFERENCES

1. Von Rokitansky, C. (1860). *Zesch. Gesselsch. Aerte. (Wien)*, **16**, 577
2. Whitfield, C.R. (1986). Endometriosis. In *Dewhurst's Textbook of Obstetrics and Gynaecology for Postgraduates*, 4th edn, pp. 609–623. (London: Blackwell Scientific)
3. Simpson, J.L., Elias, S., Malinak, L.R. and Buttram, V.C. Jr (1980). Heritable aspects of endometriosis 1: genetic studies. *Am. J. Obstet. Gynecol.*, **139**, 327–331
4. Strathy, J.H., Molgaard, C.A., Coulan, C.B. and Melton, L.J. (1982). III: Endometriosis and infertility: A laparoscopic study of endometriosis among fertile and infertile women. *Fertil. Steril.*, **38**, 667–672
5. Darbois, Y. (1987). Etiological factors of endometriosis. In Keller, P.J. (ed.) *Endometriosis: Contributions to Gynecology and Obstetrics*, vol. 16, pp. 1–6. (Karger: Basel)
6. Jeffcoate, T.N. (1975). *Principles of Gynaecology*, 4th edn, pp. 350–364. (London: Butterworth)
7. Tyson, J.E.A. (1974). Surgical considerations in gynaecological endocrine disorders. *Surg. Clin. North Am.*, **54**, 425–442
8. Schweppe, K-W. (1988). Etiology, pathogenesis and natural history of endometriosis. In Genazzani, A.R., Petraglia, F., Volpe, A. and Facchinetti, F. (eds.) *Advances in Gynaecological Endocrinology*, vol. 2, pp. 79–96. (Carnforth: Parthenon Publishing)
9. Schmidt, C.L. (1985). Endometriosis: a reappraisal of pathogenesis and treatment. *Fertil. Steril.*, **44**, 157–173
10. Thomas, E.J. (1988). New perspectives in hormonal therapy for endometriosis. In Genazzani, A.R., Petraglia, F., Volpe, A. and Facchinetti, F. (eds.) *Advances in Gynecological Endocrinology*, vol. 2, pp. 139–148. (Carnforth: Parthenon Publishing)
11. Wheeler, J.H. and Malinak, L.R. (1983). Recurrent endometriosis: incidence, management and prognosis. *Am. J. Obstet. Gynecol.*, **146**, 247–253
12. Elstein, M. and Bancroft, K. (1988). Endometriosis: the goal of treatment. In Genazzani, A.R., Petraglia, F., Volpe, A. and Facchinetti, F. (eds.) *Advances in Gynecological Endocrinology*, vol. 2, pp. 107–114. (Carnforth: Parthenon Publishing)
13. Matta, W.H. and Shaw, R.W. (1988). Endocrinological aspects of the aetiology and management of endometriosis. In Brush, M.G. and Gouldsmit, E.M. (eds.) *Functional Disorders of the Menstrual Cycle*, pp. 251–277. (New York: Wiley)
14. Malinak, L.R. (1990). In *Proceedings of the ICI Conference on Endometriosis*, Cambridge, September 1989, p. 142. (Carnforth: Parthenon Press)
15. Montgomery, J.C. and Studd, J.W.W. (1987). Oestradiol and testosterone implants after hysterectomy for endometriosis. In Bruhat, M.A. and Canis, M. (eds.) *Contributions to Gynaecology and Obstetrics*, vol. 16, pp. 241–246. (Basel: Karger)
16. Ranney, B. (1971). Endometriosis III. Complete operations. *Am. J. Obstet. Gynecol.*, **109**, 1137–1144
17. Wilson, E.A. (1988). Surgical therapy for endometriosis. *Clin. Obstet. Gynecol.*, **31**(4), 857–865
18. Ranney, B. (1970). Endometriosis I. Conservative operations. *Am. J. Obstet. Gynecol.*, **107**, 743–53
19. Studd, J.W.W. and Thom, M.H. (1981). Ovarian failure and ageing. *Clin. Endocrinol. Metab.*, **10**, 89–113
20. Thomas, E.J. and Cooke, I.D. (1987). The impact of gestrinone on the course of asymptomatic endometriosis. *Br. Med. J.*, **294**, 272–274
21. Hill, L.L. (1932). Aberrant endometrium. *Am. J. Surg.*, **18**, 303–321
22. Buttram, V.C. Jr and Betts, J.W. (1979). Endometriosis. *Curr. Prob. Obstet. Gynecol.*, **2**, 3–58
23. Studd, J.W.W., Andersen, H.M. and Montgomery, J.C. (1986). Selection of patients — kind and duration of treatment. In Greenblatt, R.C. (ed.) *A Modern Approach to the Perimenopausal Years*, pp. 129–140. (Berlin: Walter de Gruyter)
24. Hammond, C.B., Rock, J.A. and Parker, R.T. (1976). Conservative treatment of endometriosis: the effects of limited surgery and hormonal pseudopregnancy. *Fertil. Steril.*, **27**, 756–766
25. Dmowski, W.P. (1981). Current concepts in the management of endometriosis. *Obstet. Gynecol. Annu.*, **10**, 279–311
26. Andrews, W.C. and Larson, G.D. (1974). Endometriosis: treatment with hormonal

pseudopregnancy and/or operation. *Am. J. Obstet. Gynecol.*, **118**, 643–651

27. Roddick, J.W., Conkey, G. and Jacobs, E.J. (1960). The hormonal response of endometrium in endometriotic implants and its relationship to symptomatology. *Am. J. Obstet. Gynecol.*, **79**, 1173–1177

28. Prakash, S.J., Ulfelder, H. and Cohen, R.B. (1965). Enzyme-histochemical observations on endometriosis. *Am. J. Obstet. Gynecol.*, **91**, 990–997

29. Janne, O., Kauppila, A., Kokko, E., Lantto, T., Ronneberg, L. and Vihko, R. (1981). Estrogen and progestin receptors in endometriosis lesion: comparison with endometrial tissue. *Am. J. Obstet. Gynecol.*, **141**, 562–566

30. Roddick, J.W. Jr., Conkey, G. and Jacobs, E.J. (1960). The hormonal response of endometrium in endometriotic implants and its relationship to symptomatology. *Am. J. Obstet. Gynecol.*, **79**, 1173–1177

31. Tamaya, T., Motoyaha, T. and Ohono, Y. (1979). Steroid receptor levels and histology of endometriosis and adenomyosis. *Fertil. Steril.*, **31**, 396–400

32. Metzger, D.A., Oliver, D.L. and Hanney, A.F. (1991). Limited hormonal responsiveness of ectopic endometrium: histologic correlation with intrauterine endometrium. *Human Pathol.*, in press

33. Bergqvist, A., Jeppsson, S. and Kullander, S. (1985). Human uterine endometrium and endometriotic tissue transplanted into nude mice. Morphologic effects of various steroid hormones. *Am. J. Pathol.*, **121**, 337–341

34. Vierikko, P., Kauppila, A., Ronnberg, L. and Vikho, R. (1985). Steroidal regulation of endometriosis tissue: lack of induction of 17β-hydroxysteroid dehydrogenase activity by progesterone medroxyprogesterone acetate or danazol. *Fertil. Steril.*, **43**, 218–224

35. Haney, A.F., Handwerger, S. and Weinberg, J.B. (1984). Peritoneal fluid prolactin in infertile women with endometriosis: Lack of evidence of secretory activity by endometriotic implants. *Fertil. Steril.*, **42**, 935–938

36. Carlstrom, M., Bergqvist, A. and Ljungberg, O. (1988). Metabolism of estrone sulfate in endometriotic tissue and in uterine endometrium in proliferative and secretory cycle phase. *Fertil. Steril.*, **49**, 229–223

37. Kauppila, A., Isomaa, V., Ronnberg, L., Vierikko, P. and Vikho, R. (1985). Effect of gestrinone in endometriosis tissue and endometrium. *Fertil. Steril.*, **44**, 466–470

38. Greenblatt, R.B. and Tzingounis, S.V. (1979). Danazol treatment of endometriosis: long-term follow-up. *Fertil. Steril.*, **32**, 518–520

39. Lemay, A., Maheux, R. and Faure, N. (1984). Reversible hypogonadism induced by a luteinizing hormone (LH-RH) agonist (buserelin) as a new therapeutic approach for endometriosis. *Fertil. Steril.*, **41**, 863–871

40. Continho, E.M. and Azadian-Boulanger, G. (1988). Treatment of endometriosis by vaginal administration of gestrinone. *Fertil. Steril.*, **49**, 418–422

41. Moghissi, K.S. and Boyce, C.R. (1976). Management of endometriosis with oral medroxyprogesterone acetate. *Obstet. Gynecol.*, **47**, 265–267

42. Dizerega, G.S., Barber, D.L. and Hodgen, G.D. (1980). Role of ovarian steroids in initiation, maintenance and suppression. *Fertil. Steril.*, **33**, 649–653

43. Novak, E.R. and Hage, A.F. (1958). Endometriosis of the lower genital tract. *Obstet. Gynecol.*, **12**, 687–693

44. Doty, D.W., Gruber, J.S. and Gordon, C.W. (1980). 46XY pure gonadal dysgenesis: a report of 2 unusual cases. *Obstet. Gynecol.*, **55** (suppl. 3), 631–635

45. Kempers, R.D., Dockerty, M.B., Hunt, A.B. *et al.* (1960). Significant postmenopausal endometriosis. *Surg. Gynecol. Obstet.*, **111**, 348–356

46. Madgar, I., Ziv, N. and Many, M. (1982). Ureteral endometriosis in postmenopausal women. *Urology*, **22**, 174–176

47. Vorstman, B., Lynne, C. and Politano, V.A. (1983). Postmenopausal vesical endometriosis. *Urology*, **22**, 540–542

48. Abeshouse, B.S. and Abeshouse, G. (1960). Endometriosis of the urinary tract: a review of the literature and a report of 4 cases of vesical endometriosis. *J. Int. Coll. Surg.*, **34**, 43–63

49. Henriksen, E. (1955). Endometriosis. *Am. J. Surg.*, **90**, 331–337

50. Punnonen, R., Klemi, P.J. and Nikkanen, U. (1980). Postmenopausal endometriosis. *Eur. J. Obstet. Gynecol. Reprod. Biol.*, **11**, 195–200

51. Binns, B.A.O. and Bannerjee, R. (1983). Endometriosis with Turner's syndrome treated with cyclical estrogen/progestogen. Case report. *Br. J. Obset. Gynaecol.*, **90**, 581–582
52. Ray, J., Conger, M. and Ireland, K. (1985). Ureteral obstruction in postmenopausal women with endometriosis. *Urology*, **26**, 577–578
53. Pinkert, T.C., Catlow, C.E. and Straus, R. (1979). Endometriosis of the urinary bladder in a man with prostatic carcinoma. *Cancer*, **43**, 1562–1567
54. Oliker, A.J. and Harris, A.E. (1971). Endometriosis of the bladder in a male patient. *J. Urol.*, **106**, 858–861
55. Djursing, H., Peterson, K. and Weberg, E. (1981). Symptomatic postmenopausal endometriosis. *Acta Obstet. Gynecol. Scand.*, **60**, 529–530
56. Goodman, H.M., Kredenstser, D. and Deligdisch, L. (1989). Postmenopausal endometriosis associated with hormone replacement therapy. A case report. *J. Reprod. Med.*, **34**, 231–233
57. Grant, A. (1966). Additional sterility factors in endometriosis. *Fertil. Steril.*, **17**, 514–519
58. Meigs, J.V. (1953). Endometriosis: etiologic role of marriage, sex and parity: conservative treatment. *Obstet. Gynecol.*, **2**, 46–53
59. Kistner, R.W. (1958). The use of newer progestins in the treatment of endometriosis. *Am. J. Obstet. Gynecol.*, **75**, 264–278
60. Schenken, R.S., Williams, R.F. and Hodgen, G.D. (1987). The effect of pregnancy on surgically induced endometriosis in cynomolgus monkeys. *Am. J. Obstet. Gynecol.*, **157**, 1392–1396
61. McArthur, J.W. and Ulfelder, H. (1965). The effect of pregnancy upon endometriosis. *Obstet. Gynecol. Survey*, **20**, 709–733
62. Walton, L.A. (1977). A re-examination of endometriosis after pregnancy. *J. Reprod. Med.*, **19**, 341–344
63. Kistner, R. (1959). The treatment of endometriosis by inducing pseudopregnancy with ovarian hormones. A report of 58 cases. *Fertil. Steril.*, **10**, 539–556
64. Sensky, T.E. and Liu, D.T.Y. (1980). Endometriosis: associations with menorrhagia, infertility and oral contraceptives. *Int. J. Gynecol. Obstet.*, **17**, 573–576
65. Cramer, D.W., Wilson, E. and Stillman, R. (1986). The association of endometriosis with oral contraceptive use. Presented at the *43rd Annual Meeting of the American Fertility Society*, September 27–October 2, Toronto, Abstract 328
66. Buttram, V.C. (1979). Cyclic use of combination oral contraceptives and the severity of endometriosis. *Fertil. Steril.*, **31**, 347–348
67. Hamblen, E.C. (1957). Androgen treatment of women. *South. Med. J.*, **50**, 743–752
68. Hammond, M.G., Hammond, C.B. and Parker, R.T. (1978). Conservative treatment of endometriosis externa: The effects of methyltestosterone therapy. *Fertil. Steril.*, **29**, 651–654
69. Salmon, U.J., Geist, S.H. and Walter, R.I. (1939). Treatment of dysmenorrhoea with testosterone propionate. *Am. J. Obstet. Gynecol.*, **38**, 264–377
70. Schenken, R.S. and Malinak, L.R. (1978). Reoperation after initial treatment of endometriosis with conservative surgery. *Am. J. Obstet. Gynecol.*, **131**, 416–421
71. Hammond, C.B. and Haney, A.F. (1978). Conservative treatment of endometriosis. *Fertil. Steril.*, **30**, 497–509
72. Spangler, D.B., Jones, G.S. and Jones, H.W. Jr (1970). Infertility due to endometriosis. *Am. J. Obstet. Gynecol.*, **109**, 850–857
73. Pratt, J.H. and Williams, T.J. (1980). Indications for complete pelvic operations and more radical procedures in the treatment of severe or extensive endometriosis. *Clin. Obstet. Gynecol.*, **23**(3), 937–950
74. Puolakka, J., Kauppila, A. and Ronnberg, L. (1980). Results in the operative treatment of pelvic endometriosis. *Acta Obstet. Gynecol. Scand.*, **59**, 429–431
75. Brosens, I., Boeckx, W. and Page, G. (1988). Microsurgery of ovarian endometriosis. *Human Reprod.*, **3**, 365–366
76. Henderson, A.F., Studd, J.W.W. and Watson, N. (1990). A retrospective study of oestrogen replacement therapy following hysterectomy for endometriosis. In *Proceedings of the ICI Conference on Endometriosis*, September 1989, Cambridge, pp. 133–142. (Carnforth: Parthenon Press)
77. Thom, M.H. and Studd, J.W.W. (1980). Hormonal implantation. *Br. Med. J.*, **280**, 848–850

78. Studd, J.W.W., Chakravati, S. and Collins, W.P. (1979). Plasma hormone profiles after the menopause and bilateral oophorectomy. *Postgrad. Med. J.*, **54**, 25–30
79. Chakravati, S., Collins, W.P., Newton, J.R., Oram, D. and Studd, J.W.W. (1977). Endocrine changes and symptomatology after oophorectomy in premenopausal women. *Br. J. Obstet. Gynaecol.*, **84**, 769–775
80. Studd, W.W., Chakravati, S. and Oram, D. (1977). The climacteric in the menopause. *Clin. Obstet. Gynecol.*, **4**, 3–29
81. Sampson, J.A. (1925). Endometrial carcinoma of the ovary arising in endometrial tissue in that organ. *Arch. Surg.*, **10**, 1–72
82. Goldberg, M.I., Alan, B.P. and Jerome, L.B. (1978). Clear cell adenocarcinoma arising in endometriosis of the rectovaginal septum. *Obstet. Gynecol.*, **51**, 31s–40s
83. Scully, R.E., Richardson, G.S. and Barlow, J.F. (1966). The development of malignancy in endometriosis. *Clin. Obstet. Gynecol.*, **9**, 384–411
84. Ridley, J.H. (1966). Primary adenocarcinoma in implant of endometriosis. *Obstet. Gynecol.*, **77**, 261–267
85. Mostoufizadeh, G. and Scully, R. (1980). Malignant tumours arising in endometriosis. *Clin. Obstet. Gynecol.*, **23**, 951–963
86. Dockerty, M.B., Pratt, J.H. and Decker, D.C. (1954). Primary adenocarcinoma of the rectovaginal septum probably arising from endometriosis. *Cancer*, **7**, 893–898
87. Ferreira, H.P. and Clayton, S.G. (1958). Three cases of malignant change in endometriosis including two cases in the rectovaginal septum. *J. Obstet. Gynaecol. Br. Emp.*, **65**, 41–44
88. Lash, S.R. and Rubenstone, A.I. (1959). Adenocarcinoma of the rectovaginal septum probably arising from endometriosis. *Am. J. Obstet. Gynecol.*, **78**, 299–302
89. Young, E.E. and Gamble, C.N. (1969). Primary adenocarcinoma of the rectovaginal septum arising from endometriosis. Report of a case. *Cancer*, **24**, 597–601
90. Brooks, J. and Wheeler, J. (1977). Malignancy arising in extragonadal endometriosis. *Cancer*, **40**, 3065–3073
91. Shamsuddin, A., Villa Santa, U. and Tang, C. (1979). Adenocarcinoma arising from extragonadal endometriosis 14 years after TAH and BSO for endometriosis. *Am. J. Obstet. Gynecol.*, **133**, 585–586
92. Granai, C., Walters, M.D. and Sufair, H. (1984). Malignant transformation of vaginal endometriosis. *Obstet. Gynecol.*, **64**, 592–595
93. Lott, J.V., Rubin, R.J. and Salvati, E.P. (1978). Endometrioid carcinoma of the rectum arising in endometriosis. Report of a case. *Dis. Colon Rectum*, **21**, 56–60
94. Reimnitz, C., Brand, E., Nieberg, R.K. and Hacker, N.F. (1988). Malignancy arising in endometriosis associated with unopposed estrogen replacement. *Obstet. Gynecol.*, **71**(3), 444–447
95. Laslahti, K. (1972). Malignant external endometriosis: a case of adenocarcinoma of umbilical endometriosis. *Acta Pathol. Microbiol. Immunol. Scand.*, (suppl.), **223**, 98–102
96. Reintoft, I., Lange, A.P. and Skipper, A. (1974). Coincidence of granulosa-cell tumour of ovary and development of carcinoma in rectal endometriosis. *Acta Obstet. Gynecol. Scand.*, **53**, 185–189
97. Studd, J.W.W. (1989). Prophylactic oophorectomy. *Br. J. Obstet. Gynaecol.*, **96**, 506–509

16
The future

E. J. Thomas and J. A. Rock

It has been the aim of this book to provide a review of current thinking in all the major areas of endometriosis. The authors have responded excellently to their task. It is now our great pleasure to leave the discipline of writing chapters that are controlled by references and data and simply speculate on where advances in our understanding and treatment of this disease may occur over the next five to ten years. This chapter will be a combination of both our views and should give the perspective from both the United States and Europe. The main areas that we will discuss will be research and treatment.

RESEARCH

The introduction of laparoscopy and the resultant increase of our ease of access to the pelvis has created problems in our interpretation of the finding of endometriosis. Opinion ranges from the belief that it is probably a normal finding in most women to the belief that any visual endometriosis is of pathological significance. Some workers consider that invisible or microscopic disease is also important. We feel that these problems will only be resolved by exploring the fundamental problems of the pathogenesis of endometriosis and the control of its growth and proliferation. Such investigations require the use of basic science techniques, and the advent of the new biology provides powerful research tools. Using these it should be possible to determine the tissue of origin of endometriosis and the control of its cellular function and differentiation. There are three epithelia of importance: the endometrium, peritoneal mesothelium and endometriosis. Laboratory models should be able to be created using *in vitro* culture of these epithelia that should give us a clearer picture of their interaction. There are an ever-increasing number of growth factors and other molecules being identified that could have a role in the pathogenesis of the disease. If *in vitro* models of endometriosis are created they will provide an opportunity to investigate the cellular action of these compounds. The role of the immune system is likely to be important and the application of molecular techniques should reveal important information. There is still an important role for animal models since it is very difficult to perform ethical *in vivo* experiments in the human female. These models would have most relevance if they investigated the spontaneous disease in animals who have been shown to express it phenotypically, i.e. simians.

Clinical research should be used to explore the potential of new drugs. It would be very interesting to determine what factors cause the disease to become so widespread and active in certain individuals. A clearer picture of the natural history of the disease is required. This means large, controlled trials, which, although they are expensive to perform, are essential to verify that we should be continuing to prescribe surgical or medical therapy to our patients. Along with these comparative trials it is important to continue to investigate the aetiology of endometriosis. Epidemiology is a complex science and care is needed in the design of these studies. It is also difficult because we have not yet accurately defined the disease, so that there is an imprecision about the denominator in epidemiological studies. This re-emphasizes the need for research to be directed at an understanding of the fundamental aspects of the disease.

In order to increase our understanding of endometriosis it would be helpful to have a non-invasive method of diagnosis. Work by David Barlow and colleagues from Oxford has shown that it is possible to image endometriosis with the monoclonal OC-125 that has an attached radioisotope. The sensitivity of this technique means that it does not appear to be adequate for daily clinical use, but further developments are likely. One difficulty is that we can visualize tiny amounts of endometriosis at laparoscopy that are beyond the sensitivity of any imaging technique. It may be that nuclear magnetic resonance will be able to image small amounts of the disease, although that has not been shown so far. Serum markers provide potential for determining the response to treatment but their diagnostic use is limited because normal tissue can express these proteins and carbohydrates.

Although there are many difficulties, this is an exciting time for research in endometriosis. Clinicians should use the skills of their scientific colleagues to design experiments that investigate the fundamental aspects of the disease. It is inevitable that such investigations will also reveal much about physiology of the normal endometrium. We are very fortunate that in endometriosis we have a marvellous controlled model for normal and abnormal epithelium of the same type. We should take this opportunity to use the disease to explore fundamental aspects of the control of epithelial growth and proliferation. Although it is not neoplastic, endometriosis possesses many of the aspects of this phenomenon and could give much information about metastases and epithelial interactions leading to disease spread. The interaction between endometrium and the peritoneal mesothelium could provide a potent source of information about metastatic spread. As long as clinicians harness the powerful tools available today to investigate cellular function, it is possible that endometriosis will move outside the realms of the gynaecologists and excite many others.

TREATMENT

Although research may fascinate us as scientists and clinicians, it is the treatment of the disease that interests our patients. The first aim must be to define the indications for treatment. Having done that then there is the potential for developing new forms of treatment. In the United States there is already considerable use of the intra-abdominal laser and other forms of laparoscopic surgery. That is bound to extend through Europe and other parts of the world. However, training in these skills is long and the costs can be significant. Therefore, in many countries throughout the world there will be a place for a long time for laparotomy and conservative surgery. We must continue to develop and maintain these skills, since they provide an excellent solution to symptomatic endometriosis and to repair of damaged tubes and ovaries in the infertile woman.

Recently, new medical treatments, namely the LHRH analogues and gestrinone, have been developed. However, all current therapies have considerable side-effects and are contraceptive, a major problem in the infertile. The use of combination therapy to lessen side-effects should be explored. For example, it is possible that a combination of LHRH analogues and hormone replacement therapy may still be effective in treating the disease without the hypo-oestrogenic effects. It is more difficult to minimize the side-effects of danazol, gestrinone and progestagens. There are strategies that can be used, such as aerobic exercises. It would be interesting to see whether cyclical progestagen in the luteal phase could treat the disease without being contraceptive. Further work should be done to explore the possibilities of the non-steroidal anti-inflammatory drugs. There is evidence that they will treat dysmenorrhoea due to endometriosis very effectively by prescription during menses. They do not improve the visual appearance of the disease but they are effective and are not contraceptive. The place of such therapies needs to be defined clearly.

More potent and purer anti-oestrogens and anti-progesterones are being developed by the pharmaceutical companies. Whether these will have any efficacy in endometriosis is unknown, but this needs to be explored. Endometriosis is such a complex tissue with such variable receptor expression that it is quite feasible that it could be treated by a progestagen in one patient and an anti-gestagen in another. As endometriosis is an oestrogen-dependent phenomenon it is logical to assume that it could be treated by anti-oestrogens. It can be assumed that novel compounds will appear in the future, perhaps designed following the increase in the knowledge of the cellular function of endometriosis that will occur as a result of the research described above. All these possibilities are exciting but the conclusion from the current position is that we must accurately define the indications for and role of any treatment in endometriosis. Until that is clarified we will not be sure that any new treatment represents an advance.

There are interesting possibilities in exploring strategies that may prevent this disease, which appears to be occurring with increasing frequency. Anecdotally it is rare to find the disease in women using the oral contraceptive. If this observation is shown to be true, then that gives us interesting information about the pathogenesis of endometriosis and a possibility of preventing it. Currently it seems that delaying menarche, having infrequent and light periods and smoking are the main factors that will help prevent the disease. It is manifestly either impossible or inappropriate to recommend these strategies, but it would be interesting to investigate whether other factors such as delaying first pregnancy is a true risk factor for endometriosis. It may be that we will be able to give concrete recommendations about lifestyle to women in the future that may help them to avoid endometriosis.

CONCLUSIONS

There are many interesting possibilities in both research and treatment in the future. Let us hope that over the next decade we are able to extend our understanding of endometriosis so that we will be able to lessen its impact on women in the reproductive years.

Index

peritoneal, release sites 68
synthesis 69
  activators 87
  endometriosis aetiology 69–71
  and infertility 70–71
prostanoids 80, 86–90
protein kinase C, and EGF receptors 63
pseudomenopause, induction 60
pseudopregnancy therapy 60, 222, 239,
    279
  danazol comparisons 251
psychological problems, surgical results
    effects 214
pulmonary endometriosis 164, 169–71,
    177
  catamenial symptoms 164, 171
  management 171–72
pulmonary nodules, asymptomatic 164,
    171–2

race, and incidence 12
racial aspects 4, 12
Ranney classification 134–5
reactive oxygen intermediates 103–4
rectal pain 79, 80
recurrent disease
  post-GnRHa therapy 272
  post-laser therapy 205
  rate 275
  risk 144
renal endometriosis 163, 164
reproductive hormones, dependence
    13–14
research, future 291–3
retrograde menstruation see menstruation,
    retrograde
rheumatoid arthritis 101
ruby laser 199

SAMBA, oestrogen/progesterone levels
    43
Sampson classification 131–2
Sampson theory, of aetiology 154
self-antigens
  interaction 98
  tolerance 100–1
serum markers 186
sex hormone binding globulin (SHBG),
    testosterone level effects
    228–9
slow-reacting substance of anaphylaxis
    87
sperm phagocytosis, by macrophages 83
splenosis, endometriosis mimicking 172
staging
  Beecham 134, 135
  Feinstein 146
  Gonella 146
  Ingersoll 136, 137

Markham 155
  surgical 185–6
steroid autoradiography, steroid binding
    assay 39–40
steroid hormone binding globulin (SHBG),
    danazol interaction 245
steroid monoxygenases 240
steroid receptors 186, 276–7
  assay techniques 34–5
  concept 33–4
  danazol binding 243–5
  endometriotic tissue 59
  environmental factors 50–1
  exogenous hormone effects 51
  gestrinone binding 230
steroidogenesis enzymes 240–3
  monoxygenase group 240
  oxidoreductase group 240
stroma, endometriotic tissue 48–9
Sturgis and Call classification 133
subperitoneal endometriosis 21, 22, 23
sucrose gradient method, steroid receptor
    assay 34
surgery 186–7
  complete operations 194–6, 279–84
  contraindications 187
  incidence 275
  objectives 188
  see also conservative surgery
systemic lupus erythematosus (SLE) 101,
    104, 105

T lymphocytes 98–9
telelysosomes 29
testosterone
  and endometriosis 279
  gestrinone effects 228–9, 231
  implants 284
testosterone proprionate 239
thoracic endometriosis 164, 169–71, 177
  catamenial symptoms 164, 171
  management 171–2
thromboxanes 68
trabecular bone loss, GnRH agonist-
    associated 252–3, 271–2
transforming growth factor alpha (TGFα)
    64
transport theory, of aetiology 154
treatment
  fertility impact 120–2
  future 293–4
  strategy choice 186–7, 192
  see also medical therapy; surgery
tubal ligation, diagnostic 4
tubal motility, prostaglandin effects 88
tumour necrosis factor (TNF) 91

umbilical area endometriosis 172
unsuspected endometriosis 144